To all my com?
the Juvenile Court and
Child Study Institute
from whom I learned
so much

Henry L Hartman MD

Basic Psychiatry for Corrections Workers

Basic Psychiatry for Corrections Workers

By

HENRY L. HARTMAN, M.D., (L)FAPA

Medical Director
Court Diagnostic and Treatment Center

Psychiatric Consultant
Juvenile Court and Child Study Institute
Lucas County, Ohio

Clinical Professor of Forensic Psychiatry
Medical College of Ohio at Toledo

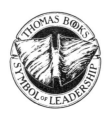

CHARLES C THOMAS • PUBLISHER
Springfield • Illinois • U.S.A.

Published and Distributed Throughout the World by

CHARLES C THOMAS • PUBLISHER

Bannerstone House

301-327 East Lawrence Avenue, Springfield, Illinois, U.S.A.

© *1978, by* CHARLES C THOMAS • PUBLISHER

ISBN 0-398-03663-2

Library of Congress Catalog Card Number: 77-2182

With THOMAS BOOKS *careful attention is given to all details of
manufacturing and design. It is the Publisher's desire to present books that
are satisfactory as to their physical qualities and artistic possibilities and
appropriate for their particular use.* THOMAS BOOKS *will be true to those
laws of quality that assure a good name and good will.*

Printed in the United States of America

OO-2

Library of Congress Cataloging in Publication Data

Hartman, Henry L
  Basic psychiatry for corrections workers.

  Bibliography: p.
  Includes index.
  1. Psychology, Pathological. 2. Interviewing in
psychiatry. 3. Psychopharmacology. I. Title.
RC454.4.H37   616.8′9′0024365   77-2182
ISBN 0-398-03663-2

This book is dedicated in all humility to the members of one of the most unrecognized and underacknowledged disciplines in this country, the professional corrections workers.

PREFACE

THIS book has grown out of in-service training programs with which I have been intermittently involved over the past twenty-five years. In 1952, I first began to conduct workshops for personnel of the Juvenile Cout and Child Study Institute (the Juvenile Detention Home) of Lucas County, Ohio. In 1953, I entered into a formal relationship with those institutions as psychiatric consultant. That relationship has continued to the present. The amount of time devoted to this aspect of my professional life has increased through those years, and in-service training of counseling and custodial staff, whether on a formal or informal basis, has been, I hope, a mutually enriching experience. I know I have learned much from my part in these sessions. From 1964 through 1972, my contacts with corrections workers increased through the many workshops I conducted for probation and parole officers in Ohio and Michigan. In 1972, I joined the staff of the Court Diagnostic and Treatment Center, a forensic clinic serving ten counties in northwestern Ohio. In addition to performing those evaluations mandated by law, the clinic aids corrections personnel in devising programs for probationers and offers therapy groups for selected probationers. From my first days at the Center in 1972, I have conducted weekly, ongoing, in-service training sessions. In 1975, the former Director of the Center, Larry Chase, M.S.W., suggested that in his opinion some of the material of those sessions would make a worthwhile volune. Hence, this book was written.

During these years, indeed since I first entered psychiatric residency training in 1937, there has been a tremendous outpouring of literature on the psychiatric aspects of antisocial behavior. Little of that has been directed specifically toward the corrections worker. I have, of course, drawn heavily on that resource in the formation of my own concepts of mental illness, particularly as those concepts may be applied in corrections. In those instances in this book where material has been drawn directly from the work of others, those individuals have been specifically credited. There is at the end of the book a reading list which is designed as a guide for those who might want to increase their knowledge of any individual topic beyond the depth to which that topic has been covered. The inclusion of any book in the reading list does not imply that that book has been consulted in preparing this manuscript. In some instances the views expressed in this book may be at variance with the views expressed in the material in the reading list.

All illustrative cases have been developed from real people, seen at one stage or another in my career. Even when this case material has been entered in evidence, and is a matter of public record, an attempt has been made to obscure the personal details. It is probable that in spite of this effort, certain individuals may feel that this is a case with which they have had contact. If that occurs, then I can only hope that the case chosen was so typical that it can represent many different individuals.

It is customary at the beginning of a volume of this sort to acknowledge one's debt to those who have assisted in its preparation. I have always felt in the past when reading such material that it was there as window dressing. It is only as I set down my own acknowledgements that I am aware of how meaningful these statements of indebtedness really are. Indeed, it is difficult to find the proper words to express the gratitude I feel.

I should like to express my appreciation to my coworkers at the Court Diagnostic and Treatment Center. The interaction of the professional staff there has been immeasurably helpful in sharpening my own concepts. The office and clerical staff have been zealous in guarding my time and providing innumerable little services cheerfully and willingly. I cannot name each person individually; there are too many involved. I should like to single out Cynthia Sikorski, M.A., the Director of the Center who has been unfailingly cooperative. I also owe a deep debt of gratitude to Carole Jones, the office manager, who has worked so diligently in order to arrange for competent secretarial help to be available for me when needed. Most of all I am indebted to Pat Tomczyk, on whom the greater part of the burden for typing, retyping, and typing yet again has fallen. No matter how great the demands made on her, she has remained unfailingly pleasant and helpful.

Finally, I should like to express my affectionate gratitude to two members of my family. My daughter, Joan Hartman, with much effort, taught me how to write simple, declarative sentences. I can only hope that she approves of this finished product. My devoted wife, Eve, has been patient and understanding throughout the long months of my writing and rewriting. Her encouragement and interest kept my own interests at high pitch. Her careful reading of much of the final draft has helped to keep ambiguities to a minimum.

H.L.H.

INTRODUCTION

FROM the days when man first started disseminating information to his fellows by means of cave drawings to the present television newscasts, the first reaction to news of some particularly heinous, incomprehensible offense typically has been, "He must have been crazy to have done something like that." Crime and mental illness always have been linked, either rightly or wrongly, in the public mind. More likely in earlier times the statement would have been, "He must have been possessed by the gods (or witches)." Indeed, in various ages throughout history, treatment of antisocial offenders and the mentally ill has been strikingly similar. At the same time pickpockets were being hanged by the neck for stealing handkerchiefs, witches were being burned at the stake for their misdeeds.

Who were the witches? They were the epileptics, the hysterical, those who saw visions or heard strange voices or professed peculiar beliefs, i.e. the mentally ill. The two groups were confined in the same jail, were subject to the same expulsion from the city, were bound with the same chains and shackles. Indeed, the practice of granting bail to those accused but not yet convicted of crime is believed to have begun with the bailors of Elizabethan England. These were the village elders who were called on by the crown to guarantee the future harmlessness of those people granted the king's grace from punishment by reason of insanity.

This tendency to regard these two groups as springing from a common stock continues today in the practice of combining Departments of Corrections and Departments of Mental Health under one administrative head. While this union continues in some states, others are dissolving the marriage, which never seems to have lived up to the expectations that contacts between

xi

these two groups would be mutually enriching.

Until recently there were those who felt all crime was the product of mental illness. Fortunately, this simplistic view is no longer tenable. There are very few psychiatrists and no criminologists left who espouse it. But, mentally ill people do commit crimes, whether because of or in spite of their illness. Offenders do have breakdowns under the stress of confinement in jails. Thus, the corrections worker constantly comes in contact with the mentally ill. There is a need, then, for correctional workers at every point in the system to have some familiarity with basic psychiatric concepts. This is equally true for probation counselors, parole officers, prison guards and, for that matter, prosecuting attorneys, defense attorneys, and members of the bench.

Not only do corrections officers come in contact with the mentally ill themselves, but in these days of institutional interdependence and interrelationships, it is inevitable they will be bombarded with material from psychiatric workers. Corrections workers, therefore, must be able to understand the diagnoses attached to the individual, the approaches employed in the description of personality types, and the terminology in which this material is couched. This need to understand psychiatric terminology and concepts will continue to grow by leaps and bounds as waves of change sweep the country in the laws governing the commitment of the mentally ill to mental hospitals.

In too many instances in the past, the word "hospital" has been a euphemism for "warehouse." The word hospital implies treatment, yet most of the patients in state hospitals are not getting treatment, at least not treatment adequate to their needs. The reasons for this are extremely complex and beyond the scope of this book. The significance for corrections workers lies in the manner in which attempts to correct this situation are being made. Rather than working toward improving conditions in the hospitals, attention has been focused on changing the treatment location to the community.

In the past, the mentally ill could be kept against their will in hospitals because they needed treatment, whether or not they received that treatment. Starting in 1969 with the Lanterman Petris Short Act in California, these new laws say, in effect, that people may not be kept in mental hospitals against their will unless it can be demonstrated that these people pose a very obvious threat either to themselves or to those around them. (In other words, the patient is either suicidal or homicidal.)

While at the moment of writing relatively few states have passed such laws, a 1975 decision of the United States Supreme Court makes the spread of these laws to all states almost inevitable. The Court's decision in the case of *Donaldson v O'Connor* says, in effect, that it is unconstitutional to keep in a hospital, against his or her will, a patient who is not a danger to him or herself and who is not receiving adequate treatment. The exact definition of adequate treatment is still up in the air. However, it is doubtful state legislatures will come up with the tremendous sum of money needed annually for adequate treatment. The net effect, therefore, will be to lower markedly the population of state hospitals.

The results of these statutes are beginning to be seen already. As noted, California was the first state to pass such a law. Since, then, admission rates in California jails have increased in direct proportions to the decrease in the population of the state's mental hospitals. This does not mean that former patients of mental hospitals are dangerous or that we are going to see a wave of violent crime as a result of this action. (It is true that some patients on release from mental hospitals have committed serious crimes, but their number is negligible in proportion to the number of patients discharged.) What we are seeing is a tremendous increase in charges of vagrancy, indecent exposure, petty theft, public nuisance, and other offenses of this nature. In attempting to write presentence reports on these individuals, probation officers will have to depend on material received from state hospitals. They will be confronted constantly with terms such as "schizophrenic reaction, chronic undifferentiated type" or "epileptoid personality disorder" and should have some concept as to what these terms mean and what they imply as to the future behavior of the individual about whom a recommendation must be made.

At the same time more former mental hospital patients are showing up in jail settings, more and more forensic centers are being founded. These are centers which are being established for the specific purpose of determining the mental status of offenders and making recommendations for their future. In some instances, the centers also serve as treatment facilities for these individuals. A minority of them have both inpatient and outpatient facilities. Many of these centers will receive monies from various mental health funds. Hence, their reports will have to be couched in diagnostic categories acceptable to these funding agencies. For the most part, this means the corrections worker must be familiar with the second edition of the *Diagnotic and Statistical Manual of Mental Disorders (DSM II)* prepared by the committee on nomenclature and statistics of the American Psychiatric Association. This does not mean the corrections worker has to become a diagnostician, although there may be times he or she feels forced into that role. It does mean the corrections worker, particularly the probation and parole officer who deals with offenders outside of institutions' walls will have to be familiar with these terms and what they imply.

But, psychiatry as a discipline has more to contribute than an understanding of psychiatric jargon. In common with other social sciences, it can add a great deal to the technical armamentarium of the corrections worker. Interviewing skills and communications mastery are particularly helpful in corrections, where a large part of the interviewee's effects are devoted to conning the interviewer and where the time spent at any one meeting is often much shorter than optimal.

Again, in common with other social sciences, psychiatry has much to say about various ways of looking at people, particularly where such personality evaluations may furnish rough rules of thumb as to what to anticipate in behavior. Such personality evaluations also may lay the foundations for getting along with various and varied individuals with a minimal amount of friction. Finally, the probations worker should have some familiarity with the treatment modalities of psychiatry, particularly where drug therapy is concerned, since he or she will become exposed more and more to people who are taking these medications and should have some awareness of their influence on behavior.

Psychiatry also can offer lessons of practical importance which it has learned through long experience. Without any claim to infallibility, psychiatrists have learned the main indicators for potential suicide through bitter experience. They can jelp jail or prison leaders pick out those individuals who demand greater attention in this regard than do most. Similarly, the insights of psychiatry can help to pinpoint for the corrections worker those people who are apt to become violent or to express their feelings in impulsive, aggressive ways.

We live in what has been call a drug-oriented society. Therefore, it would seem to be important that the corrections worker know about mind-altering drugs, both the street variety and those which the physician prescribes for therapeutic purposes.

It is with the hope of furnishing this sort of helpful information that this book was written. It is not a description of work which has been done, complete with controls, degrees of statistical significance, factor analyses, and outcomes. It was not written to develop any theory of why people become criminals or to delineate any other theory of the same sort. It is not a first aid manual of what to do until the psychiatrist comes, nor an attempt to indoctrinate corrections workers to the psychiatric point of view, nor to turn them into mail order psychiatrists. It makes no pretense to being an erudite and scholarly tome covering the entire field of everything that has been written about the relationship between psychiatry and corrections. For this reason, you will not find footnotes with references to articles validating every statement that is made.

This book is an attempt to sort out from the twenty-four years of contacts with corrections workers, both on the job and in countless hours of both formal and informal in-service training, those things which seem to be of the most practical significance for the correctional worker to know. These have been drawn from many sources over the years, and there is no intent to present this as an original work. Any time a statement is made which represents a seemingly unique or idiosyncratic viewpoint, it will be so labeled. Although the book is not annotated, there is a bibliography of various reference work to which the interested reader may turn to amplify the boundaries of the book.

The first part of the book deals with various diagnostic categories of mental illness alluded to above. It is true that offenses have been committed by people who have been diagnosed as suffering with almost every single subtype of mental illness which exists. However, only those entities which are seen more commonly by the corrections worker will be discussed. As each of the diagnostic categories are described, we will discuss, when possible, the sort of offenses most commonly associated with this type of mental illness. It is worth repeating that in describing these associations there is no attempt to imply that a causal relationship exists between the mental illness and the offense. Likewise, in giving these classifications, there is no attempt to get bogged down in the quagmire of "not guilty by reason of insanity." Whenever it is possible, in connection with each of these categories, specific recommendations will be made to facilitate the worker's relationship with this particular sort of individual.

The second section of the book deals with interviewing and communications, with particular reference to the sorts of communications which are indicators of potential violence directed either inward against the self or outward to others. Attention will also be paid to the specific nature of dealing with the "con" as well as methods of dealing with the delusional individual.

The final section concerns itself with drugs and the offender. This will cover not only the common therapeutically used drugs, but also the more common street drugs encountered. Hopefully, this section will cover interactions between various sorts of drugs as well as discussing rough norms for behavior while under the influence of a particular drug.

CONTENTS

PART ONE
Mental Disorders and Corrections

PART TWO
Interviewing and Corrections

PART THREE

Drugs, Alcohol, and Corrections

Basic Psychiatry for Corrections Workers

PART ONE
MENTAL DISORDERS AND CORRECTIONS

Chapter 1

FUNDAMENTALS

BASIC ASSUMPTIONS

 THERE are three basic assumptions which have dictated the content and format of this book. One of these has to do with corrections and corrections workers; the other two concern psychiatry and psychiatrists. Unless the implications of these assumptions are thoroughly understood, there is a definite danger that the intent will be misinterpreted, the material misconstrued, and the suggestions misapplied. It is hoped that this section will lay the foundation for a clearer understanding of the remainder of the book.

 The first assumption is that corrections is one of the helping professions, and that being a probation or parole officer, a jail or prison counselor, a guard or section leader, means more to most people in those positions than just having a job. Certainly, the size of the paycheck is not an adequate explanation as to why people spend their lives in these positions. Admittedly, there are a few people who enter this field out of a need to exercise power. With rare exceptions, they do not stay very long. The majority of corrections workers have a basic interest in people. They share a belief that behavior can change or be changed. At the same time it has been demonstrated that the starry-eyed idealist does not last long in corrections unless that idealism is tempered with realism. Many corrections workers assume an attitude of cynicism. Implicit in the premise of this book is that this attitude is a protective mask which still covers a desire to be of help.

 There is a sign in the office of the floor leaders of the girls' section of the Lucas County Child Study Institute (the Juvenile Detention Home for Lucas County, Ohio) which portrays this mixture of cynicism and concern present in most corrections workers. The sign says, "We the willing, led by the unknown, are doing the impossible for the ungrateful. We have done so much, for so long, with so little, we are now qualified to do anything with nothing." Nothing demonstrates the ambivalence of this attitude better than the fact that this sign is printed in very large letters but is hidden on the back side of a filing cabinet, where it is rarely seen.

It is with the basic premise that workers are interested in knowing more about their charges as people that this book is written. Implicit in that assumption is another one, that this knowledge will help the worker to avoid spinning his or her wheels when dealing with the people described in this book. It is in this spirit that specific recommendations are made for dealing with certain types of individuals. Many of these suggestions seem time consuming, almost to the point that they appear to impose an impossible burden on the overladen worker. Also, they will not always work. There is no way in which a cookbook approach can work in human relations. It would be nice to be able to advise the worker for each depressed person who is a shoplifter, "Spend twenty minutes talking about deprivations of childhood, and devote ten minutes to 'you can do better.' Do this for three sessions. For the next three sessions spend ten minutes on sexual behavior and five on the power of positive thinking." This would be fine, but it would not work. It implies that all people who are depressed are the same, or all people who shoplift are the same. Those statements of course are false. At the same time these suggestions frequently will demonstrate that the longest way round is the shortest way home. Hopefully, they are attuned to the circumstances of the worker's community resources as well as to the basic need to have enough successes to be willing to continue to confront the ever-increasing caseload. Finally, they embody the never dying hope that in some utopian day there will be a caseload small enough that all the necessary helpful steps may be taken by the worker.

The second assumption is that psychiatry is still an inexact science. The constant addition of more precise observations leads to an ongoing revision of the theoretical constructs of the reasons for maladaptive human behavior. It is obvious that until now no one theory has been devised which is capable of explaining all of human behavior, adaptive or maladaptive. If there were such a theory there would be no need for a diversity of systems, each claiming to have the ultimate truth. It is probable that as observations continue to be accumulated, particularly in the areas of genetics, neurochemistry, neurophysiology, and neuropharmacology, it will become obvious that there is no unitary cause for mental disorder, just as there is no unitary cause for crime. (Because this is a book on basic psychiatry, there has been no mention of the social, cultural, economic, or political roots of behavior, even though they are of tremendous importance in the development of maladaptive behavior, particularly antisocial behavior.) This recognition that psychiatry is an inexact science implies that any statements that are made as to causation, no matter how dogmatic they may sound, are only tentative and are subject to revision as new facts emerge.

This also implies that for the present the most accepted way of imposing order on the tremendous diversity of human behavior is by observation and description. This description must be not only cross-sectional, that is a slice of observable behavior at a particular moment in time, but also be longitudinal, that is historical. Otherwise a misleading picture may emerge.

For example, *A* and *B* are examined separately. Each shows roughly the same behavioral picture. Each is disturbed, excited, agitated, and mildly confused. Each looks rather wild-eyed and disheveled. Each talks of hearing others talking, others who cannot be seen by the observer. Each feels that these others are attempting to do something unspeakably horrible, to *A*, in *A*'s case, to *B*, in *B*'s case. On cross-sectional examination of behavior, they are indistinguishable.

Longitudinal examination presents different pictures. *A* gives a family history of having a maternal aunt currently in a mental hospital, a grandfather who died there, and a brother who is alcoholic. *A* has been a withdrawn, rather timid person all his life. He has worked for the past two years, but for the past two months he has expressed more and more fear of going to work, hinting that his fellow employees do not like him and are going to do something to him. For the past week he has refused to go to work. For the past three nights he has not slept. He would open a little chink in the drapes to look out to see if enemies were prowling around outside the house. He became more and more upset, confused, excited, and suspicious. Finally, he attempted physically to restrain his family from leaving the house for fear that unknown enemies might harm them. At that point he had to be forcibly taken to a hospital for help.

B on the other hand has not worked. From early high school days he has run around with a group which is heavily into alcohol and drugs. He has had occasional periods when for a few hours he has not been completely in contact with his surroundings. These episodes have not been of very long duration. Twenty-four hours before being seen in the hospital he had taken a large quantity of an unknown drug (later found to be PCP). He did not come out of his confused state and he too was brought to the hospital.

These histories serve to differentiate *A*'s condition from *B*'s. A diagnosis can be made on the basis of the cross-sectional plus the longitidinal description of their behavior. *A* would probably be diagnosed as **Schizophrenia, Paranoid Type** and *B* as **Psychosis with Drugs or Poison Intoxication (PCP Psychosis)**. These diagnoses carry with them implications of practical significance. They dictate a different *prognosis* for each of these two people, that is a different prediction of what the eventual outcome will be in each case. They also indicate different follow-up care once each person is released from the hospital.

The third assumption is that there is such a thing as mental illness or disease to which the so-called medical model can apply. The medical model states that there are specific entities called diseases. These are identified by symptoms of which the sufferer or his family complain, and objective signs which can be observed, named, and even measured, either directly or by laboratory examination. Each disease has a specific pattern, which helps to differentiate it from similar conditions. Each case of a specific disease runs a generally similar course and has a similar outlook (prognosis) if untreated. This concept also implies that eventually a specific cause and a specific treatment will be found for each disease.

This does not imply that each condition discussed in this book is a disease. The personality disorders have become a part of the character structure of the individual and can scarcely be called illness. In the light of present knowledge, this is true also for many sexual deviations. This does not imply that these conditions are necessarily congenital, desirable, or untreatable.

CLASSIFICATION IN PSYCHIATRY

It has been obvious since man first observed his fellows that certain symptoms of disordered behavior occurred in clusters that could be differentiated from other symptom clusters. (Such clusters are called *syndromes*.) It later became obvious, as in the example above, that the same syndrome could arise under different circumstances. It also became apparent, depending on the life history and the symptom cluster, that the condition would progress along certain lines if untreated, and definite outcomes would result. This combination of developmental history, behavioral symptoms, clinical course, and outcome could be viewed as constituting a specific disease entity.

Many attempts have been made to name these illnesses and to classify them in such a way as to make sense. As more has been learned about both the manifestations and causations of mental disorders, it has been necessary to change and modify these classifications. The first section of this book is organized around the classification which is currently most widely used in this county. This classification is presented in a booklet published in 1968 by the American Psychiatric Association entitled *The Diagnostic and Statistical Manual of Mental Disorders* (second edition). This is known familiarly as *DSM II* and conforms to the *International Classification of Mental Illnesses,* as edited by the World Health Organization. The history of the development of this classification system corroborates the statement that psychiatry is an inexact science. The first edition of the *Diagnostic and Statistical Manual of Mental Disorders (DSM I)* had been published sixteen years earlier in 1952. The second edition came out in 1968. A start has now been made on the revision of DSM II and it is expected that DSM III will be introduced in 1978. It is regrettable that labels have to be applied to people as they carry the false expectation that people always behave in accordance with their labels. Yet without labels, categories, and classifications it would be an impossible task to attempt to communicate about mentally disturbed individuals.

Another great drawback to labels is the human expectation that once we have named something we understand it. This, of course, is not true. This assumption about labeling is particularly misleading in human behavior. It has become an axiom that human behavior is not motivated; it is over motivated. There is not only one reason for behavior; there are many. This would seem to make it even more important that classification depend only on behavior rather than on attempting to include causation. Yet as the example of *A* and *B* would demonstrate, this would lead to even greater confusion. In *DSM II* an attempt is made to divide conditions in general into those with known causes, generally either organic or toxic, and those whose causes are still unknown. Subdivisions are then made under these two main headings.

There are difficulties inherent in any attempt at classification. Even this basic division into organic and functional disorders is not a simple one. For example:

> Mr. C was referred to this agency in a presentence status, after having been found guilty of discharging a firearm in a menacing manner. He had been in a small neighborhood restaurant having a cup of cofee. He suddenly said to the counterman, "Hey, they can't do that," and left abruptly. He went outside and was seen to argue briefly with two or three young men who were lounging around there. He then walked off to return in a few moments carrying a shotgun, which he discharged in their general direction, shattering a window in the restaurant. He pled guilty after arrest and was referred to this agency, the Court Diagnostic and Treatment Center, prior to sentencing, because he had an obvious disability.
>
> Mr C was twenty-nine years of age. He had been in the military service, stationed in Germany in peace time, where

he was involved in an automobile accident. He received a severe head injury. He was unconscious for several days and was discovered to have sustained a depressed fracture of the skull. He was operated on at that time and had had a large metal plate inserted in his forehead. On his return to this country he had gone to work. He had married and done moderately well for about nine months. At that time he complained of increasing headaches at work (he worked in a noisy factory) and finally had to give up work altogether. He spent varying periods of time in Veterans' Hospitals receiving many tests and examinations. He was finally declared 100 percent disabled and was given a disability award, which at the time of the offense was something over $900.00 a month.

For approximately three months before the episode which brought him to the court he had started to have blackout spells. These were increasing in frequency, and he had had one while mowing the lawn on the day before the episode. On neurological examination at this center he was found to have definite evidence of after-effects from his injury. In addition to the plate in the skull, he had difficulty in talking, both in finding the proper words *(aphasia)* and in his pronounciation. His speech was somewhat slurred and jerky *(dysarthria)*. He showed very definite evidence, on examination of the retinae in his eyes, that there was an increase in the pressure of fluid inside his head. This would be a ready explanation for his blackout spells and his apparent irritability and loss of control. Obviously the diagnosis was **Nonpsychotic Organic Brain Syndrome, with Brain Trauma, Post-traumatic Personality Disorder.**

But was it?

On talking to Mr. C it was discovered that his parents' marriage had been quite unhappy. They had stayed together "for the sake of the children" Mr. C had felt that his father had gotten the bad end of the stick. He not only felt closer to the father, he identified with him. His father had been a classy dresser; Mr. C liked nothing better than to get dressed up in snappy clothes and go out where he could be seen. His father had been a heavy drinker who "carried his liquor like a man." His father said, "A man who can't be drunk all night and not go to work the next day is not a man." Mr. C had tried to be a heavy drinker, in spite of his head injury. (He had been told he should not drink.) Since he believed his headaches were due to hangovers and not due to his head injury, he had continued to work for as long as he could take it. "A man should be able to work no matter how much he had had to drink the day before." His father's idea of a good time was to get dressed up, take his wife to a nightclub, always act like a gentleman, and never get into an argument with another patron. If Mr. C were out with his wife and there was some sign of an argument, he would excuse himself, go to the men's room, and go out the back door. His wife would then join him.

The father had died six years before the offense. Mr C held his mother responsible for the father's death. The father had high blood pressure and the doctor told him he had to take it very easy. The mother insisted that she wanted to visit her relatives in a distant state for her vacation, and the father had to take her. The father did so. He loved to dance. So did the relatives. In spite of the doctor's orders, he danced steadily on this particular night of the trip. He fell dead on the dance floor.

Following the father's death, the mother lived with Mr. C and his wife. Six months before the episode in question she had remarried. She had brought her new husband to live with them. In spite of constant statements that she was looking for a home, she did not make any attempts to move out. Mr. C did not think that she was carrying her share of the financial load. He felt that he could not make it on his disability pension, and he was worried about his financial future.

Mr. C had only one thing which had belonged to his father; that was his father's 1967 car. Mr. C treated it as a shrine. He had spent over two thousand dollars in refurbishing it, including new wheel caps, engine, and upholstery. He kept it constantly clean and polished. He rarely drove it, so that it would remain a memorial. He finally felt that he was so much in debt that he could not afford to keep two cars, so he sold the 1973 car which was the one he customarily drove. On the day of the offense he had been on some errands and had parked his father's car in front of the restaurant while he went in to have a cup of coffee. The, "Hey, they can't do that" was his exclamation on seeing one of the young men sit on the trunk of the car. His father's image was being defiled. As he shot the gun, he said, "Next time this will be at *you*."

This then was not either/or; it was both/and. Surely the signs of increasing intracrainal pressure needed immediate medical attention. Undoubtedly, this factor diminished his control. At the same time, no amount of surgical or medical intervention would prevent a recurrence of this maladaptive behavior without attention to the human problems which were present.

Despite this example of the inadequacy of classification and labeling, it remains the only practical way in which one professional can communicate with another in a direct and concise fashion. It must always be understood, however, that no label ever completely and adequately describes a human being. This book is written in declarative sentences. It contains very few statements which say "with the exception of," "but Henderson disagrees," "in Thompson's study it was found 0.5 percent had a different outcome." It must be understood that these declarative, at times almost dogmatic statements, are not absolutes. They must be read as they are written. They are attempts to abstract the essence of those beliefs which are the most widely held at the present time. The accumulation of new knowledge with the passage of time may force a change in those statements, just as *DSM III* may dictate differences in the particular way labels are applied.

There are 218 different mental diseases listed in *DSM II*. No attempt will be made to cover all 218 disorders. Only those conditions will be discussed which have some practical significance to the corrections worker, in that people to whom these labels have been affixed are more apt to commit antisocial offenses than are equally disturbed people to whom other lables have been applied, labels which will not be discussed in this book. This does not imply that the antisocial offense is necessarily the direct result of the condition, although it may be.

Conditions are labeled in *DSM II* under a number system. Each main heading is assigned a three digit code. For example, **295, Schizophrenia.** Each division under this main heading is designated by a single digit following the main number. For example, **295.2 Schizophrenia, Catatonic Type.** If this division is subdivided a two digit number is used after the period. Thus, **295.23** is **Schizophrenia, Catatonic Type, Excited.** The first time any designation is introduced in this book, it will be in bold face type, followed by the proper code. This designation, without the number, will then be used consistently throughout the book.

Chapter 2

MENTAL RETARDATION

GENERAL CONSIDERATIONS

THE first condition to be discussed is **Mental Retardation (310-315).** Psychiatrically, mental retardation is described in two ways: according to degree and according to cause. The term mental retardation is so familiar that one probably rarely stops to ask what is meant by it. This is a term which designates those people whose general intellectual functioning is below that considered to be normal. An integral part of this concept is that this subnormal functioning is a result of difficulties originating from the developmental period, either that part of it during which the child is carried within its mother's body or that part of it embodied in the early years of life.

While one generally thinks of mental retardation in terms of intelligence quotient, or IQ, what is actually being discussed is an impairment in the ability to learn, an impairment in the ability to adjust socially, or a developmental failure in growth, sometimes all three. The intelligence quotient itself, while a convenient measuring rod, never should be the only standard used in making the diagnosis of mental retardation, or in evaluating its severity. Also to be taken into account are the ways the individual has progressed in school, in work, and in social adjustment. Indeed, there is a diagnosis of **Unspecified Mental Retardation (315).** This classification was created to account for those people in whom, for some reason or other, it is impossible to evaluate fairly and precisely the exact limits of intellectual functioning; however, even the most casual observer would know it is subnormal.

Thus, the intelligence quotient can be expressed in definite figures more easily than some of these other factors which go into producing the total picture of mental retardation. The degree of retardation is generally expressed by this quotient. According to *DSM II*, the general class of mentally retarded is divided into **Profound Mental Retardation**, IQ under 20, (**314**); **Severe Mental Retardation**, IQ of 20-35, (**313**); **Moderate Mental Retardation**, IQ of 36-51, (**312**); **Mild Mental Retardation**, IQ of 52-67, (**311**); and **Borderline Mental Retardation**, IQ of 68-85, (**310**). As far as coding in mental retardation is concerned, the index number indicates the degree of retardation, the subhead, the cause. Thus, **311.8** indicates **Mild Mental Retardation Due to Psychosocial (Environmental) Deprivation.**

It is rare in corrections to be concerned with other than the borderline or mildly mentally retarded. Those with an IQ under fifty function so poorly that most of their lives are lived in a sheltered environment where they have little opportunity to come in conflict with the law. Once in a great while, an individual in the moderate mental retardation subclass will be goaded by the teasing or bullying of peers or others into direct violent retaliation. With little or no knowledge of social or legal expectations and with impaired behavior control and judgment, he or she might attempt to satisfy primitive drives, such as hunger or sex, without due regard for the rights of others. Actually, these groups are much maligned by the public. Only rarely do they have this sort of difficulty. More commonly, they are exploited by society. The correctional worker is much more apt to be involved with those whose IQ is over fifty, those classified as mild or borderline mental retardation.

MENTAL RETARDATION DUE TO PSYCHOSOCIAL (ENVIRONMENTAL) DEPRIVATION (.8)

The causes of mental retardation are legion; *DSM II* lists sixty-one, although many of these are quite rare. The majority of mentally retarded whose behavior might bring them into conflict with the law are those whose mental retardation is caused by what *DSM II* classifies as **Psychosocial (Environmental) Deprivation (.8)** (usually **310.8** or **311.8**). This group makes up the greatest bulk of the mentally retarded. In these instances, a careful history and clinical and laboratory examination fail to reveal any evidence of organic disease or metabolic factors which might have caused the mental retardation. This general heading is divided under two subheadings. The first of these is **Cultural-Familial Mental Retardation.** To be placed in this category, it is necessary that at least one parent and one or more sibling(s) also show evidence of retardation. It was believed until recently that this was definitely an inherited condition; up to this point it has been impossible to identify the specific genes which carry the presumably inherited defect. The current belief is that the cultural level of the home environment which mentally retarded parents provide is apt to be quite low. Hence, the developing child does not receive all the necessary environmental stimulation to foster maximum potential growth in intelligence. The greatest part of these individuals classify in degree under the heading Mild or Borderline Mental Retardation.

The second group under this heading of psychosocial (environmental) deprivation are those **Associated with Environmental Deprivation.** Those people who belong to this group have been reared in an impoverished environment which failed to give them the necessary degree of environmental stimulation in infancy and early childhood. Such environments might include Appalachia or the ghettos of larger cities. As in the preceding group, such cultural deprivation robs the developing child of the ability to acquire the knowledge and skills needed to perform at normal standards. Also included in this group are those born blind or deaf, or both. Such defects cause a severe limitation on sensory input, even though the environment might be otherwise rich in stimulating factors. Unless there is an attempt to overcome these handicaps, the resultant retardation, although more severe than the first type, still falls into the mild range. With rehabilitative efforts, such children may even reach the borderline level. Indeed, some of them may even attain a superior intellectual level. Helen Keller is, of course, a prize example.

OTHER CAUSES

There are numerous other causes of mental retardation. It has been established that 75 percent of all cases fall into the categories already mentioned. Malnutrition, either of the mother during pregnancy or of the child as an infant, may contribute to mental retardation. This may be due not only to poverty, but to food faddism as well. Intrauterine infections may cause mental retardation in the child. Birth injury may lead to cerebral palsy; not all children with cerebral palsy are mentally retarded, but many are. The same thing holds true for the so-called minimally brain damaged child or hyperkinetic child. A definite congenital defect leads to Down's Syndrome, or mongolism. Inborn errors in metabolism with resultant inability to properly utilize certain elements in food may lead to mental retardation. Phenylketonuria (PKU) is the most widely known of these. Mental retardation can be prevented if the condition is discovered in infancy and corrected by the proper diet. Prolonged, very high fever accompanying infectious disease in infants may lead to mental retardation, as may complications of certain infectious diseases. Untreated epilepsy in a very young child may lead to deterioration in mental functioning. (This is not meant to include those children who occasionally have convulsions during periods of high fever.) Poisoning by lead and other heavy metals in infancy is sometimes seen in the history of the mentally retarded. For the purposes of the corrections worker, it is not necessary to inquire about the presence of these conditions in all cases of mental retardation. It is wise to note them when they are volunteered during history taking.

Any discussion of the relationship between mental retardation and crime must include at least some mention of the so-called XYY Syndrome. In *DSM II*, this would be classified as **Mental Retardation with Chromosomal Abnormality (.5).** Under this category, there is a special class, **With Sex Chromosome Anomalies.** Genetically, it is the presence of a Y chromosome which determines if the embryo becomes a male. Because of anomalies in chromosomal development and maturational splitting and mating, it possible to have a male who instead of having one Y chromosome has two, and hence the XYY Syndrome develops. Studies of large numbers of births show that the incidence of this XYY Syndrome is one in one thousand live male births. Such individuals are almost always taller in height than average and are generally mildly mentally retarded. Because they have been found in larger numbers in prison populations than in the general population, there was formerly felt to be some connection between the XYY Syndrome and crime. Many carefully conducted studies now seem to indicate that there may be some connection between the presence of the XYY Syndrome and antisocial offenses, but there is definitely no increase in aggression or violent crime in this group. Work in this field is still being done. Until the final answer is found, it would appear to be the better part of judgment not to associate a criminal career and the extra Y chromosome.

The connections between mental retardation and antisocial behavior are fairly obvious. Because of their deficits, the mentally retarded do not function in the educational sphere as well as their more fortunate peers. As youngsters they are usually placed in special schools for the mentally retarded or in special classes in regular public schools. (In many communities, these facilities do not exist.) These children are placed in the lowest track in their classrooms, continuously singled out as being different and not as bright as other kids. They become the target of taunting and teasing very early in life. In spite of popular myths to the contrary, those who are mentally retarded do not, as a general rule, equal their more fortunate peers in physical capacity and dexterity. They are apt to be as blundering and awkward on the playground and athletic fields as they are in the classroom. There is no way in which to excel or come to the fore, so they grow up with very low self-images.

This lack of ability of some mentally retarded people to cope adequately with the demands of the environment may cause other aggressive, antisocial offenses. The frustrations which build up may lead to an explosive type of behavior. Sometimes this behavior is directed against those perceived as tormentors or as responsible for the frustrations. At other times this behavior may be directed in a nonspecific fashion against the environment. It cannot be stressed too often that, in spite of this, a minority of mentally retarded individuals come into conflict with the law. Indeed, considering the handicaps that they struggle against, it is remarkable that this number is proportionately so small.

THE ROLE OF THE CORRECTIONS WORKER

What is the role of the corrections worker in his attempt to work with the mentally retarded who have been involved in the criminal system? It goes without saying that one of the first tasks is to help restore a feeling of self-worth and dignity to the mentally retarded. This means a strict avoidance of such terms as "dummy, stupid, nitwit" when dealing with them. Efforts should be made to assist them in reaching their maximum potential educational level, particularly insofar as vocational education is concerned. Perhaps nowhere in the whole field of criminology is rehabilitation to gainful employment as important as it is in dealing with the mentally retarded who are apt to form the dregs of the labor market. Another important part of the corrections worker's job, where it is practical, particularly in probation or parole, is to enforce strictly the section of the probation or parole conditions which deal with the nonassociation with known criminals. This is because the mentally retarded are so easily dominated and are in general so suggestible. The probation or parole officer should almost become the key person in the support system which these people need, and should see to it that other community agencies are mobilized to help them. Work with mentally retarded individuals is frequently frustrating and, on the surface, nonrewarding. However, with patience and perserverance, it is amazing what can be taught and learned. Suggestions must be phrased in the simplest terms possible, repeated as frequently as possible, and in as many different ways as possible. It is always necessary to be sure that one problem, direction, or suggestion is clearly understood in a most direct, concrete, practical way before proceeding to the next one.

The mentally retarded person is apt to be suspicious when caught in the toils of the law. In order to allay these suspicions, a relationship must be formed through a combination of firmness, fairness, respect, and the desire to be of help. The loyalty to those who are seen as genuinely trying to be of help may be the worker's most potent tool.

Chapter 3

ORGANIC BRAIN SYNDROMES
(290-294)

GENERAL CONSIDERATIONS

THIS and the following chapter will be concerned with **Organic Brain Syndromes (290-294).** In general, organic brain syndromes are of two types. The first consists of those in which the functions of the brain (and hence presumably of the mind) are overwhelmed by poisoning, whether acute or chronic. The second includes those in which actual anatomical damage to the brain can be demonstrated. This change may be due to disease, degenerative process, new growth, or injury. All organic brain syndromes have certain symptoms in common. Whenever these symptoms appear, the possibility of organic brain syndrome should be considered. The question can then be answered by further tests. These symptoms may be present to a marked or to a much lesser degree, but at least many of them should be present.

There are five such sets of symptoms:

1. Impairment of Orientation. The individual has difficulty in orienting himself in time and place, occasionally even as to person, that is, "Who am I?"
2. Impairment of Memory. This may involve only the more recent past, the remote past, a specific circumscribed period of the individual's life, or all of these.
3. Difficulty in Cognition. This involves such functions as learning, the retention of skills such as reading and writing, proper interpretation of input from the environment, problem solving, etc.
4. Defective Judgment. Included here are both practical and abstract judgment. The former has to do with the realities of the life situation; the latter includes the answer to ques-

tions like, "What would you do if you found a stamped, self-addressed envelope?"

5. Disorders of Feeling Tone. Chapter 6 deals with the major mood disorders. What is under consideration here are the changes in emotional responsiveness which may be seen in organic brain damage. In many of these conditions, the emotions are very much on the surface. They may change with any change in stimulus. At times, irritability is very common. At other times, a childish type of silliness, sometimes called *witzelsucht* is seen. One mood may follow another in rapid succession.

The disordered mental state is the direct result of the damage to the brain, but the degree to which that disorder expresses itself and the nature of the expression may, at times, have more to do with the underlying personality traits of the individual than with the actual damage to the brain itself. Thus, a degree of brain damage which may cause serious symptoms in one person may cause much milder symptoms in another. The location of the damage is an important factor in symptom production. At times, relatively large *lesions* (areas of damage) may occur in so-called silent brain areas and give no evidence of their presence. It should also be noted that organic brain syndromes may be acute or chronic in nature. Sometimes it is only the passage of time which reveals, with any certainty, that this is a chronic brain syndrome. In other situations, it is obvious from the outset that the condition will never improve. One other fact in relationship to organic brain syndromes deserves mention. That is, that an individual suffering from such a syndrome may or may not be psychotic. When classification is done, the individual is described as having a psychosis[1] with a particular organic brain syndrome, or as having the organic brain syndrome without psychosis.

There are very definite connotations implied when the term psychosis is used, whether in relationship to an organic brain syndrome or to those disorders for which no specific cause can be found. These connotations hold true no matter what aspect

[1]Psychosis implies that mental functioning has been so seriously impaired that the individual is no longer able to cope successfully with the ordinary demands of life.

of personality function has been disordered by the underlying condition. Distortions of reality may result from an improper input of environmental stimuli or from an improper processing of what is taken in. Swings in mood may be so severe that they completely impede the individual's capacity to react and respond adequately to a situation. For example, the loss of a ten-dollar bill is seen in a completely different light by those to whom at that particular moment this is the best of all possible worlds than it is by those who are neither unduly happy or unduly sad, or by those that are so overwhelmed by a despair so black that everything seems hopeless. Memory no longer functions properly if words no longer have meaning. Once there is no way of establishing cause and effect relationships, the grasp on reality may be completely lost.

ALCOHOLIC PSYCHOSES (291)

The most common of the organic brain syndromes are those due to alcohol. **Alcoholic Psychoses (291)** must be differentiated from simple drunkenness, even though many individuals when drunk manifest some, if not all, of the five symptoms which were listed as being characteristic of organic brain syndromes. Several of the alcoholic psychoses are of significance to the corrections worker and hence, will be described. The focus in this section is on those alcoholics who have become psychotic. The extremely important question of alcoholism, as such, will be taken up in Chapter 19.

The first of the alcoholic psychoses to have any significance for corrections workers is **Delirium Tremens (291.0)**. This is that alcoholic condition popularly known as DTs, the "shakes", the "horrors", the "willies", the "heebee-jeebies", the "terrors", the "screaming meemies", etc. There is almost always a long history of heavy alcoholic consumption before delirium tremens develops. As a general rule, delirium tremens is initiated by abstinence over a period of several days. Generally, this abstinence has been enforced because the sufferer is in a hospital or is in jail. For this reason, many authorities look upon it as a withdrawal phenomenon. There is usually a history of having substituted alcohol for food over a considerable period of time. As a result, deficiency of vitamins occurs. Delirium tremens commonly start with a preliminary period of one to three days of marked shakiness and tremor of the hands. This is particularly apt to occur in the morning. As the condition develops, the tremor encompasses the entire body. At times, it gets so severe that speech is indistinct because of tremors of the tongue or throat. During this same two or three day preliminary period there may be extremely bad nightmares from which the sufferer wakes up screaming and bathed in sweat. This so-called *prodromal* (preliminary) period is followed by a persistence of symptoms whether awake or asleep. The tremor is accompanied by profuse sweating. Extreme confusion is seen, with loss of orientation; characteristically this is both to time and place. It may occasionally be to person.

The most typical feature of the condition is the presence of extremely vivid, visual hallucinations. It is most characteristic of delirium tremens that the hallucinations are tiny in nature, although they do not have to be. There may be whole parades of little men climbing in under the crack of the door, or spiders walking up and down the wall, even climbing over the sufferer. Indescribable monsters are even more horrifying because they would fit in a thimble. Even the traditional "pink elephants" are generally no larger than a small house cat. All of this is panic-inducing for the sufferer, who cowers in a corner, trembling and sometimes pointing shakily at the source of the torment. Progressive weakness follows. The sufferer may be reduced to simply lying on the bunk; muttering, shaking, and from time to time feebly lifting a hand.

Naturally, such an individual is not about to commit a crime, but every corrections worker should be absolutely sure of the ability to recognize delirium tremens as soon as possible. "Pink elephants" may sound funny, but this is truly a deadly illness. Corrections workers have more than their share of clients with delirium tremens since alcoholism is so common in the lives of these clients. This condition is an acute emergency. As soon as the corrections worker even suspects its presence, medical help should be summoned. Transfer of the offender to a hospital is an urgent necessity. The mortality rate of untreated delirium tremens ranges up to 15 percent; that is, one out of every six people who have the disease will die. Even with the best treatment, the mortality rate has never been lowered below 3 percent in any reported series.

It might be well to add that other forms of the condition are seen. There may be delirium tremens without tremor, in which only the confusion, perspiration, and hallucinations are present. Or, there may be delirium tremens without delirium, in which only marked perspiration and tremor are present. The last carries the most favorable outlook, but such people deserve careful attention because this may represent simply an early stage of the disease which may develop fully within a few days.

The next alcoholic psychosis to be considered is one of which every corrections officer should be aware, although it is much more apt to be a law enforcement officer who comes in contact, sometimes disastrously, with the individual who has developed this condition. This is called **Other Alcoholic Hallucinosis (291.2)**. For some reason, this has been very rarely reported in females. It differs from delirium tremens in almost every respect. First, the sensorium is completely clear; that is, the individual is fully oriented and completely aware of what is going on around him. As a general rule, he is not tremulous. Also, as a general rule, his food intake has been good. The one thing in addition to longstanding, excessive alcohol intake that he has in common with those suffering from delirium tremens is that he too is hallucinated. From the moment of onset, he is bombarded by voices. These tell him, in no uncertain terms, what a louse he is. They say he is the scum of the earth and does not deserve to live. According to the voices, this opinion is so universally held that society is about to retaliate for all his misdeeds by subjecting him to the most painful and lingering tortures which the mind of man can devise.

Under these circumstances, since his sensorium is clear, since he is not confused, there is no reason for him to doubt the validity of these sensory experiences which he is having. Hence, he prepares to defend himself against this imagined fate. He surrounds himself with an arsenal of weapons, barricades himself in one room of his home with an ample supply of whiskey and food, and waits for society to come and get him. He is determined that before he gives up his life others are going to pay dearly for it. Not uncommonly, such individuals are killed in shootouts with the police, but if arrested are no less dangerous because they have been incarcerated and their weapons taken away. The hallucinations persist. These people, too, belong in a hospital, though it may be some time before the true state of affairs is discovered and proper steps are taken to control the symptoms medically. Some will clear up after about thirty days of abstinence without treatment. In others, the condition appears to be chronic and permanent. With present day chemotherapy, there is hope for control if not absolute cure. Certainly, some of those described as alcoholic psychoses, other alcoholic hallucinosis, represent some of the most dangerously disturbed people with whom the law has to deal. Although during the acute stage they are better known to police, the probation or parole officer should know that this condition may recur with only limited alcohol intake and should be ready to take the proper steps should the client show evidence of beginning to drink again.

Also listed under alcoholic psychoses is the condition know as **Alcoholic Psychoses, Paranoid State (291.3)**. This, too, is a condition in which acts of violence may occur. This is seen most commonly in males, although an occasional female will develop this form of psychosis. Marked delusions about the fidelity of the spouse occur in such an individual. The jealousy of such a male is literally unbridled. The mechanisms behind these delusions range from the quite obvious to the relatively obscure. The deterioration in judgment, usually present as one of the symptoms of organic psychosis, certainly has a lot to do with them. Shakespeare, that very astute observer of human frailties, puts into the mouth of the porter in Macbeth this observation concerning alcohol and sex, "Lechery, Sir, it provokes and unprovokes; it provokes the desire but it takes away the performance." A chronically heavy drinker has more and more difficulty in attaining and maintaining an erection when he is drunk. Eventually, in many chronic alcoholics the same state of impotence is present even when not drunk. Furthermore, the chronic alcoholic has probably been much more interested in alcohol than in sex. It has even been suggested that in some of these individuals there is an unconscious homosexual component. As time goes on and the alcoholic neglects his wife more and more, he begins to feel guilty. As a defense against these feelings of guilt, he projects the responsibility onto his wife. He feels that she is accusing him of not being a man. He does not say to himself, "I'm not filling her needs, I'm not satisfying her," but rather, "She's cheating on me." As a result, he becomes more paranoid and accuses his wife of being unfaithful. He may attack or kill any man who stops at his house, be it the Fuller Brush man, the milk man, the mailman, or any other male who happens to be there. He may assault his wife, quite frequently on the grounds that she is being unfaithful to him. Either way, he ends up in the arms of the law.

Once a paranoid condition to this extent has been established in the alcoholic, it is very difficult to treat. Even if he becomes completely abstinent, his impotence may persist, and with it, his paranoid ideas. (There is some suggestion that, at this point, the impotence has become organic.) This persistence of the paranoid ideas should be taken into consideration when assessing the probatability of such an individual. Even if the condition improves there is evidence to indicate that the psychosis may return in full flower if drinking is resumed. This, of course, implies that the probation or parole officer must insist on absolute abstinence as a condition of probation or parole, and the subject should be told he will be considered in violation if he again begins to drink.

Another form of alcoholic psychosis, which lacks the dramatic manifestations of those conditions discussed up to this point, is seen frequently. It is called **Alcoholic Deterioration (291.5).** This condition also develops as the result of habitual alcohol abuse, although a rare case is seen after relatively small intake. It is manifested by the deterioration of higher mental functioning. This is believed to be caused by actual death of nerve cells as they are poisoned by the products of repeated excessive alcohol intake. The chief manifestation of alcoholic deterioration is a marked, although patchy, memory loss. There is frequently increasing muscular incoordination which goes along with this syndrome. (A specialized form of this is known as *Wernicke's disease*, in which the afflicted individual walks on his heels, so to speak, looking much like a punch-drunk prizefighter. This is caused not only by the generalized death of cells, but also by tiny hemorrhages located in areas of the brain which have to do with coordination of sight and locomotion. These hemorrhages are believed to be produced by deficiency of vitamin B.) Along with the defect in memory and the lack of coordination, there is an impoverishment of judgment and creativity. The individual cares less and less about personal appearance and becomes very slovenly. Not uncommonly, the diet for the previous week can be deduced from the various stains on the outer clothing. Mobilizing adequate help for these people can prove extremely difficult for the worker. Hopefully, the situation will improve when the care of the alcoholic is diverted from the justice system and turned over to the public health system where it more properly belongs. Even though there is a continuing spread of decriminalization of alcoholism, many deteriorated alcoholics make up a disproportionately large share of the people seen in the lower courts.

Occasionally, an individual with **Korsakov's Psychosis (Alcoholic) (291.1)** will find himself in jail or in a lock-up as a vagrant. The chief signs of this illness are disorientation, impairment of memory, and involvement of the nerves of the extremities, with resultant weakness of the hands and feet and pains in the calves. The thing which characterizes this illness from other alcoholic conditions is the fact that the individual attempts to make up for his impairment of memory by a device known as *confabulation*. Although memory is almost completely gone, the individual who confabulates acts as though it were completely intact. Thus, sitting in a jail cell before breakfast is served, and asked if he has had his breakfast, he is apt to reply, "Yes." Asked what he was served, he may start off with "bacon and eggs, french-fried potatoes, sausage, toast, and coffee," or "hominy grits and chitlings," or any other culinary delicacy of which he is aware. He will go on and on in great detail as to how much he enjoyed the meal. Three minutes later, he can be approached by the same guard, not recognize ever having seen the guard before, and if asked if he has had breakfast, will say, "No, but there isn't any need to give me food, because I only finished my supper an hour ago and I haven't even had my night's sleep." The prime significance of this condition is that the guard, or any other person who comes in contact with him, should not misinterpret the situation and think that the prisoner is making jokes with him or trying to mislead him, and hence, react with irritation. This, too, is an individual who belongs in a hospital. Although this is a chronic condition, sometimes if it is spotted early enough and treated with massive doses of vitamins, particularly of the B variety, recovery is possible.

The discussion of alcoholic psychoses is brought to a close by consideration of two conditions which are quite identical symptomatically but are differentiated by the quantity of ingested alcohol necessary to produce them. One is known as **Acute Alcohol Intoxication (291.4)**; the other is **Pathological Intoxication (291.6)**. Both of these are acute brain syndromes. Both must be differentiated from simple drunkenness. Drunkenness does not imply psychosis although it may resemble it. The outstanding characteristic of each of these conditions is the wild outburst of psychotic behavior brought on by the consumption of alcohol. These are the fighting drunks who smash up bars, sometimes a whole series in one night. They intimidate and overwhelm individuals who are caught in their destructive path. Frequently the next day they have no recollection at all of the wide swath of destruction that they wrought the night before. What differentiates the two from each other is the quantity of alcohol consumed. Pathological intoxication comes on after only minimal alcoholic intake; sometimes just one drink is enough to release the entire picture. As a usual rule, this happens the very first time an individual takes a drink and continues to happen anytime any alcohol is consumed thereafter. In a lesser number of people who demonstrate pathological intoxication, there is a history of diminishing tolerance to alcohol. Originally, and for quite some time, they could consume large quantities of alcohol, sometimes without any problems over and beyond simple drunkenness. As time goes on, it takes less and less alcohol intake on any particular occasion to make them drunk. Finally, one drink will not only make them drunk, but will bring about this destructive psychotic outburst. In some individuals who manifest pathological intoxication a very careful history and diagnostic work-up may reveal the presence of an underlying temporal lobe epilepsy (see Chapter 4), the manifestations of which are released by alcohol. Another abnormal state which is sometimes released by alcohol consumption is the **Episodic Dyscontrol Syndrome** (see Chapter 9).

In Acute Alcohol Intoxication, the same symptomatology occurs but only after the individual has consumed a great deal of liquor. Rarely, temporal lobe epilepsy is also found to underlie acute alcohol intoxication. Much more commonly, the basic problem in this condition is an underlying personality disorder, either an **Explosive Personality (301.3)** or **Passive Aggressive Personality (301.81)** (see Chapter 10). If either of these conditions, that is, temporal lobe epilepsy or personality disorder, can be demonstrated to be the basic problem, then this classification should be used.

From a medico-legal standpoint, individuals with either of these two alcoholic psychoses present a very troublesome problem insofar as responsibility is concerned. First, the differential diagnosis between these conditions and plain lying about not remembering is at times very difficult to make. Sometimes, the only way it can be made is on the historical basis that every time such an individual drinks such an episode follows. In addition to this the question of responsibility comes up. Certainly, after one or two attacks of pathological intoxication, an individual might be expected to have enough forewarning of what might happen so that alcohol is avoided. Thus, any further drinking implies responsibility. Not uncommonly, these people will seek medical help before there are problems with the law. Anyone who has had three or four experiences of taking one or two drinks, and then remembering nothing about the evening is apt to become quite concerned about the possibility of something being wrong. This is particularly true if friends tell a long tale of fights and flights about which nothing is remembered. This question of responsibility becomes far more complex in the case of acute alcohol intoxication occurring as an episode in a chronic alcoholic, because then the interesting question arises as to whether or not the drinking is under the individual's control.

From the viewpoint of the corrections worker attempting to work with such a person, total abstinence is an absolute requirement of probation conditions. This should be fortified by every means within the probation worker's command. Where abstinence is a condition of probation, it is wise to obtain independent appraisals of the öffender's continuing sobriety. This frequently poses a real dilemma for the worker. If he is detected checking up without the offender's foreknowledge, there is almost always an immediate reaction of, "You don't trust me," which serves as a good excuse to go out and get drunk. It is far better to put this on the table at the beginning of the relationship. Some statement can be made like, "I know how difficult it is for alcoholics to lay off completely. I will be checking on your abstinence from time to time as a way of helping you."

The probation officer should reinforce the demand for abstinence by every means at his command.[2] Although direct confrontation with the consequences of continued drinking sometimes has an adverse effect, it may have to be employed. Alcoholics Anonymous can be a powerful help to many alcoholics. Supportive reinforcement of abstinent patterns, first by recognition and praise, and then by progressively relaxing other conditions of probation is a helpful adjunctive technique. When an epileptic basis or an underlying personality disorder is suspected, medical consultation should be utilized. Even in the absence of these states, medication prescribed by the physician may be useful. This may take the form of specific vitamins and minerals or of Antabuse®. As long as the latter is in the

---

[2]While this material has been in press, a Supreme Court decision has rendered it inoperative. The Court has held that if an individual drinks because of chronic alcoholism, abstinence may not be a condition of probation, since the drinking is beyond the person's control.

system, the individual will become violently ill if he takes a single drink. Except for the treatment of withdrawal symptoms, or the period immediately thereafter, the use of any of the minor tranquilizers is not indicated as an aid in the long term management of the alcoholic who demonstrates either pathological intoxication or acute alcohol intoxication.

PSYCHOSES ASSOCIATED WITH OTHER PHYSICAL CONDITIONS (294)

There is another condition which is closely allied to the alcoholic psychoses. This is known as **Psychoses Associated with Other Physical Conditions (294)**. From the point of view of the corrections worker, the most important of these is called **Psychosis with Drug or Poison Intoxication (Other Than Alcohol) (294.3)**. All those psychotic conditions which are either triggered or caused by intake of drugs are listed under this heading. Discussion at this point does not consider the question of drug use or abuse, which is certainly important to the corrections worker. These will be discussed in the appropriate chapters in Part Three of this book. This section concerns those psychotic conditions caused by certain psychedelic drugs and by poisons. The situation here is very similar to that seen in the alcoholic psychoses: an acute condition may be caused by ingesting a particular drug one or two times or by overdosing with it; or a chronic condition may be brought on by long-term abuse. There were a series of very interesting cases of acute psychotic reaction occurring with the first or second use of marijuana by servicemen in Viet Nam.

> In one such instance, a soldier was doing guard duty immediately following his first experience with marijuana, and another serviceman in his outfit came by wearing a Mickey Mouse® T-shirt. The guard said, "Halt, who goes there?" and the T-shirt wearer said, "You know me, I'm your buddy, what do you mean 'Halt, who goes there?' " The guard shot and killed him. He stated he was convinced, at that moment, that because he was wearing a Mickey Mouse T-shirt he must be a Communist, therefore, he was "in league with the Gooks, and bang, eliminate him."

Naturally, of course, the question is raised whenever anything of this sort occurs, "How is it known that this is not simply malingering to escape punishment?" The whole matter of malingering is a very complicated topic, but a thorough investigation at the time convinced those in charge of the investigation that the man was legitimately psychotic because of having smoked marijuana. His condition improved within forty-eight hours and he was utterly horror-stricken and repentant because of what he had done. The relatively large number of incidents of this sort occurring in Viet Nam, in contrast to the almost complete absence of this sort of behavior while under the influence of marijuana in this country, is explained in the terms of the relative weakness of street marijuana here as compared to that available in South Viet Nam during the war years. Other drugs particularly known to produce an acute psychotic reaction are LSD ("acid"), "speed", and PCP ("elephant pills", "angel dust"). While a psychotic condition may be caused by these drugs, it is rare that antisocial behavior will result while in that psychotic condition, although by now several cases have been reported in which the severe excitement and agitation led to physical assaults on those in the environment.

What has been described to this point are conditions resulting from an acute intoxication by a specific drug. There are, in addition, psychoses caused by chronic drug abuse. It is almost characteristic of the present day chronic drug user that he does not limit himself to the use of any one drug but takes drugs of a number of different classes, sometimes simultaneously and sometimes sequentially. For this reason, it is very difficult to single out psychoses which are characteristic of the abuse of any one specific drug. One exception to this statement concerns the ingestion of the amphetamines, more commonly known as speed. Speed is a very common drug of abuse since it produces a high which many find very exhilarating. Many users were first introduced to speed by a physician. In the past, it was frequently used because of its appetite suppressant qualities. It is, therefore, widely used in so-called diet pills. Chronic overuse of speed not uncommonly leads to a form of paranoid psychosis in which persecutory ideas are quite common. Once such a psychosis is established, it tends to persist over long periods of time, even with abstinence from the drug and with treatment. While under the influence of such delusions, fantasized enemies may be harmed or even killed. (Examples of this sort of psychotic reaction due to chronic use of cocaine are beginning to be reported.)

> An illustrative case study concerns Mr. D, an eighteen-year-old man, about to graduate from high school, who had been heavily into drugs for about two years. For the six months preceding the onset of his difficulty he had been heavily into speed. During a Christmas vacation, accompanied by a friend, he started to drive to a college in which he felt he might be interested. It was a cold, rainy day and the road was icy. Some forty miles from home he decided that he did not have the guts to continue to drive on. He had the friend drop him by the side of the road and the friend continued on alone. Mr. D went into a nearby gas station to phone home. He began to have a very peculiar feeling that everyone in the gas station was staring at him because of his long hair. He began to get panicky. By the time someone from home came to get him, he was in an acutely agitated state. When his father walked into the home that night, he went berserk, thinking that the father was going to kill him, and attacked his father rather viciously. It was necessary to restrain him and take him to a hospital.

The psychoses which are seen with mixed drug usage tend to be far less specific. Many of them take on a schizophrenic (see Chapter 5) quality, while others show symptoms of apparent deterioration in judgment, thinking capacity, and self-esteem. There is very commonly an emotional dulling or flattening, sometimes progressing to almost complete apathy. These psychoses are of interest to the corrections worker as entities in themselves. Because of the psychosis, such misdemeanors as vagrancy, loitering, exhibitionism, public nuisance, and other offenses of this character may occur. Traffic offenses and felonies, not related directly to the drug usage but to the psychotic behavior which the drug use has led to, may also occur. The psychosis may be reversible and the corrections worker then has to deal with the rehabilitation of the individual once the psychosis has responded to treatment. As will be stressed in the chapter on drug abuse, rather than psychosis due to drug usage, the primary function of the corrections worker is dealing with the underlying personality problems which led to the drug abuse in the first place. This will be dealt with in detail later in this volume.

There is one other condition included in this general category of psychoses associated with other physical conditions which is quite rarely linked to antisocial behavior. When this linkage does occur, it is dramatic, almost always featured in the news media, and poses a real problem ultimately for the corrections worker. This is **Psychosis with Childbirth (294.4).** This is one of the conditions referred to in Chapter 2 in which there *is* a specific relationship between the mental illness and the antisocial offense. It is common, if not universal, for some mild degree of depression to be seen following childbirth. This is generally referred to as the *postpartum blues.* It comes on about the third or fourth day after the birth, is characterized by an illogical feeling of depression and very easily induced tears, lasts from twelve to twenty-four hours, and is gone. In some instances, however, this condition persists and worsens to a degree that it takes on the characteristics of a full-blown psychosis. Frequently, the mother seems fine when leaving the hospital, but within two to ten weeks becomes psychotic. As a general rule, the diagnosis will be made that this is a case of schizophrenia, reactive depression, or a depressed phase of manic depressive psychosis (see appropriate chapters) which has been triggered by childbirth. In relatively rare instances, such a psychosis occurs in a female in whom the most rigorous search fails to produce any indication that anything other than the childbirth itself was responsible for the illness. It is the nature of the resultant depression, rather than the cause, which is important for corrections.

At times, this depression takes the form of an agitated depression. In this state the woman begins to believe that this is the worst of all possible worlds, that she is the worst creature in this worst of all possible worlds, that nothing is ever going to be better, and, that because of her, her newborn child and her other children, if she has others, are going to have to suffer the tortures of the damned throughout their lives. As a result of these psychotic beliefs, such a woman may, and not too infrequently does, attempt to kill herself and her children. The intention is good. It is meant to spare the children needless suffering — a sort of mercy killing. Statistics show that for some reason, presumed to be correlated with basic personality factors, when women attempt suicide they do it more frequently by poison or gas than by one of the more violent methods such as stabbing, shooting, or hanging. One of the most commonly used gases is carbon monoxide, either from an automobile exhaust or from cooking or heating gas. When such a murder-suicide attempt is made, often the children, being much more susceptible to the effects of carbon monoxide, die, whereas the mother is found in time to be saved. The mother may attempt to kill only the children because she feels she is guilty and she has to continue to suffer, whereas she is sparing the poor innocents the pain of further suffering. In either case, the individual now faces the charge of murder.

In the usual course of events, such a woman would be recognized as mentally ill, not competent to stand trial, hospitalized until restored to competency, tried, and then either found not guilty by reason of insanity or found guilty but sentenced to immediate probation to a court officer. Under the latter circumstance, the attitude of the probation counselor will be one of the most significant factors in determining whether permanent rehabilitation is possible.

The presence of psychosis with childbirth may sometimes lead to a lesser type of offense, namely child abuse. Under these circumstances, the depression, rather than leading to self-depreciation and condemnation, may instead lead to feelings of being overwhelmed, unable to cope, and being ineffectual. There is a subsequent loss of positive self-image accompanied by irritability. These feelings may be taken out on the child. Here, too, if the situation is properly understood, the natural sentence will be probation, and again the attitude of the probation officer is of utmost significance in rehabilitation.

These offenses are so blatantly and obviously contrary to human experience and expectations that the perpetrator is very apt to arouse feelings of disgust, anger, and rejection from those people with whom she has to deal. Proper understanding should lead to empathy, understanding, and helpfulness. In rare instances, punitive attitudes may aid in the woman's expiation of guilt, but in the long run the more empathic attitudes are the ones which are most apt to be productive of rehabilitation. In those instances where the probation officer does become involved, it is, of course, these latter attitudes which are most effective in helping the probationer to come to grips with the very painful reality of resuming her life. It is frequently desirable, and at times necessary, particularly in the latter stages of the rehabilitative process, to involve the husband. This allows him to deal honestly with some of his own feelings of anger and dismay. He may well have suppressed these feelings in an attempt to aid his wife. Unless he is able to ventilate these adequately, they may well come to the surface in disguise and sabotage whatever efforts the probation officer is making. At times, it will be extremely helpful to involve the woman in some form of community activity in which she may feel that she is making a contribution. Such things as volunteer work in a nursing home or a hospital can be quite helpful. Once the acute stage of mourning the loss of her own child or children or working through the guilt of child abuse is passed, volunteer work in a nursery or day care center may also be helpful. Usually, there will be a physician involved with the offender in these instances and the probation counselor will want to be in close touch with the person administering the medical care.

Not infrequently, the probation officer will be asked as to the advisability of having another child to replace the one who was lost in this fashion. Of course, no hard and fast rules can be laid down to cover every situation; close consultation with medical personnel is advisable. In those instances where childbirth has precipitated a manic depressive, depressed type, illness, the birth of another child will trigger an identical depression in approximately 50 percent of the cases. The question of having another child should be referred to the appropriate medical person.

Another area in which the probation officer will have to furnish a tremendous amount of support is in terms of reentry into the community. As unobtrusively as possible, the officer should attempt to make a very careful appraisal of the mood of the community, particularly the immediate neighborhood. As noted above, very negative feelings are sometimes aroused by such an act. If these have not been changed when the offender returns to the community, it may sometimes be necessary to advise the couple to move to a new location. It must be stressed that only a very small number of women who suffer from psychosis with childbirth are involved in this sort of antisocial behavior. The number is significant enough, however, so that the corrections worker must always be aware of it.

Chapter 4

ORGANIC BRAIN SYNDROMES — PART TWO

PSYCHOSIS ASSOCIATED WITH INTRACRANIAL INFECTION (292)

THE next general heading under organic brain syndrome is **Psychosis Associated with Intracranial Infection (292)**. The greater number of the conditions listed under this heading in *DSM II* will not be discussed. Individuals so afflicted may be acutely or chronically ill. They may have some brain deterioration which may be accompanied by neurological signs, but for the most part, they are not involved in antisocial behavior. The most significant exception to this occurs in a form of syphilitic involvement of the brain. This is called **General Paralysis (292.0)**. This was the first so-called mental condition which was shown to be due to a specific infection and which responded to a specific treatment. It is labeled general paralysis because people with this condition, if left untreated, eventually become completely paralyzed to the point where they are bedridden. Fortunately, mental symptoms usually precede the onset of paralysis by several years. This allows time for adequate treatment if the condition is diagnosed. In rare instances, there may be only a relatively brief period of time, six months to a year, between the onset of symptoms and death.

There is a long time lag, usually from ten to fifteen years, between the original infection with the *spirochete*, the organism which causes syphilis, and the onset of symptoms of general paralysis. In the past, many individuals, particularly females, but occasionally males, could be infected with syphilis and not know that they had contracted it until many years later, when they begin to develop the symptoms to be described.

The present day treatment for syphilis in general, as well as for general paralysis, is by penicillin. An intensive campaign was waged against syphilis immediately following World War

II, and it had been felt that the disease was almost completely eradicated. For many years very few cases of general paralysis were seen. Recently, there has been an increase in reported cases of syphilis. This is due to a combination of the relaxation of the intensive drive against the disease, because of the complacent feeling that it was well under control, and the general change in sexual morality which has led to a marked increase in the number of sexual contacts of any one person. As a result of the increasing incidence of syphilis more cases of general paralysis are being seen. If the present trend continues, that number will continue to increase over the next several years, again assuming importance for the corrections worker.

Everyone who is infected with syphilis and who does not have treatment does not necessarily develop general paralysis. There are many other manifestations of syphilitic infection which may occur. Of all untreated cases of syphilis, only 28.9 percent develop syphilis of the nervous system. Of these, only 12 percent will develop general paralysis. Thus, approximately 3.5 percent of untreated syphilitics develop general paralysis. Because it has lain dormant in the body over all those years, syphilis is generally not suspected when the brain illness starts. Syphilis has been known as the "great imitator" because syphilitic disease of any part of the body can mimic almost any other disease. This is also true of syphilis of the brain. The original symptoms may appear to be those of almost any of the psychoses. However, a typical case approximates a course as follows:

> An individual, generally in the late forties, mental health seemingly unimpaired, now begins to make more and more gross errors of judgment. Along with this, there begins to develop some mildly grandiose ideas. The feeling grows within the individual of being a lot richer than in actuality. There are delusions of possession of all sorts of magic or superhuman powers. Dress becomes bizarre, and personal hygiene and cleanliness are disregarded. The general appearance deteriorates quite badly. At the same time, mental processes begin to slip gradually. An individual who might have been very sharp mathematically now finds, for example, that multiplying two digits by two digits in the head is an impossible

task. Simultaneously, certain motor and sensory difficulties may appear. One of these may be difficulty in speech, a condition which has been called *dysarthria*. The speech begins to be slightly slurred, almost as though the individual had been drinking. Syllables begin to be transposed. As this progresses, speech becomes almost completely disorganized. At this same time, there may be beginning disturbances in locomotion and in eye-hand coordination. The full-blown psychosis is usually characterized by markedly grandiose delusions and gross errors in judgment. It is here that the significance of this illness for the corrections system is concerned.

If an individual has delusions of being the richest and most powerful person in the world, and coincidentally, judgment has been badly impaired, then that individual can see no harm in walking into a store, picking up an expensive piece of merchandise and walking out with it. "It's mine. I own everything." There is nothing wrong in driving a car ninety-five miles per hour or trying to run over the policeman who attempts to interfere with this behavior. After all, no one should dare to try to stop the most powerful person in the world.

The following excerpt from an intake interview done at the Court Diagnostic and Treatment Center illustrates the sort of data which should immediately arouse suspicion of possible general paralysis:

Mr. E was being seen in presentence status on a charge of aggravated assault. At this point, the interviewer tried to focus on the present offense and asked the client what his charge was. He responded that he had no charges against him and he stated that his case was thrown out of court. It had not been thrown out of court. He was then asked why he had gone to court earlier that morning. He stated that he had been to court because a woman had gone into his house and taken some meat out of his refrigerator without asking him. In the actual episode, the woman, who lived in another apartment in the same apartment building in which he resided, had been sitting on the porch. He approached her and committed the offense with which he is charged.

He was then asked if he knew the woman and he responded, "Yes" He stated that he was outside talking to her

husband at the time she went into the house. He stated that
he walked into the house and observed her in his refrigerator
and asked her what she was doing. At that time he stated that
she did not respond but hit him with an object instead. After
she hit him, he became angry, "So I cut her with my knife."
He was then asked what kind of a knife it was. "A pocket
knife." The client was then asked if he usually carried knives
in his pocket and he stated he owned both knives and guns.
The client stated that after he cut the woman he returned to
the porch were her husband was. He was then asked if he
thought he had done the right thing by cutting her for her
having gone into his refrigerator. He stated that he did not
cut the woman for going into his refrigerator, but when she
hit him with that object that made him angry. And, furthermore, she did not have to go into his house and take meat
from his refrigerator without asking him because he would
have given her anything she wanted had she asked for it.
When asked what happened to the woman, he stated, "the
police didn't do anything to her."

Mr. E further told the interviewer that, even if his case had
not been thrown out, the police could not do anything to him
because he was only defending himself. He further stated,
"they would have thrown it out even if I wasn't the FBI." He
was asked how far he went in school and he responded, "I
was the first school teacher ever been down here. I taught
every-body how to read and write." He further stated that he
taught in a place called "Crystal City." When he was asked
where Crystal City was, he stated it was a city "located on the
other side of heaven." The interviewer then asked the client
how many times he had been married and he again became
quite grandiose and stated he had wives all around the world.
He further stated, "all the FBI and all the women that ain't
married belong to me." He ventilated some of his other grandiose ideas, stating he was the federal government, the FBI,
that he owned all the penitentiaries and everything else in
this country.

This is a typical picture of a patient suffering from general
paralysis. It is of extreme importance that the corrections
worker be alert to the possibility of the existence of this illness,
because this is a condition which can be treated specifically and
cured. If the disease has progressed only to the point that symp-

toms are due merely to irritation and swelling in the brain, then antibiotic treatment may reverse all the symptoms and cause the entire picture of the illness to disappear. If more extensive brain pathology has already occurred, then the progress of the disease may be stopped, but the patient will never return completely to normal. Differentiation of general paralysis from other conditions which may cause grandiosity, such as schizophrenia or paranoid states (see Chapters 5 and 7) is made on the basis of laboratory tests done on blood and spinal fluid and through neurological evaluation. It should be reassuring to know that general paralysis is not a communicable stage of syphilis. The worker does not have to be afraid of contracting the illness.

Other infections of the central nervous system, even when associated with psychosis, are seen so rarely by the corrections worker that there is no need to include them in this volume. Rarely, an individual in the early stages of encephalitis (popularly known as sleeping sickness) will behave in a bizarrely aggressive fashion. On rare occasions, similar behavior may be seen in some stages of an uncommon hereditary disease of the nervous system called Huntington's Chorea. (In this condition there are incoordinated involuntary jerking movements similar to those in St. Vitus Dance.)

DISORDERS OF THE AGING PROCESS

The next group of organic conditions which has significance in terms of antisocial behavior is associated with the aging process. While a distinction is made, diagnostically, between **Psychosis with Cerebral Arteriosclerosis (293.0)**, and **Senile Dementia (290.0)**, and **Presenile Dementia (290.1)**, they may most conveniently be discussed under the head of Aging Processes. The term *cerebral arteriosclerosis* refers to hardening of the arteries which supply the brain. Probably the commonest analogy which is used to describe what goes on in this process is to compare it with the rusting in lead and iron pipes. In both instances (the pipe and the arteries), this leads to a narrowing of the inner diameter. This narrowing in the arteries leads to a diminished flow of blood to the brain. This in turn leads to a diminished supply of oxygen and nourishment. These lead first to malfunctioning, then to death of brain cells. In addition, because of the narrowing of the smaller blood vessels, there is a tendency for the blood cells to pile up one on another and to form blood clots in the affected blood vessel. These blood clots shut off the flow of blood completely. There will quite frequently be loss of consciousness at this time. This is referred to as a *stroke*. Depending on the size and location of these clots, there may or may not be noticeable physical consequences such as paralysis or weakness of an arm or a leg or difficulty in speech. As these episodes increase in number, behavioral changes will be noted. The same "rusting" process leads to weakening of the blood vessel with a possibility of hemorrhage through it and the destruction of tissue in the area of the hemorrhage. This also leads to a stroke and to eventual deterioration, but in a much more rapid fashion.

In senile dementia, for reasons which are not quite so clear, there is also a progressive death of individual brain cells with resultant behavioral changes. There is some difference in the two condition. In cerebral arteriosclerosis the downward progression is apt to be irregular. There are periods of return to almost normal functioning, alternating with periods of disturbed functioning. Sometimes these alternations occur in the course of a twenty-four hour time period, sometimes over a longer interval of time. There is a gradually progressive downhill course. In senile dementia, the downhill course is not interspersed with periods of normal functioning.

It is also of a good deal of practical significance that, although there is an organic basis for both of these conditions, the behavioral symptoms are not apt to appear until there is an environmental stress. Such a stress might be the loss of a spouse, the necessity to move from a home to a smaller apartment because of changing financial circumstances, the death of a close friend, or hospitalization for some unrelated illness. It is almost as though the personality was able to compensate for the progressive loss of brain substance until some crisis situation occurs. Then compensation becomes more difficult and decompensation of the personality takes place. Presenile dementia involves the same sort of downhill course as senile dementia and is attributable to similar sorts of loss of brain substance. Differentiation between them is that they occur at different ages and run different courses. Presenile conditions have an onset between fifty-five and sixty and have a much more rapid downhill course than do the senile dementias. It is not at all unusual for death to occur from eighteen to thirty-six months after the onset of a presenile dementia.

There are many behavior problems associated with these disorders of the aging process. The two most commonly seen are progressive difficulty with memory, and mood changes. Increasing irritability is the most common mood change in the early phases. Depression is also frequently an early alteration of mood and is generally seen at one stage or another of the illness. Suspiciousness is another commonly encountered mood difficulty and is particularly apt to occur if one of the senses, such as vision or hearing, particularly the latter, begins to fail. The reason for the suspiciousness associated with hearing loss is fairly obvious. If one is not clearly taking in what is going on around one, it is very easy to misinterpret events in a frightening way. Another less frequently seen changing mood is that of a rather silly sort of cheerfulness, quite out of keeping with the situation. The failing memory and difficulty in thought processes lead eventually to disorientation and marked confusion. Interestingly, although delusions may result from the suspiciousness and the confusion, hallucinations are very unusual in the senile disorders.

If only the end stages of these conditions were being considered, it would be difficult to understand why they are included as being of significance to corrections workers. Those very demented individuals, who may or may not be paralyzed and may or may not be confined to bed, obviously do not commit crimes. It is in the earlier stages of the disorders that antisocial behavior occurs. The elderly individual, who is apt to be alone and lonely, whose judgment is impaired because of the impairment in thought processes, is apt to get involved in sex play with young children. The kindly old man who has the neighborhood girls and boys into his house is looking for company as much as anything else, but there are vague stirrings of sexual desire which he may not, at times, even recognize as such. He is incapable of fulfilling these desires along socially acceptable lines because he cannot attract a suitable female and because, in many instances, he will not be able to carry out successful sexual relations if he could. Thus, he is quite prone to start sex play with these children. Such play is most apt to be limited to fondling and caressing the child, possibly exposure of his own genitalia, and sometimes handling of the children's genitalia. This last is more uncommon. On even rarer occasions, there may be some oral sexuality involved. At times, when younger teenage boys are involved, there may be some blackmail on the part of these youngsters. The elderly individual may become as much the victim as the victimizer.

The corrections worker may frequently be of marked help in rehabilitation if aware of the role of environmental factors in the production of this condition. Mobilization of community resources in terms of Golden Age Groups and attempts to involve the individual in community activities of the sort which give him some feelings of being of use and of worth again may do a good deal, not only in preventing recidivism, but actually in reversing some of the seeming organic changes. The depression which so often accompanies this condition frequently responds to chemotherapy on the part of the physician. The physican and the corrections worker, by joint effort, may restore an individual to a really meaningful life pattern. Above all, these people do not belong in jail. Hospitalization should be used as a last resort because it may lead to life-long institutionalization.

The case of Mr. F is cited to illustrate this condition and its management. This seventy-four year old, white, male widower was referred to the Court Diagnostic and Treatment Center for presentence examination and recommendation. He had been accused by two teenaged boys, aged thirteen and fourteen, of having asked them to perform oral sex on him under the pretext of educating them sexually. On examination, he was a depressed, lonely, garrulous man, who was able to give only a sketchy account of his life, which had to be supplemented from other sources. He had always been an active individual, had worked with his hands, and had been a very steady worker. He had been married at the age of twenty, but had been childless. He had, however, practically become a foster father to a young man to whom he was distantly related. This young man had lived with him while going through college and graduate school, but then as he had married and started raising a family of his own, had moved out of the house. He continued to maintain his interest in his uncle at that level which his own life pattern would permit.

Mr. F. had been forced to retire at sixty-eight. When he was seventy-one his wife had died. For awhile, the work necessary to maintain the home kept him going. As time passed, he was aware of becoming increasingly lonely. His interests became more and more limited. He stopped his shopping trips, began to take less care of his personal appearance and of the home. At this point, some of the neighborhood boys, with whom he had always been friendly, started congregating in his house and, to all intents and purposes, ripped him off. They smoked his cigarettes. At first they cadged money from him. Later, they began to pick up anything that was left around loose. They stole objects from the home and sold them for money. He tolerated this behavior just because of their companionship.

The record is not completely clear as to who actually instigated the sexual behavior, but sexual play started. It never got beyond the talking and showing stage. One of the boys, in a fit of pique because Mr. F would not give him money on demand, reported the behavior to his parents, who notified the police.

A recommendation for probation with intensive casework and medical help was made on this man. Antidepressant medication was prescribed by the physician. The probation officer was instrumental in two areas: (1) He reinforced the efforts of the foster son to have the uncle become more involved with him; and (2) He aided Mr. F to involve himself in activities at a retiree center. Even with all this, Mr. F's judgment was poor enough so that on one or two occasions the worker again found the boys in question in Mr. F's home. When he remonstrated with him he was told that it was just so lonely that he had to have someone around. Gradually, Mr. F began to be more and more involved in other activities so that he was able to put a firm foot down, and keep the boys out of his house. He developed many interests and even the seeming memory loss and confusion began to clear. Some eighteen months after the offense, he was continuing to do well.

Another type of antisocial behavior which is sometimes seen in these individuals is the result of the development of suspicious delusions. These delusions are most apt to center around marital infidelity on the part of the spouse. With the poor judgment and the lack of control that goes with organic brain damage, these individuals may become acutely disorganized and attempt physical harm, either to the spouse, who they feel is unfaithful, or to individuals in the area whom they believe to be persecutory. This may sometimes end in real tragedy as firearms or other dangerous weapons may be involved. The condition seen is very much like alcoholic psychosis, paranoid type, to which the element of confusion has been added.

PSYCHOSIS WITH EPILEPSY (293.2)

Epilepsy is a very significant disorder to the corrections worker for two reasons. The first of these is that the opportunity is given to dispel the widely held notion that all epileptics are dangerous, surly, and explosive. This is simply not true. It has been demonstrated that the **Epileptoid Personality (301.3)** (see Chapter 9), with wild outbursts of rage on slight provocation, is far more common in the general population than it is in epileptics. The second significant aspect for the corrections worker is that there are some epileptic disorders in which criminal offenses, sometimes serious ones, can be committed. Again, the admonition that this applies only to the minority of the epileptics must be kept in mind when, in the presentence report, the investigator is trying to evaluate past history and relate it to current events.

Epilepsy is a temporary disturbance of the functioning of the brain which is manifested by attacks occurring at recurrent intervals. There are many varieties of these epileptic attacks.

Those factors which link them under one heading, *epilepsy,* are the following: the presence of a hereditary factor; a repetitive, episodic, behavior pattern which is different from the normal behavior pattern of the individual; disturbance in the electro-encephalogram, more commonly known as the EEG. (The EEG measures rhythmic changes in the brain, just as the electrocardiogram, or EKG, measures rhythmic changes in the electric potential in the heart.) Not all convulsions are caused by epilepsy and even in the presence of a definite family history, caution must be taken to rule out such things as seizures following brain injury, seizures due to brain tumor, seizures due to mild cerebrovascular disorders, and seizures caused by drugs or poisons.

With the exception of petit mal epilepsy, any other form of the condition may be thought of as occurring in six phases. These are the prodromal phase, the aura, the attack or seizure, the postattack phase, the confusional phase, the resting or interval phase. It is not necessary for each phase to occur in each cycle. At times, many seizures may occur in rapid succession without any interval of clear consciousness between. Such a condition is called *Status Epilepticus.*

The *prodromal phase* is manifested by a marked change in personality which lasts from a few minutes to a few days preceding an attack. Some people never experience a prodromal phase. The change in personality is generally in the direction of increased restlessness, irritability, and aggressiveness. A simple request, normally evoking smiling acquiescence, may bring on a verbal tirade of abuse or may even be accompanied by physical resistance. Once the entire attack has run its course, there is generally a feeling of great embarrassment with genuine expression of penitence. Many times, the connection between the abnormal behavior in the prodromal phase and the underlying illness is not made until brought to light by a careful history.

The next phase, the *aura,* when present, is a definite warning that a seizure is to follow. The aura is almost always perceived as a sensory experience. The nature of this experience varies widely from individual to individual. It may be a strange odor, a buzzing in the ears, a feeling of lighheadedness, a tingling in the fingers, a feeling of depersonalization or disembodiment. Sounds may appear unusually loud, or surroundings may seem to retreat to a great distance. An aura has been reported consisting of a feeling of "there is something terribly important which I must remember, but I don't know what it is." There is no end to the various forms which aurae may assume.

Generally, a particular aura is idiosyncratic for any one individual. That is, having once experienced an aura before a seizure, the same one will always appear. At times, the aura is extremely brief and the seizure follows immediately thereafter. At other times, there is a relatively long interval between the beginning of the aura and the attack itself. During this interval the person may have time to find a place of relative security. Some individuals may avoid an attack by conscious effort after having experienced the aura. Some people find it impossible to predict on any particular occasion whether or not an attack will follow an aura, or whether the aura alone will occur. Obviously, it must be quite trying to have a strange sensory experience and not know whether or not it is going to develop into unconsciousness or peculiar behavior. At times, confusion during the aura itself leads to disturbed and even antisocial behavior.

The nature of the *attacks* or *seizures* varies with the type of epilepsy and will be described as each variety is discussed.

A period of *confusion* follows each attack. (This is not true for petit mal attacks.) This confusion will last from a few seconds to several hours or even days. All sorts of bizarre behavior may appear in this period of clouding of consciousness. In some patients, this is followed by an irresistible urge to sleep. On awakening, clarity has been restored. The periods of confusion which occur during the aura, during the attack itself, or immediately after the attack have been called epileptic *twilight states, fugues,* or *clouded states.*

The final phase of the epileptic cycle is the *interval period.* Depending on the degree to which the condition has been amenable to control, this may last from a very short period of time to months or even years. As a general rule, in the interval phase, the behavior of the epileptic is no different from that of any other individual. Exceptions to this will be noted at the appropriate times.

Epilepsies are classified according to the nature of the behavior disorder and the nature of the electroencephalographic change. *Grand mal* seizures are the most common, the most dramatic, and the best known of all the varieties of epilepsy. In the grand mal attack, with or without an aura, there is a sudden onset of loss of consciousness. All the musculature of the body suddenly stiffens. At this point, the eyes generally roll up because the muscles rolling the eyes upwards are stronger than the other eye muscles, hence, they take predominance. There may be, coincidentally, a loud scream, because in the stiffening of the muscles the breath is forced out through the constricted vocal cords. Almost invariably, the individual drops to the ground like a block of wood. Severe injuries may result from this fall. This phase of stiffened muscles is called the *tonic* period and lasts from thirty to sixty seconds. It is followed by the *clonic* phase in which there is alternate contraction and relaxation of the muscles, during which the individual jerks rhythmically in all extremities and may bounce around. The mouth opens and closes. The tongue may be badly bitten during this period. Also, during this period, there may be relaxation of the bowel and bladder sphincters, and the individual might either soil or wet. The clonic phase lasts for approximately two minutes during which time the person becomes blue because of lack of oxygen. As this phase passes, respiration is resumed, the color returns to normal, and the subject usually breathes in a snoring, stertorous fashion. There may or may not be foaming at the mouth. The individual then remains unconscious for four to five minutes, awakens in a dazed and confused state, and may, at this time, be extremely restless. It is during this confused stage, following recovery of consciousness, that a small minority of people with grand mal seizures may become quite dangerous. It is at this time that they are apt to be explosive. They thrash about restlessly, resisting all attempts to hinder their movements. Again, it must be stressed that this represents a very small percentage of all epileptics. On rare occasions, following a grand mal seizure, what is called an epileptic fugue may result. In such a condition the individual wanders for several hours. Behavior may appear purposive, but it is actually aimless and confused. Under such conditions, crimes may be committed without the person's awareness.

The second type of epileptic episodic behavior disorder which is seen is *petit mal*. As a usual rule petit mal begins in childhood. It may persist throughout life. However, more commonly, the attacks stop at around the age of fourteen. It is rare for an individual to develop petit mal initially after that age. Both petit mal and grand mal seizures can coexist in the same individual. In petit mal, the individual simply goes into what seems to be a state of lack of awareness or blankness for a period of two to thirty seconds. There is no stiffening of muscles, the eyes do not close, there is no special motor movement, there is no fall. The person may freeze in the middle of doing something. At times, extremely minute motor movements may be noted. There is generally an almost imperceptible moment of confusion following the attack and the person then goes on as if nothing had happened. During such periods, of course, individuals are much more apt to be hurt than they are to hurt someone else.

Petit mal status does occur. This consists of one attack occuring within a very rapid sequence following another. If this sequence lasts, the behavior seen by the observer is quite similar to that in an epileptic clouded state or twilight state. Since most individuals with petit mal do not have a history of grand mal seizures, and since it is difficult to attribute the confusion that they illustrate to an organic factor, the status may go unrecognized unless an electroencephalogram is taken during this period. People with petit mal status, as in other epileptic clouded states, have been known to carry on very complex psychosocial behavior, sometimes quite antisocial in nature, *apparently* well aware of what they are doing, but without any *real* awareness. Other than these rare instances of status, individuals with petit mal epilepsy are not commonly seen in court settings, at least not in situations which are due to their epilepsy.

Another type of epilepsy is the so-called psychomotor seizure or psychomotor equivalent. These have also been called temporal lobe seizures. Since both terms are used the corrections worker should be familiar with both. It is quite possible both describe a form of focal epilepsy; that is, the seizure discharge originates from one specific focus in the brain. The differentiation between psychomotor and temporal lobe epilepsy may rest on whether this seizure discharge originates in the temporal lobe, or even on whether it spreads to include temporal lobes. In a psychomotor seizure, an individual goes through a stereotyped behavior pattern without falling and without apparent loss of consciousness. It is quite easily seen that such an individual is not "with it" during an attack. The particular behavior pattern is markedly stereotyped for each indivudal, but may not in any way resemble an attack that another person with the same illness may have. A woman may constantly get out her purse, open it, fumble with its contents, take them out, and put them back until the attack is over, then look up blankly and start talking as though nothing had happened. Another person has been constantly observed to remove his clothing during such an attack. As soon as the attack is over and the confusion has passed, he will look, almost in a panicky way, for the clothing and don it almost immediately. The stereotyped behavior may be even more complex than this, or as simple as merely plucking at an earlobe with a thumb and finger until the attack is over. These individuals are generally not dangerous. Anyone, of course, with a psychomotor seizure which involves removal of clothing is liable to be arrested for exhibitionism.

Those in a psychomotor seizure *do* resist any attempt to stop the normal pattern of the seizure being carried to conclusion. They may become quite violent in such cases, even though they are quite unaware of what they are doing. One such patient manifested a psychomotor seizure in a very unfortunate way, namely a stereotyped drive to kill herself. In her attacks she would shatter windows in an attempt to drive the shards of glass into any part of her body. She would be perfectly harmless as far as an onlooker was concerned, unless that onlooker, out of humanitarian impulses, attempted to restrain her from trying to slash herself in this fashion. Then the onlooker would be subject to a vicious attack with glass.

In temporal lobe epilepsy, the aura is frequently that of a bad odor, acute or obtunded auditory perceptions, or occasionally by feelings of *déjà vu*, that is, a sensation of already having experienced something which is really unfamiliar. Sometimes its opposite, *jamais vu*, not recognizing very familiar objects serves as the aura. Stereotypic behaviors in some temporal lobe seizures in their early stages are snuffling movements of the nose, smacking movements of the lips, or more rarely repetitious handling of the genitalia.

Twilight states, either in the prodromal, aural, or postictal states, are most commonly associated with psychomotor or temporal lobe seizures. Extremely complex, well organized, and apparently meaningful behavior can be carried out in these conditions, which may last for hours or days.

Mr. G, a twenty-one-year-old male, was arrested because of interstate transportation of a stolen vehicle. He was found on a snowy night in a field in Michigan, some three miles from the Ohio border, sitting in a stolen car in a dazed state. State troopers apprehended him because it was very easy to follow the tracks from the road into the field and to see the car just sitting there. Mr. G claimed to have no memory of stealing the car. What made this seem very strange behavior was that at the time of the episode, he had in his possession the keys to three other cars. One was his own. This was parked in the parking lot of a bowling alley. His last memory was of being there. The second and third sets were of the cars of his father and mother. These cars at the time of the theft were parked in the family garage, not more than two blocks from the bowling alley. They were available to him at any time he wanted them. The stolen car had been taken from a used car lot next door to the bowling alley. The young man insisted that he remembered nothing about having taken it.

A detailed history revealed the presence of three earlier episodes in which he had behaved peculiarly, although not antisocially. At the expiration of these episodes, he also could

not remember them, and indeed denied having been involved
in them. In one instance, as a boy of thirteen, he had gotten
on his bicycle and stayed away for several hours, finally calling from a different part of the city to say he was lost and
asking to have someone pick him up. The family at that time
refused to believe that he could not remember. They felt only
that he was using it as an excuse for having stayed out so late.
On this occasion, the theft of the car, electroencephalographic
tracings were done for the first time, and showed the presence
of seizure discharge in the temporal lobe. Fortunately, he
responded very well to medical treatment and no brain
surgery was necessary.

There is another type of seizure discharge with which the
corrections worker should be familiar. This is known as the
fourteen and six p.c. seizure. It is named fourteen and six p.c.
seizure because in the electroencephalographic tracing bursts of
six per second cyles are seen to alternate with bursts of fourteen
per second cycles. It is believed that this form of epilepsy originates in the area of the brain between the pituitary gland and
the *thalamus,* that part of the brain which receives primitive
sensations. This area, the *hypothalamus,* is particularly concerned with the function of control of the endocrine glands by
way of its connections to the pituitary. It is also richly connected with areas of the brain having to do with many emotional responses. Typically, fourteen and six p.c. epilepsy starts
with an aura of uneasiness in the stomach, or of even actual
stomach pain, which may last for a reasonably long period of
time and which may be quite severe. Indeed, some of these
people undergo all sorts of gastrointestinal x-rays and tests
before the true cause of the difficulty is found. The aura is often
succeeded by a sort of twilight state in which rather violent,
aggressive, antisocial behavior of a complex nature occurs.
This condition is uncommon enough so that the average corrections worker may never see one. On the other hand, it is
dramatic and clean-cut enough that if the thought of such a
condition existing occurs to him and he requests, through a
physician, that an electroencephalogram be done, he may be
instrumental in reversing the entire pattern of the individual's
life.

It was mentioned that in the interval phase the epileptic is apt to be no more involved in crime or antisocial behavior than is the average individual. Rare aggressive acting out or psychotic behavior has been reported in epileptics in the interval phase. When this does occur, careful observation and questioning may bring out the fact that actual minute psychomotor or temporal lobe seizures were occurring at the time of the psychosis and that this was really not an interval phase at all. In some individuals under good medical control a period of increasing irritability and feelings of malaise may build up in the interval phase. They then deliberately do not take their medications for two or three days. The resultant seizure seems to clear the air, and on recovery they feel well and go back to taking their medication. This is relatively uncommon, but something that the corrections worker should be attuned to.

One other syndrome occurring in epilepsy frequently comes to the attention of the corrections worker. This condition is known as *epileptic deterioration*. Although marked advances have been made in the treatment of epilepsy, there are some epileptics whose seizures can not be brought completely under control. Such people may have from one attack per week to one attack per year. When epilepsy is uncontrolled in this fashion, there seems to be a tendency as time goes on for deterioration in mental functioning to occur. Thinking capacity, drive, and judgment are all impaired. In many instances they present almost the same picture which is seen in simple schizophrenia to be described in Chapter 5. Occasionally, this epileptic deterioration will be seen in individuals whose seizures are under good control. It has been reported even with people who have no more than one or two seizures in their lifetime. As a general rule, however, it occurs most frequently when the number of seizures has been great. Such individuals are prone, because of their lack of judgment and the general deterioration in their thought processes, to commit petty offenses. On occasion they may experience loss of control and demonstrate impulsive aggressive behavior.

Ms. H was a case in point. This twenty-nine-year-old woman had had epilepsy most of her life. In spite of intensive

ailment from fallen arches to sexual acting out to the effects of low blood sugar. Under careful scientific scrutiny, none of this work has proved to be valid. This contention of the behavioral effects of low blood sugar is as hard to dispel as the myth of the prevailing dangerousness of the epileptic. Each time one ardent proponent's claims have been thoroughly disproved, another arises to trumpet this same theory as though it were brand new and valid.

The corrections worker has several tasks insofar as epilepsy and the corrections system are concerned. The first task is getting a careful history from the family so that the various epileptic syndromes as a contributing cause of any antisocial behavior may not be overlooked. The second task is working in close conjunction with the family and the family physician to ensure that any medication which is prescribed is taken. Medication for the epileptic is just as necessary and, indeed, in some instances, as life-saving as is insulin for the diabetic or vitamin B-12 for the person with pernicious anemia. In cases of epileptic deterioration, the corrections worker can be of great help to the client by urging the family to provide close supervision or by trying to make other arrangements, such as day care treatment in a nearby regional mental health center.

The typical epileptic offender is most likely to be dangerous when in one of the confused states. These generally occur either in the prodromal period, the period of the aura, or in the postseizure state. It is during these times when the epileptic is generally unaware of what he/she is doing that aggressive behavior may occur. In an institutional setting, such as a jail or prison, it is important to be aware of this possibility. All controls should be applied as gently as possible during this period. It may be necessary to use restraints. In psychomotor attacks occurring within an institution, no attempts should be made to stop the psychomotor attack unless it is dangerous to the individual or those around him. Such potential dangerousness is rare. As noted, there will be a very brief period of confusion following the equivalent, although generally this is so short that it would be inconsequential. The chief problem, then, comes either during an epileptic fugue with accompanying

excitement or during the irritable buildup stage before temporal lobe seizures, and during the confused stage following
such a seizure. Control is almost entirely by medication, but
until such medication can be administered, adequate help to
effectuate control without a wild fracas is essential.

Even though the repetition of this warning may be boring, it
is essential to stress that the overwhelming majority of epileptics are not involved in crime or antisocial offenses. At one time
it was held that there was an epileptic personality which accompanied this disorder, but even this belief is no longer tenable for the greatest number of epileptics. Old beliefs die hard.
One of the most important functions which the corrections
worker may perform in his role as professional is to foster the
dissemination of knowledge that the epileptic is generally a
harmless, inoffensive person, as interested in being a good ci-
tizen as anyone else. Only by concerted effort can this mistaken
notion be dissipated and the epileptic begin to return to the
mainstream of community life.

PSYCHOSIS WITH INTRACRANIAL NEOPLASM (293.3)

It is not at all surprising that tumors of the brain should give
rise to abnormal forms of behavior. The corrections worker will
have little opportunity professionally to see people with brain
tumors. Characteristically, tumors of the brain cause specific
symptoms and neurological signs which allow the diagnosis to
be made and treatment administered. Antisocial behavior rarely
occurs after the tumor has progressed far enough for the proper
diagnosis to have been made. The tumors which are of significance to corrections are the so-called silent tumors. These are
either (a) so small in size during their early stages that they
have not caused any of the usual manifestations and/or (b)
occur in areas of the brain where, until they grow to large size,
physical symptoms are not seen, but behavioral problems may
result. These areas are the so-called silent areas of the brain:
parts of the prefrontal lobes and areas in the temporal lobes.
On rare occasions, what appears to be a temporal lobe seizure,
characterized by an aura of an unpleasant odor and the experience of a dreamlike state with very complex behavior, may

indeed be a first sign of a tumor of the temporal lobes. Such an attack is generally referred to an an *Uncinate Fit,* so-called because it arises in the *uncus,* a part of the temporal lobe.

At other times, tumors in either the temporal area, which has a good deal to do with aggressive and sexual drives, or in the prefrontal area, may cause bizarrely aggressive behavior. It is a strange but well-documented phenomenon that occasionally the first symptom of the presence of such a tumor is a fear of killing. This fear is not of killing any one particular person, but just the fear of going beserk and killing senselessly. Probably this should be stressed more to the medical profession than to the corrections worker, although certainly in no discussion of organic disorders of the nervous system which have to do with crime can it be neglected. Probably the best known example of this situation was the notorious "Texas tower killer" who held a whole city police force at bay for several hours and massacred innocent citizens. He had consulted physicians because of this urge to kill. Apparently, even though such an urge was out of keeping with the personality picture which he presented, no thorough investigations had been done. An autopsy was performed and he was found to have a tumor not much bigger than a pea, located in a significant area of the brain.

PSYCHOSIS ASSOCIATED WITH BRAIN TRAUMA (293.5)

In these days of mechanization of industry and of all forms of transportation, the accidental production of injury to the brain is a not uncommon thing. One of the factors which differentiates nerve cells from any other type of cells in the body is that once a nerve cell is destroyed it is never replaced, nor can it regenerate. All the actual nerve cells or *neurons* which will ever be present are there at birth. No more are grown in a lifetime. Intellectual development depends not on the addition of more neurons but in the development of rich connections among them. Once any of those cells are destroyed, they are not replaced; there are certainly enough present at birth so that a great number have to be destroyed before there is any significant loss of functioning. In the last section, small tumors in silent areas of the brain which caused a great deal of difficulty were discussed. Here, almost the opposite statement is being made, namely, that it is possible to have large areas of the brain destroyed without personality functioning being greatly impaired, even though motor or sensory function may be. On the other hand, many changes in personality due to injuries to the brain can, and do, occur.

The change which is most apt to occur immediately following a brain injury is unconsciousness. This may last from a few brief moments to weeks or even months. The length of time that the unconsciousness persists is generally dependent on the severity and the location of the injury. Conversely, it is sometimes possible to determine the severity of a former injury by the length of time unconsciousness had lasted. Probably everyone has experienced minor head injuries of one form or another throughout life. The odds are good that every child has dropped from mother's hands during the early years of life. Most people try to climb trees and fall out of them. More and more people are bumped in auto accidents. Fortunately, most of these injuries are completely without significance. While they may damage the head, they do not, in any way, damage the brain. When the brain has been damaged, there are unquestionably certain effects which follow. Just as in a brain tumor, however, there are only certain of these effects which are of concern in the corrections field. Three of these should be mentioned.

All of them involve personality changes. The first of these is what has been referred to as the *Post-Traumatic Personality State*. It is characterized by increased loss of control, increased irritability and aggressiveness, and loss of judgment. It does not, necessarily, affect other mental or physical functions. There was quite a furor during World War II when a well-known hockey star, at the height of his career, was turned down for the armed services by his draft board because of having developed a post-traumatic personality. This had become manifest as the summation of the many minor head injuries, and with them brain injuries, which he had sustained as a result of his long career in hockey. In contrast to his previous personality, he was now extremely quick on the trigger. He was beginning to spend almost as much time in the penalty box for fighting as he was on the ice. He showed heightened reflexes, an increased tendency to go to pieces under stress, and faulty judgment. He would have been a disaster in any conceivable army unit. These individuals, like some epileptics, show an increased susceptibility to the effects of alcohol and very easily become fighting drunks. Their contacts with the courts are usually due to acts of aggression and violence. They may pose a very difficult problem to the corrections worker since they have no insight into the situation, consider themselves to be perfectly normal, and resent the implication that they are in need of supervision, or possibly medication, to help them to control themselves.

The second type of post-traumatic personality disorder having implications for corrections is seen most usually when the head injury has occurred in childhood and adolescence. These individuals may appear to show an almost complete psychoemotional recovery from very severe head injuries, even though there may be evidence of physical damage in the form of paralysis, weakness, or loss of sensation of one or another limb. Some time after the injury, a time span extending from two to three years to as long as ten to twelve years, a very definite personality change begins to be noted. This change is in the direction of the so-called *antisocial personality* which will be described at length in Chapter 9, under the Character Disorders. These people show a complete change in the personality which existed prior to and for several years following the accident. They now seem to have no feelings for the rights or feelings of other people. They seem to be completely unable to learn from experience. They commit antisocial acts, largely of a nonviolent nature, with no compunctions. They are rather hurt in their feelings when they are apprehended and asked to take responsibility for their own behavior.

A typical case is that of Ms. I, a twenty-three-year-old woman who had been described as being an extremely extroverted, stable girl, well-liked by all, an exceptionally good student, active in sports, with no asocial or antisocial tendencies, indeed a responsible, feeling, sensitive person. At the age of fifteen, she had been thrown by a horse and received a very severe brain inury. She had been unconscious for several weeks and on regaining consciousness at first went through a clinical picture which was indistinguishable from that which was described under alcoholic psychosis, Korsakov's Syndrome (see Chapter 3). She was confined to bed for several more weeks and slowly improved. No evidence of any psychosocial effects of the injury could be detected at the expiration of a year, even though she still had a weakness in one leg and a decided limp because of the shortening in the bone in that leg. However, starting at age twenty, she began such activities as "bad check" writing, collecting door to door for charities but never turning the money in, forging her parents' signatures to checks, and bilking stores. When arrested, she could see absolutely no reason why she should be arrested. She felt that people were stupid to have been taken in by her. She formerly evidenced a great deal of love for her parents, now she treated them as objects rather than people.

She was given a suspended sentence and placed on parole, but within a short period of time had violated her parole conditions; she left the state and was arrested in a neighboring state where she had assumed a false name, and had wormed her way into the confidence of a businessman as a trusted employee. In a very short period of time she had embezzled a large sum of money. It is not known why this change in personality is delayed when the head injury occurs in childhood and adolescence. There is no evidence of increasing brain cell damage through the years.

The third type of disorder associated with the so-called post-traumatic personality is a deterioration very similar to that which has already been described in epileptic deterioration or in senile deterioration. Petty misdemeanors, rather than any more severe forms of antisocial behavior, are characteristic of this group. The corrections worker, in attempting to help these people, must see that careful supervision is provided. Very often, case work services in various agencies must be enlisted to help the individual continue to adjust.

THE ROLE OF THE CORRECTIONS WORKER

The corrections worker has a very important role to play in the instance of those people with organic disorders of the central nervous system who come into contact with the courts. Many times it is only by a carefully taken social history done as part of the presentence investigation that the suspicion is raised that there may be some disorder of the central nervous system underlying the antisocial behavior. Medication, and even at times neurosurgery, while often necessary, may show only partial success in the rehabilitation of the offender. Even where these treatment modalities are used, it is frequently a part of the corrections worker's tasks to see that the doctor's orders are adhered to. Abstinence from alcohol, as has been repeatedly stressed, is essential in the successful management of any organic brain condition. No one enjoys riding herd on another's habits, yet helping the offender to remain abstinent is one of the most crucial points of the worker's job in these conditions. In many instances, particularly with the aged and with the deteriorated epileptic, mobilization of community resources can be a tremendous aid in resocialization. With this there may come a return of function, previously thought to be permanently lost. Only too often community agencies seem threatened and almost paralyzed when dealing with antisocial offenders. The corrections worker may be forced by default to assume the role of the case manager. It is possible for him to do an effective job, particularly if he maintains a close liaison with the physician and employer.

The worker dealing with the offender with organic disorder of the central nervous system must always keep in mind the basic symptoms in those disorders. Confusion and loss of memory do occur; the result may be missed or late appointments. Change in mood is a common manifestation of these conditions. It was pointed out that irritability is the most common of the mood changes. Care must be taken not to react to irritability with irritability. It is necessary to be soothing without being patronizing or treating the person as a child. That last can be most annoying and increase the irritability. The difficulty in cognition may require that the simplest procedures be gone over may times before they are understood. (Only too often an irritable, "What are you telling me that so many times for, I'm not stupid," is heard.) Patience, gentleness, yet firm controls, supplement the necessary socialization and vocational reeducation.

At the same time it is important that the corrections worker try to counteract the tendency of the person with organic brain disorder to attribute all of his difficulties to that disorder or to refuse to tackle new situations on the grounds that "I can't do that" or "I'm not allowed to do that." This attitude can be paralyzing to any effort toward rehabilitation. The worker should get a clear picture (preferrably from the physician) of the actual deficits and limitations present. This understanding should be used gently and constantly to counter excuses.

Chapter 5

SCHIZOPHRENIA (295)

GENERAL CONSIDERATIONS

THE remainder of Part One will discuss those psychiatric conditions which, at least as far as is known up to the present time, are not primarily organic in nature. These are the **Psychoses not Attributed to the Physical Conditions Listed Previously (295-298)**. The first one of these is **Schizophrenia (295)**. A vigorous debate has been going on in the field of psychiatric criminology as to whether a signicant number of people diagnosed as having schizophrenia are involved in antisocial behavior. There have always been isolated case reports of particularly bizarre and grotesque murders and murder-suicides committed by schizophrenics, but there are those who say the numbers involved are relatively infinitesimal. However, it has been shown that there is a proportionately high rate of schizophrenics among offenders examined at a large forensic clinic. The greater number of these are said to be arrested for misdemeanors rather than felonies. A recent study in a large municipality indicated that the rate of violent and potentially violent crimes was slightly higher among a sample of discharged mental patients than for the the country at large. Schizophrenics made up 47 percent of this total group. They were responsible for 49 percent of patients involved in violent offenses and 38 percent of those involved in nonviolent offenses. Further, of those patients arrested for violent offenses involving bodily harm, schizophrenics had the highest number of mean offenses per patient, more than two times that of any other diagnostic category. These figures would suggest that schizophrenics do become involved in antisocial behavior, and that their offenses may be of a serious, as well as of a nuisance, variety. Since the current trend in mental health practice is to treat as many people as possible in the least restrictive psychiatric settings, there will be an increasing number of individuals with schizophrenia in the community-at-large. This is in spite of the fact that there is no absolute increase in the incidence of schizophrenia. It would appear, then that schizophrenia will be of increasing significance to the corrections worker, whether or not there is a direct cause and effect relationship between that illness and crime.

There is still a question as to whether schizophrenia is one condition or is a whole series of differing conditions which resemble each other and are grouped together because many of the symptoms are the same. There are many ways of discussing schizophrenia. The definite causes of this condition are still unknown. Like the argument about the causes of crime, this is a subject which tends to generate as much heat as light. An uncritical reading of the numerous papers written by the ardent proponents of one particular theory or another can only lead to the conclusions reached by the blind men on their first encounter with an elephant. Certain factors do seem to be implicated. There would appear to be a hereditary factor present, but it seems improbable that schizophrenia itself is inherited. What does appear to be inherited is a tendency for schizophrenia to develop under conditions of lesser stress than in those who do not have this hereditary tendency. If stress is intense and prolonged enough, no hereditary factor is necessary. There are many types of stress which appear to be significant for the development of this condition. Many writers emphasize the importance of disturbed family interactions in the patient's childhood. The pattern of parental double messages is felt to be a particularly important factor in breaking down coping mechanisms in the child. The parent sends one message with words, "Don't you dare get into any fights," and another message by behavior, either indulging in fights or praising someone who does. As a result, the child is never sure what is expected. Another family pattern which has been implicated is that of the double bind. One parental request can be satisfied only at the cost of another. The mothers of some schizophrenic children have been described as schizophrenogenic, namely, schizophrenia-producing. Such mothers are said to be extremely cold and rejecting, as well as utilizing faulty communication and the double bind. The fathers of schizophrenic children are said to have been extremely dominating and subjugating. On the other hand, there are many who feel that the personalities of parents have little to do with the ultimate development of schizophrenia.

The problems of sexuality which normally come to the fore at adolescence are particularly bothersome to those with a tendency to schizophrenia. Such adolescents are particularly apt to worry about meeting the demands of their gender roles. "Can I be masculine (feminine) enough?" Thoughts about possible homosexual tendencies are also particularly troubling. Since coping mechanisms have been impaired, the attempt to solve these problems may lead directly to the development of illness. Cultural, social, and economic factors have also been implicated at one time or another in the genesis of this disease. Currently, there is a fringe movement which would attribute the development of schizophrenia to faulty nutrition with particular attention to lack of certain vitamins and trace minerals.

At present, the most exciting finding is that some form of disordered brain neurochemistry is present. This holds true regardless of the presenting symptoms or the theoretical cause. The subject of the exact nature of these neurochemical disorders is much too complex to be discussed in a book of this sort. The significance of this research lies in the fact that, as the nature of this disordered neurochemistry is more clearly understood, it becomes possible to develop more specific medications. This is a two-way street, in that the analysis of the nature of medications currently found to be effective in dealing with the symptoms of the illness further clarifies the nature of the disordered neurochemistry. It is particularly important to be aware of the presence of this underlying physiological and chemical disorder because of the mistaken belief, held by so many, that the medications used in treating this illness are simply tranquilizers. While it is true that they are frequently used because of their calming effect on excited patients, they do have a definite antipsychotic effect. Indeed, in many instances, the tranquilization is an undesirable side effect, and more and more medications are being developed which have the antipsychotic effect without tranquilization.

It would appear then, that the etiology, or cause, of schizophrenia may be described as follows: Because of heredity, certain people are more susceptible to the stresses which arise when they are brought up under pathological family situations, under disturbed social, cultural or economic situations or are exposed to naturally occurring environmental stress. These stresses result in neurophysiological-chemical changes in certain areas of the brain. These changes in brain chemistry are expressed as a particular form of disordered behavior which is labeled schizophrenia. In other words, schizophrenia is a complex biological, sociological, physiological, psychological process. In this respect, the situation in schizophrenia is very analogous to that in criminology, where the answer to "Why does any one person become an offender?" is a complex multisystem, an interlocking, socioeconomic-cultural-psychological mechanism rather than a simplistic, unitary situation.

The diagnosis of schizophrenia is made from both the longitudinal picture of the life history of the individual and the disturbance of behavior seen at the time of examination or examinations. The longitudinal history is particularly important in attempting to differentiate Schizophrenia from Psychosis Due to Drugs and Endogenous Toxins. In this life history, one would expect to find some of the following elements:

A family history of mental illness.

A lifelong disturbed relationship within the family.

A cold, rejecting mother.

A dominating, subjugating father.

The use of double messages in family communication.

A common occurrence of double-bind situations in the family.

A tendency to being a loner.

The use of daydreams and fantasy as attempts to cope with painful reality.

Difficulties in sexual adjustment, beginning in adolescence, particularly centering around fears about homosexuality.

Cultural conflicts, such as those which occur in children of immigrants or in children brought from one area of the country to another, etc.

Although schizophrenia may occur in individuals with relatively commonplace life histories, the brief discussion of the case in Chapter 1 presents a quite typical picture of the life course seen in the majority of schizophrenics. The majority of schizophrenics, particularly males, tend to have a tall, slender body build, with flabby muscles and a droopy posture. (This does not mean that thick-set muscular males with good posture never develop schizophrenia.) The actual onset of the acute illness may be prolonged (sometimes for months) or relatively sudden (over a few days). One other aspect of the history is of benefit in making the diagnosis of schizophrenia. This is the course of the illness. If untreated, schizophrenia tends to persist. As time goes on the individual becomes progressively worse, until eventually there is obvious deterioration. The rate of this progressive downhill course varies with the type of schizophrenia. Hebephrenics deteriorate most rapidly; paranoids have the slowest course. In some individuals treatment slows, but does not stop the progressive deterioration. In some patients the disease presents as isolated attacks, separated by periods of time. It is then seen that the recovery following each attack is not quite so complete as from the previous one. In time this leads to a deteriorated state, even in the intervals between attacks. It might be noted that it is not uncommon for an individual to have one episode of Acute Undifferentiated Schizophrenia in adolescence, and then to be well adjusted for years, possibly for life, with no residual symptomatology.

In the cross-sectional clinical observation of behavior, what is seen most typically is a disturbance in the thinking process itself. The patient tends to think in nonlogical, or what has been called *paralogical,* ways. This basic disturbance in thought process leads to the many symptoms which are seen in schizophrenia. One of the easiest ways of categorizing and making some sense of the symptoms seen in this illness is that described by Bleuler who coined the term schizophrenia (schizo-split; phrenia-mind). Bleuler felt that this condition represented a split in the mind. What should be stressed is that *this* splitting is not the splitting which is typical of the split personality, so loved by fiction writers and made a household word by novel length case reports of treatment of real cases. *That* split personality refers to the individual being one person one moment and someone else the next, with neither personality having any awareness that the other exists. The splitting in schizophrenia has to do with a much more fundamental split, namely a splitting between thought and feeling. Some degree of this splitting or dissociation is found in every schizophrenic.

Bleuler laid down four criteria for the diagnosis of schizophrenia. These four criteria are referred to as the four *A*s. The first *A* refers to Association and has to do with that basic disturbance in thought process which is the basis of all schizophrenic pathology. This disturbance in thought processes is first manifested by a *loosening of associations* between one thought and the next. As a normal thing, when one person is talking to another, even though the conversation may switch from one topic to another, a careful reconstruction of that conversation leads to a discovery of the associations between one thought and the next, which led the talk to move from one topic to another. A corrections worker talking to a parolee, a probationer, or prisoner, whomever that person may be, as a rule can generally tell why that person's thought moves from one topic to the next. What led from one to the other is quite clear. If it is not immediately clear, this connection soon becomes evident as the topic is elaborated. In the schizophrenic individual, there is a progressive disorganization of those natural connections. A new topic appears in the conversation, and somehow the listener is unable to establish how it got there from the last topic. For example, if the topic were horseracing and the matter of the small size of jockeys comes up, that would be quite a natural association. If, however, while talking about horseracing with no reference to the size of jockeys in general, a speculation were raised as to the relative size of the penis of a specific jockey and that of the speaker it could be considered a loose association. Sometimes, the listener's own fantasy will lead to an awareness of the association between A and B, but it is a pretty farfetched one which would not commonly be made.

As the pathological condition progresses, however, it becomes more and more difficult to trace the association from A to B and then to C. Even if the speaker is asked to explain it and tries to do so, the listener cannot see any connection between these two events. The association is one that is unique for that individual. It is something that is somehow bound up in the unconscious thought processes. When the cognitive disorder in schizophrenia has progressed far enough, the listener, in trying to follow such a conversation, feels as though grasping for a handful of smoke, with one disconnected thought pattern after another just oozing out through the fingers. Pushed to its extreme, what is liable to emerge from a schizophrenic's mouth is what has been called *word salad*. This is a collection of words which have no understandable association, one with the other, and which convey no meaning whatsoever to the listener. When talking with one of these individuals who shows looseness of association, the listener's reaction is one of bewilderment, a feeling of something strange happening, something that cannot be quite pinned down. On analysis, it is apparent that this feeling of strangeness stems from some defect in the other's thought process. It is this defect which we call *looseness of associations*. If this flow of thought is allowed to proceed without interruption, the individual will not come back to the original starting point. The flow of thought continues to wander in an ever bewildering maze which goes nowhere. This, then, is Bleuler's first *A*, difficulty in the Associative process.

The second *A* has to do with the Affect or the emotions. There is always some disturbance of the emotions in schizophrenia. The most primary disturbance, the one Bleuler considered to be quite specific for schizophrenia, is the dissociation between emotion and cognition, the *splitting* previously referred to. The *affective* (emotional) tone the individual displays has absolutely nothing whatever to do with the subject of conversation. Extreme examples might be "My mother died yesterday, ha ha ha ha. . . and I'm going to the funeral, ha ha ha ha. . . tomorrow" or "That was a marvelous party we had last night; I can't remember when I have had a better time" while tears are streaming down the cheeks. Obviously, these are extremes. This dissociation between content of thought and emotion induces a feeling of bewilderment in the listener. This feeling can be a help in diagnosis. Frequently, diagnoses are made, not only from what is actually observed about the person under consideration, but from the emotional resonance which is set up within the observer. Almost always, when a feeling of something strange, distant, peculiar, bizarre is provoked by an individual, that person will prove to be schizophrenic. Subjective feelings in the observer which may occur in relationship to other conditions will be noted as those conditions are discussed.

Commonly, in the schizophrenic, sometimes even before the dissociation of affect, a general blunting or *flatness* of affect is seen. If the mood is happiness, then happiness is not as great as might be expected from the circumstances. If the mood is sadness, the sadness is not to the expected degree. This, eventually, leads to what appears to be withdrawal and coldness. Another term that is sometimes used for this coldness or flatness is *poverty of affect*. Eventually, this flattening or poverty of affect may suddenly disappear and the extreme dissociation just noted may replace it to a degree sufficient to suggest severe deterioration. The second *A* then, deals with Affect, the emotions and their disturbance.

The third *A* is Ambivalence, or simultaneously contrasting feelings, attitudes, or desires. The ambivalence of the schizophrenic is an exaggeration of that ambivalence which all the world feels to a lesser extent. The schizophrenic is ambivalent about almost everything. "I hate you, I love you," "I will, I won't," "I am interested, I am disinterested," "I want to, I don't want to." This applies to almost every wish or experience, which may be simultaneously felt as both positive and negative. It has been suggested that this ambivalence is the result of the double messages with which the schizophrenic has been raised.

Ambivalence is one of the reasons that schizophrenics are notoriously so indecisive. The extreme example of ambivalence in schizophrenia is the condition which is called *blocking*. The schizophrenic suddenly seems to freeze, either when asked a question, which from the viewpoint of the examiner seems to pose no problem, or spontaneously at some point in the conversation. The observer is aware of the tremendous effort that is being made to say something and yet no words come out at all. The mouth is held tensely open, the Adam's apple may even be moving up and down, the whole bodily set is that of someone about to speak and yet no sound emerges. One explanation of this is that the ambivalence has led to two directly opposed thoughts trying to be expressed at the same time. Neither one of them can clear the channels of communication with the result that blocking occurs. The two opposed thoughts commonly carry love—hate implications. The block may persist for some time. When conversation resumes it will almost always be about a topic different from the one which led to the block. The schizophrenic may also exhibit blocking when motor behavior is involved. This, too, is an expression of ambivalence. The picture of a patient standing in a doorway unable to go either forwards or backwards is certainly not an uncommon one in the mental hospital. The third *A* then stands for Ambivalence.

The fourth *A* that Bleuler referred to was Autistic thinking or Autism. This is thinking which is unique to the individual and not readily sharable with others. Autistic comes from the root *auto* meaning self, such as in automobile, a self-propelled machine, or autonomous, a self-directed action. Autistic means concerned with thought of the self. It is out of this autism that we get the hallucinations[1] and delusions,[2] the experiences that are unique to that particular individual. Hallucinations and delusions are popularly thought to be the core of schizophrenia, but are just a part of the autistic thinking. These autistic experiences are the result of the specific disturbance of the thought process. The schizophrenic's world is self-centered and everything else is tangential to it. The extreme of autistic thinking is seen in the autistic child, who does not even use a

---

[1]A hallucination is a perceived sensory experience, a sound, a sight, a smell, a tactile sensation unique to the person experiencing it and not caused by a stimulus from the world of observable reality.
[2]A delusion is a mistaken belief, held contrary to all logical argument, and unique to the person experiencing it.

language common to the rest of the world, but invents an idiosyncratic speech and talks and operates within it. The schizophrenic adult also creates a unique world and has difficulty in communicating that world to an outsider. These are the primary symptoms of schizophrenia, according to Bleuler: disorders of the Associative process and of the Affect, Ambivalence, and Autistic thinking.

While not stressed by Bleuler, it might be well to mention that a fifth *A* might be cited as typical of schizophrenic thought. This is difficulty in Abstraction, with a resultant tendency to think concretely. Anything that is heard is taken very literally by the schizophrenic. Such an individual has marked difficulty when asked to interpret proverbs, such as "A bird in the hand is worth two in the bush," "All that glitters is not gold," "A rolling stone gathers no moss." A concrete explanation for example might be, "If you have a bird in your hand, don't squeeze it too hard or it will die" or, for the second question, "If you have a gold coin and you don't polish it, it won't shine." Likewise, there will be difficulty in thinking abstractly about such concepts as a chair and a table, or pity and sympathy. Common answers about how a chair and a table are alike might be, "They both have four legs," or, for pity and sympathy, "You pity someone who is poor and you sympathize with someone who has hurt his hand." Both of these answers miss completely the abstraction that "they are both furniture" or "they are both feelings." This tendency toward concrete thinking may underlie what sometimes appears to be a very strange sense of humor on the part of the schizophrenic.

The diagnosis of schizophrenia, then is made on the longitudinal developmental history, cross-sectional observable behavior, and the course of the illness. There is, as yet, no laboratory test which can prove or disprove the diagnosis. It is confirmed by the clinical course of the disease and by the response to treatment.

SCHIZOPHRENIA, SIMPLE TYPE (295.0)

The first subtype listed is **Schizophrenia, Simple Type**

(**295.0**). The designation of simple schizophrenia is attached to this subtype largely because there is nothing dramatic about it. It is a very slowly progressive, dementing process. Beginning in late adolescence or very early adult life, the individual withdraws attention more and more from the outside world and focuses it more and more internally. The affect, as was noted for all schizophrenics, becomes dull. Personal appearance becomes less and less important. What little ambition and drive were present initially vanish as the illness progresses. The sharpness of higher cognitive functioning becomes dulled. Relatives and close friends become disturbed by what they consider shiftlessness, listlessness, and apathy. Deterioration slowly progresses even beyond that point. Withdrawal becomes more and more apparent. The male may become a vagrant. He does not hold a job, he wanders from one place to another. Quite commonly, simple schizophrenic females end up as prostitutes, drifting into The Life in an apathetic fashion. Some simple schizophrenics become exhibitionists. They become so almost more by default than by intent. That is, the mechanism of the exhibitionism is just as apt to be carelessness in rearranging clothing after having urinated in some more or less public spot as it is a deliberate attempt to expose. Antisocial behavior is more apt to take the form of misdemeanor than of felony. Vagrancy, shoplifting, prostitution, and at times chronic alcoholism, exhibitionism, and public nuisance are the sorts of offenses that simple schizophrenics commit. The end result of all the deteriorating conditions which have been discussed is very much the same. In advanced cases, only a good history will differentiate among simple schizophrenia, post-traumatic deterioration, senile dementia, epileptic deterioration, and the deterioration due to alcohol and drugs.

Only too often in the past, simple schizophrenics have been disposed of by the expedient of determining them to be not competent to stand trial. They have been sent to hospitals for the criminally insane to spend the rest of their lives. This is probably one of the most difficult of all forms of schizophrenia to treat because there are so few target symptoms to treat. Since they do not have the more florid manifestations of hallucinations or delusions that other schizophrenics show, antipsychotic medication has little to offer. Motivation for change is lacking, and neither group nor individual therapy holds out much promise. Supervision, with environmental manipulation in terms of finding simple jobs, helping them to manage their budgets, and close follow-up to see that they stay with the job and get the necessities of life for themselves, is probably all that the corrections officer has to offer. Even this little is more attention than many of these people may have had in some time. It may be instrumental in giving them a focus around which to begin to reorganize their lives. Enlightened communities will furnish well-run half-way houses for these people who are no longer equipped to make it on their own.

SCHIZOPHRENIA, HEBEPHRENIC TYPE (295.1)

Individuals suffering from **Schizophrenia, Hebephrenic Type (295.1)** begin to show symptoms very early in adolescence. These symptoms consist of increasing withdrawal, precipitous increase in first *loosening* and then *fragmentation* of associations, and rapid development of hallucinations and delusions, which take on a very bizarre and unsystematized character. It is in the hebephrenic schizophrenic that one sees the widest split between emotion and cognition. Classical cases deteriorate very rapidly so that within six to eighteen months from onset they are the stereotypic back ward patients of the older mental hospital, clothed in rags at which they continue to pick, frequently drooling, masturbating openly, giggling or weeping somewhat uncontrollably, their speech a veritable word salad. As might be guessed from this description, such people very rarely come in contact with the law.

From some reason, the picture of a full-blown hebephrenic schizophrenic is uncommon today. A large part of this change may be traced to the fact that such individuals are given antipsychotic medication at a very early stage in the illness, and illness apparently never progresses to the full-flowered state that has just been described. Beyond this, however, there seems to be some factor operating, whether it be nutritional, social, or biological, that has cut down on the real incidence of this illness as well as its relative incidence. It is mentioned here because once in a great while this term will come up in material which the correction worker obtains from previous hospitalizations of his client and the worker should be familiar with it when it occurs. Many hebephrenic patients will be seen whose clinical course has been changed by medication and hence, differs from that just described.

A case in point is that of Mr. J. This not only exemplifies the pattern of hebephrenia, but is also indicative of the fact that with medication, the full-blown picture does not develop or may not develop as quickly. This twenty-year-old male began his criminal career at the age of thirteen when he was charged with operating a motor vehicle without the owner's consent. At the age of sixteen he was found guilty of assault with intent to rob, and placed on probation as well as being fined. At seventeen he violated probation twice with offenses of assault and battery and disturbance but was continued on probation. Later in the same year the charges of possession of marijuana and unarmed robbery were placed against him. He was finally given a suspended sentence to the Ohio State Reformatory after being found guilty of breaking and entering. Within a few months, he was picked up for assault with intent to rob; the suspended sentence was imposed, and he served thirteen months of a one to fifteen year commitment.

J's father was alcoholic. His mother had had two hospitalizations for mental illness (type unknown), first when he was two and again when he was twelve. Although as a boy he had many acquaintances, he had had no close friends. He was not close to any of his siblings. Despite the arrest for possession he was not heavily into the drug culture. He had a reputation for being moody.

A psychiatric disorder was first noted on release from the reformatory. One month after his release he was placed in the psychiatric unit of a general hospital with a diagnosis of acute undifferentiated schizophrenic reaction. He was under the care of a private physician. J was placed on antipsychotic medication to which he responded rapidly and was referred for aftercare to his local mental health treatment center. It was only with great difficulty that his parole officer could get him to keep his appointments at the center. It was later learned that he did not take his prescribed medication most of the time. Within three months he was arrested and brought to jail. He had accosted a fellow employee with the accusation that the employee was crawling up inside his head, and he wanted to know how he got there. When the employee became frightened by his demeanor and assumed a defensive posture, the defendant struck him. He was admitted to the local mental health center, at which time he was severely hallucinated and deluded and showed marked fragmentation of thought. Again he was placed on psychotropic drugs, improved, and released. Shortly after his release he was picked up for driving in a stolen vehicle and charged with receipt of stolen property. Interestingly, he was apparently unaware that this was stolen property. He had a receipt for his purchase, but had his judgment been good it would have been obvious that this was hot merchandise. The price he paid for the car was so low that it obviously had to be stolen.

When seen for examination at the Court Diagnostic and Treatment Center at the request of the court, he showed the following symptoms and signs markedly suggestive of hebephrenic schizophrenia. This is a quotation from the report, "He is a tall, slender, willowy male. He has an extremely bland facial expression, occasionally illuminated by a silly grin which bears no relationship to the subject under discussion. He shows marked loosening of his associative processes, jumping from one topic to another with great rapidity and no logical connections. When the examiner attempts to make some sense out of his talk and follow the associations he is wrong far more than he is right. In talking, J tends to be very repetitive in that he will repeat the same phrase three or four times, almost as though he stutters in phrases rather than syllables. (This repetition is called *perseveration* if the same topic is constantly repeated, *stereotypy* if the same words are used over and over, and *echolalia* if the examiner's words are continuously repeated.) He talks about being extremely worried and perturbed, but there is absolutely no evidence that this is so. His entire emotional quality has an almost otherworldish, "Alice-in-Wonderland," feel to it. He is both hallucinated and deluded. Hallucinations are present in both the visual and auditory spheres. He sees people who move from behind him to in front of him and then disappear. He hears people talking with him when no one is there; at times these people will disappear and then reappear.

"He is deluded in that he has the feeling that these people who disappear actually disappear by getting into his mind, not that they are controlling his thoughts from the outside, but that these people are actually inside his head. While there they control the tempo of his thoughts as well as what he is thinking. Thus, he states that if he is reading a book, at times he will read at speeds far greater than he is intellectually capable of reading; at other times he will read at speeds so retarded that he can't understand how he can even keep the topic in mind. Yet he understands everything that he reads. At other times the person in his mind makes him say and do things that he doesn't want to do. He gets quite puzzled and upset over the fact that such a person is there and he worries constantly about how he ever got there. At night he hears insinuations that he is going to be turned into a woman. As he talks about these insinuations his voice becomes high pitched and takes on a feminine quality."

Thus, his disorder of speech, his dissociation of affect, and the bizarre quality of his nonsystematized delusions and hallucinations lead to a tentative diagnosis of hebephrenic schizophrenia, the course of which has been interrupted by medication. I encountered Mr. J again by chance on a hospital ward some weeks after the initial interview. He was ambling up and down the ward with a fixed smile and when he recognized who I was he said, "Hey man, what was all that canoodeling was going on when you saw me? You were sure mixing it up and moving around and canoodeling, and I knew you were up to something."

SCHIZOPHRENIA, CATATONIC TYPE (295.2)

The next category under the general diagnosis of schizophrenia is **Schizophrenia, Catatonic Type (295.2)**. This is further divided into **Schizophrenia, Catatonic Type, Excited**

(295.23), and **Schizophrenia, Catatonic Type, Withdrawn (295.24)**. One of the characteristics of this disorder is that it tends to occur in discrete attacks, which even before present day treatment tended to be self-limited. The length of time that any attack lasts without treatment can vary from several days to one or two years. Successive attacks may be of alternating types or of the same type. The onset of catatonic schizophrenia is usually at a somewhat older age than that of the *simple* or the *hebephrenic* types. The first symptoms are generally seen in the mid-twenties.

While these individuals may come to the attention of the criminal justice system in the intervals between attacks, the corrections worker is most apt to see them when in the excited phase of catatonic schizophrenia. In the early course of this illness before institutional medical controls are applied, the individual may harm others in an impulsively assaultive fashion. In this respect catatonic schizophrenia resembles the conditions already discussed such as acute alcoholic hallucinosis, pathological intoxication. The onset of catatonic excitement is extremely rapid. Usually, within a period of three to five days from the time the first symptoms are noted a full-blown catatonic excitement will have developed. Originally, this may be very difficult to distinguish from manic excitement (which will be discussed in Chapter 6). The differentiation is marked by looseness of association progressing rapidly to fragmentation of speech, by marked dissociation of affect, by the extremely bizarre nature of the excitement, by the presence of almost constant auditory hallucinations, and by the presence of a very poorly organized delusional system. Such people are apt to run about aimlessly, striking at both animate and inanimate objects in their way. At times the assaultiveness may take on a more purposive appearance. In untreated excitement, very bizarre dress and ornamentation may be observed. These people frequently are out of contact with their environment. As a general rule, before the condition has reached this state, someone will become alarmed enough by the peculiar behavior to have had the patient sucessfully hospitalized. At other times, before the necessary steps can be taken to effectuate this, the patient will succeed either in self-mutilation in some bizarre fashion or in having attacked others in what appears to be a brutal and senseless way.

The opposite picture is seen in catatonic schizophrenia of the withdrawn type. The individual rather than becoming excited is immobile. The body posture is rigid; sometimes the fetal position is assumed. The nature of the thought processes cannot be judged because of the presence of *mutism*. Negativism is frequently seen. (This implies not only the refusal to comply with requests, but sometimes to do the exact opposite.) Advanced stages may resemble stupor. Not infrequently at this time a striking condition is seen which is referred to as *cereas flexibilitas*, which translates literally to waxy mobility. If the arms of such an individual are arranged in a bizarre pattern, for example one is extended straight out, the other over the head, they will remain in that position for hours. The great majority of catatonic schizophrenics who arrive at this stage of withdrawal will not eat and have to be fed either by gastric tube or intravenously in order to be kept alive. Their bodily excretory functions have to be monitored, otherwise they develop marked bladder distension and bowel impaction. Just as in the excited type, if left untreated except for measures designed to preserve life, these attacks may last from one week to one or two years. Interestingly, although the withdrawn catatonic seems not to be at all in contact with the environment while this is going on, once the attack is over everything that has happened may be recalled in striking detail. It has been postulated that the extreme immobility of the catatonic is an attempt to control murderous impulses from coming to the surface. The excitement may result from the failure of such controls. It is certain the end result is ambivalence, whatever its source.

The intervals between attacks last from months to years. In these intervals the afflicted individual returns pretty much to the same degree of relative well being present before the episode. However, after each successive act definite residual symptoms begin to be noted. There is more flattening of the emotional reactions, more withdrawal tendencies, less interest in personal appearance, less drive and motivation to do things, and eventually the same state of deterioration is reached as in the untreated hebephrenic. With modern psychotropic medications, attacks may be brought under control relatively rapidly; the time interval between attacks may be prolonged almost indefinitely. This is of the greatest importance to the corrections worker because if such an individual comes in contact with the court, either because of antisocial behavior in the course of an acute excitement, or because of antisocial behavior in the interval between attacks, one of the worker's chief functions may be that of a mental health worker, namely to persuade the individual to continue to take his medication.

Many correction workers seem to have a built in bias against this aspect of their professional duties. They believe mistakenly that such a patient is drugged, not medicated. It is true that in the acute stages of these processes, particularly in excitement, the patient may be medicated to the point that a drugged state seems present, but once this acute phase is passed there is no reason why the medication should not be adjusted to the condition. The maintenance dose, which serves to prevent a recurrence, need not be in quantity to produce any discernible effect on the individual's functioning. Certainly, the responsibility for adjusting dosage rests with the physician and not the corrections worker, but the corrections worker can be essential in seeing that the offender takes the medication or in informing the doctor when it is not taken. Recent developments in psychopharmacology are stressing a type of injectable medication which has to be administered only once every two to four weeks. The medicine thus injected is released at a gradual but steady rate so that the required dosage level is always present in the patient's blood stream. Contrary to what might be expected, there is no rapid rise in the level at the time the injection is given. One of the most promising developments in the whole field of psychopharmacology is the fact that it is becoming increasingly possible to monitor the level of medication in a patient's blood at any time, and thus to arrive at the minimal level of medication necessary to maintain improvement for that particular patient.

The case of Mrs. K illustrates catatonic schizophrenia as well as the significance of taking medication.

Mrs. K was seen at the request of the court to determine her competency to stand trial. At 11:30 one evening, without any prior warning and apparently without any provocation, she had taken a pistol and shot her four-month-old son through the chest. The bullet went through the baby, the mattress, the bottom of the crib, and into the floor. She had first sought psychiatric help seven years before this episode. At that time she complained of feeling tense, unable to settle down, and very suspicious of her husband. She was said to have had this past symptom for many years. She saw her physician intermittently for two years and then presented herself in acute psychotic excitement, with marked agitation, tremendous overactivity, and bizarre delusions. At that time she was hospitalized and was given seven electroconvulsive treatments (ECT). She rapidly returned to her usual self and was discharged from the hospital on medication. It is not known whether she continued her medication at this time, or how often she was seen in follow-up treatment.

Her second hospitalization came one year later. For several days before this admission she had become more and more uncommunicative, pointing like a pre-verbal child to what she wanted. She was hospitalized when she threw all of her food, clothing, and personal articles out of the house. It was reported by the physician who saw her at that time that she was almost completely withdrawn. She was absolutely mute; she lay on her bed in a prone position with her eyes closed, her hands clasped in front of her face as though in prayers. She refused to be touched or moved, and when food was placed in her mouth she spat it out. On this occasion she was given thirteen ECTs and was discharged one month after admission as being markedly improved. Again, she was discharged with orders to stay on her medication.

Apparently these orders were disregarded and she had to be readmitted for a third time six months later. Once again at the time of admission she was completely mute and completely immobile. This changed very rapidly during the first few days of hospitalization to a period of extreme agitation, with confusion, delusional thinking, marked negativism, and refusal to do anything she was asked. On this occasion she again received seven ECTs and was again discharged as being improved. At that time she was placed on a combination of psychotropic medications. Although she did not see her psychiatrist for the next two years she reported to him by phone, had her medications refilled, and was taking them steadily under supervision.

Two years later she became pregnant. The possible bad effects of the medication on the developing fetus were not known. For that reason she was taken off her medication by the obstetrician during the time possiblity of harm existed. It is to be noted, however, the medication was not resumed once this danger period had passed. A relative reported that following the baby's birth she seemed quite normal for about two weeks and then started to behave in a strange way. She kept the window blinds down; she refused to answer the door; she would not let anyone in the house. She seemed to take very good care of the baby who "grew like a weed' to quote the informant. She insisted on keeping the baby unclothed, saying it did not need all that binding stuff.

On the tragic evening in question, the family had been in the living room watching television and she had withdrawn to her own bedroom, something which she apparently did frequently. The baby was whining a little. The father took it out in the living room with the family until it fell asleep. He then placed it back in its crib in the mother's bedroom. The other children went to bed. The father dozed off by the television until he was roused by the sound of the shot.

When Mrs. K was seen for the competency examination about three months after the event, she had again received a series of ECTs. She was still in the hospital. The following observations were made as to her general behavior. "The patient sat in a rigid, fixed pose. She volunteered no information spontaneously. When she smiled it was an almost artificial smile; it came and went in response to social demands of the situation. At other times the same smile would appear under very inappropriate circumstances. For the most part her facial expression was downcast. It too was rigid and fixed. She was oriented in all spheres. No present delusions or hallucinations could be elicited. Her answers to questions were almost monosyllabic, and she volunteered almost no information spontaneously, so that she might very well have been deluded during the examination."

This case has been presented to illustrate the relationship between schizophrenia, catatonic type, and antisocial behavior. This is a woman who had shown both catatonic excitement and catatonic stupor in the past. Apparently, from what history was known at the time of the examination, she had again become rather suddenly psychotic following a preliminary period of peculiar behavior. Apparently in that psychosis she had killed her youngster.

SCHIZOPHRENIA, PARANOID TYPE (295.3)

The subtype of schizophrenia to be discussed next is the one which is probably brought to the attention of corrections workers more frequently than are any of the other subtypes. This is **Schizophrenia, Paranoid Type (295.3)**. The thing that characterizes a paranoid individual in general, regardless of what subclassification may be involved, is suspiciousness, and this is certainly true of individuals showing symptoms of paranoid schizophrenia. It is the suspiciousness, the feeling that someone is out to get me, is going to harm me, which generally leads to antisocial behavior in terms of, "I will get my persecutor before he gets me." This was the situation in the classic McNaghten case[3], the case in which the formula for determining whether an individual could be acquitted by reason of insanity was first laid down in Victorian England. McNaghten suffered quite obviously from what today would be classified as paranoid schizophrenia. He believed that members of one political party in the British Isles were out to get him; they were doing all sorts of things to him such as poisoning his food, spreading false stories about him, following him from one place to another, causing degrading things about him to be

---

[3]Under McNaghten rules as they are customarily applied in this country, an individual may be found not guilty by reason of insanity if at the time of the offense the individual is suffering from such a defect of reason due to mental illness as not to know the nature or consequences of the act which he is alleged to have performed, or to know that the act was wrong. In some states the stipulation is added that even though knowing that the act was wrong the individual was, because of the mental disease or defect, unable to abstain from doing the wrong.

published in the papers. Finally in an attempt to stop this persecution he tried to assassinate the leader of the party, Sir Robert Peale, the Prime Minister of England. (Sir Robert Peale has also gone down in history as the man who has given his name to the British policeman, the bobby.) McNaghten, having come to the logical conclusion that the only way to stop this persecution was by ridding himself of the leader of his persecutors, shot, whether because of mistaken identity or accident, not Peale but Peale's private secretary.

The basic mechanism underlying development of a paranoid condition of any sort is what is called *projection*. In other words, an individual tends to project out onto the environment thoughts which arise from within but are unacceptable. For example, a male brought up to believe that sexual thoughts about someone of the opposite sex are extremely sinful and not to be tolerated may, in spite of himself, begin to be troubled by the thought, "I sure would like to go to bed with that girl." Since this thought is taboo to such an individual, it may be translated into "that girl sure makes eyes at me; I'll bet she'd like to go to bed with me," or it may go all the way to, "Everyone I pass on the street is thinking, 'Oh he wants to go to bed with her,' " or "Listen to the voices saying I want to go to bed with her." Sometimes these voices appear to come from within the individual. They then may be recognized as distorted products of the imagination, or there may be bewilderment at how they got inside the head (see case of Mr. J.). At other times they sound convincingly real and unmistakable, as though they came from the external world. No amount of common sense discussion will make the person believe not only that they are not coming from the outside world, but that other people do not hear them as well. From here it may be a simple step to, "I hear them broadcasting this about me over the radio," or, "They're enacting my story on television," or even, "Men from outer space are coming down in flying saucers and spreading this story all over the world about me." (It is of some interest to note that paranoid delusions tend to follow the latest scientific developments). What differentiates schizophrenia, paranoid type, from other paranoid conditions is the concomitant presence of Bleuler's four *A*s. The delusion is, of course, the exemplification of autism. In time the difficulty in associative processes, the ambivalence, and the affective disorder also will appear.

As a usual rule Paranoid Schizophrenia develops at a later age than the other forms. Onset is generally in the late twenties or mid-thirties, although on rare occasions it may not be seen until sometime in the early forties. During the early stages of the development of the disease the sufferer mistakenly thinks that word is being disseminated by whatever means about despicable personal faults. The resultant persecution is then believed to be due to these mistaken beliefs of others. This persecution may then go on to almost unspeakable tortures. In the desire to be rid of this torment, the individual may turn on the fancied foes and attempt to put this procedure to a stop once and for all. When this occurs, tragedy may result. Fortunately, before this drastic step is taken something else generally happens. There is a sudden flash of insight in which the real reason for the persecution becomes crystal clear. "These stories aren't really believed about me; they are just a cover. I am really the next president of the United States (or the former king of England, or whatever) and the persecution is a step meant to deprive me of my rightful place. However, since I am such a grandiose and exalted person, I am naturally much more powerful than my persecutors and so I have nothing to fear from them. Thus there is no reason for me to turn on them because they are no longer capable of harming me." When antisocial behavior occurs in this stage it is more apt to be due to mistaken judgment. "If I am the king, then everything in the country belongs to me, and it is perfectly all right for me to go into a store and walk out with anything I want, because it is mine anyway." This compares in many respects with the grandiose stage that has already been discussed in Chapter 4 occurring in general paralysis due to syphilis. Because there is less rapid deterioration in thinking capacity in Paranoid Schizophrenia than there is in Syphilitic Paralysis, the individual is less apt to strike at those who would prevent him from having what is rightfully his, although it is possible for controls to break down to that extent.

In the past the corrections worker had very little contact with Paranoid Schizophrenics, because shortly after their condition was discovered they would be placed in a mental hospital. Recovery or even improvement in this condition was quite rare. Now with the advent of psychopharmacology, and before that ECT or even insulin therapy, marked improvement in the condition may be seen. Once the insidious process has begun, however, the most psychopharmacology can do, at least in the present state of medical knowledge, is to arrest the progress of the disease. The basic process remains unchanged. If the individual stops taking his medication, it may manifest itself in both bizarre or antisocial behavior. At times such behavior may occur while still taking it. As has been stressed before, this is one place where the corrections worker can be most helpful, namely in stressing the importance of taking medication. He can also help in many more concrete ways: by helping to secure employment,[4] by helping to smooth over some of the friction which is apt to occur with others because of basic suspiciousness which the individual has, by furnishing a strong, always present, base to which the individual can return when in need of encouragement.

In the practical handling of these people it is a waste of breath to attempt to convince them that their delusions, or their hallucinations, are not real. They are just as real to them as the corrections worker's arms or legs are to the worker. What is more helpful is the acceptance of the fact that these beliefs are real to them, but their reality is not accepted by others, including the worker. It must be stressed that in spite of this they have a perfect right to their beliefs, but that if they want to avoid friction they must keep them to themselves. Once this statement has been made the worker should ignore any men-

---

[4]It has now become illegal in many states to deny an individual employment, whether public or private, solely on the grounds of present or past treatment for mental conditions.

tion of these beliefs, but should respond positively in a reinforcing way to any other topic introduced by the client. (Naturally if there is obvious distress and specific threats of retaliation the worker cannot ignore these.) Where possible the worker should contact the client's friends and coworkers in an attempt to elicit their cooperation in this pattern of ignoring "craziness" while concentrating on responding actively and interestedly to healthier topics. While ideally this is the job of the mental health worker, the corrections workers will only too often have to assume this role because there is no one else to take it. In spite of the pessimistic remarks about the course of this illness, I am of the opinion that a combined approach with chemotherapy, vocational therapy, recreational outlets, and the sort of support just outlined helps to maintain treated paranoid schizophrenics in society over long periods of time as functioning people.

OTHER FORMS OF SCHIZOPHRENIA

The remaining types of schizophrenia are being discussed solely because as labels they exist, and it is important that the corrections worker have some knowledge of what these labels refer to. For the most part, making the specific subtype diagnosis is a matter of splitting hairs and is of concern presently only to the research-oriented psychiatrist in his effort to determine specific etiologies (causes) for specific types of schizophrenia or specific treatment for specific types of schizophrenia. These remaining types, therefore, will be discussed very briefly. **Acute Schizophrenic Episode (295.4)** is indistinguishable originally from an acutely developing Hebephrenia or from an acute catatonic excitement. Most cases which are so diagnosed have the diagnosis changed with the passage of time to one of the other conditions. Most commonly the condition improves rapidly with medication. There is always a tendency for it to recur unless preventive measures are carried out. The same sort of antisocial behavior can be expected here as during the early stages of hebephrenic, catatonic, or paranoid schizophrenia.

Currently, one important differentiation must be made. Sometimes this can only be done with the passage of time. This is the differentiation between Acute Schizophrenic Episode and Psychosis Due To Drugs and Other Exogenous Poisons. Many times these are indistinguishable even when there is a clear cut history of drug ingestion present.

Schizophrenia, Latent Type (295.5) is extremely difficult to differentiate from **Schizophrenia, Residual Type (295.6)** and **Schizophrenia, Chronic Undifferentiated Type (295.90)**. In schizophrenia, latent type, while schizophrenic symptoms such as dissociation of affect and thought, looseness of associative processes, difficulty in judgment and flattening of affect are seen, there has never been an acute psychotic outburst noted in the individual's history. In schizophrenia, residual type, what is observed is an individual who has shown symptoms of one of the other types, but who, whether because of treatment or spontaneously, is currently showing no evidence of psychosis. Careful examination may uncover some changes in mood and some early disorders in thought, particularly a tendency toward concretistic thinking. In schizophrenia, chronic undifferentiated type, there is such a mixture of schizophrenic symptomatology, lasting over a period of time, that more precise classification cannot be effectuated.

As a final word for the corrections worker, schizophrenic individuals as a rule are inoffensive, although eccentric. The deteriorated, regressed individual may commit petty offenses, but well-preserved personalities, particularly if catatonic or paranoid, may change quite rapidly and be potentially dangerous. Such individuals should be seen frequently when on a probation or a parole officer's caseload. There should also be continuing close contact with the family. The family should be encouraged to report changes in behavior as soon as they are noticed. The worker should attempt to have adequate medical support. With the rapid development of knowledge in brain chemistry, physiology, and pharmacology, very hopeful strides have already occurred in the understanding and amelioration of these baffling and formerly hopeless conditions. A great breakthrough may not come tomorrow, but the hopeless attitude which formerly pervaded all discussions of schizophrenia is no longer completely justified.

Chapter 6

MAJOR AFFECTIVE DISORDERS

GENERAL CONSIDERATIONS

SCHIZOPHRENIA was described as being primarily a disorder in the *process of thought.* All the symptoms could be viewed as arising from this basic disorder. The **Major Affective Disorders** (296) might be described as being primarily disorders in *mood,* and all the symptoms displayed arise from this basic disorder. Mood is that feeling tone which permeates the individual's life at any particular period. Mood is distinguished from emotion by its duration. The analogy has been drawn in which emotion is compared to the weather, i.e. it is hot or cold, wet or dry *today;* mood is compared to climate, i.e. spring in New England is cool and wet. The behavior disorder in the conditions to be described in this chapter is determined by the predominance of one major mood which permeates the current life situation of the individual. This mood may be predominantly depressive, happy or euphoric, suspicious, or any combination thereof. The other important factor in the diagnosis of one of these conditions is a lack of any obvious triggering or precipitating cause in the individual's environment to which the mood disorder can be attributed. For this reason, these conditions are frequently referred to an *endogenous* disorders (*endo* — within, *genous* — giving rise to, generation). That is, they arise within the individual.

If depression is taken as an example of one of the affective disorders, there is a continuum from normal grief, through the mild illness, reactive depression, to the serious disorder, endogenous depression. Everyone, in the course of a lifetime, suffers from loss: A man's wife dies quite suddenly; a woman carries a child through nine months of pregnancy, and then the child is stillborn; periodic financial dips occur, and a man who has slaved all his life building up a business loses it through no fault of his own. For such an individual, to be sad in reaction to one of these losses seems to be quite ordinary and expected. This reaction is called *grief,* or if prolonged, *mourning.* These responses are normal. If the sadness is protracted enough so that the depression had interfered with the individual's life to a greater degree than is commonly experienced, or if the depths of the reaction seem to be out of line with the severity of the loss, it is called a **Neurotic Depressive Reaction** or a **Reactive Depression.** It has progressed beyond grief and is illness. If the depression intensifies to the point where, in reaction to this loss, the individual loses contact with reality, it is called a **Psychotic Depressive Reaction.** If a similar depression, severe enough to interfere with the individual's perception of reality, occurs without any precipitating cause, then it is called an *Endogenous Depression.* Both Psychotic Depressive Reaction and Endogenous Depressive Reaction are classed under the major affective disorders; neurotic depression and grief are not.

INVOLUTIONAL MELANCHOLIA (296.0)

Involutional Melancholia (296.0) is the first of the major affective disorders to be discussed. The term *involutional* refers to the change of life. This change takes place in both men and women, although it is more obvious in women. The most characteristic event of the change of life in women is the gradual, or rapid, cessation of the menstrual periods. This is usually accompanied by episodic, sudden sensations of extreme bodily warmth, usually called *hot flashes.* Along with this there may be changes in the distribution of body fat, atrophy of the breasts, changes in the vaginal mucosa, and, occasionally, increased growth of hair on the face and extremities. There may be an increase in sex drive at this time. All of these changes are brought about by diminution in levels of circulating hormones. These are natural processes. This change in women generally occurs between the ages of forty-two and forty-nine, although it may occur anywhere between thirty-five and fifty-five. It may be brought about earlier by surgical removal of the reproductive organs. The change of life in men is not demonstrated by such obvious symptoms. It generally occurs at a later age, although some more recent writers tend to believe the change of life occurs earlier in men than in women. Men may have hot flashes but the general pattern is that of loss of interest, appetite, sleep and weight, along with bodily complaints.

Involution takes place in everyone and it is a normal part of the aging process. Involuntional melancholia is not, but is an illness. The striking feature of involutional melancholia is the severe depression which affects some people at this point in their lives. While it might seem logical to assume that involutional melancholia is the result of the hormonal imbalance which characterizes this period, this is not so. Only the listed physiological symptoms are so caused. The cause of the depression itself is still in question. It does not respond to hormonal treatment, even though the physiological symptoms may.

Just as in psychosis following childbirth, involutional melancholia may represent a depressed phase of manic-depressive illness, manifesting itself for the first time at the involutional period of life. In those instances where no evidence can be found to suggest a manic-depressive reaction, other factors would seem to be operative. The involutional period marks the gateway to old age. To many childless women, married or unmarried, this means that the hope of bearing a child must now be relinquished. To the vain, self-centered woman, whose physical beauty has been her whole life, there is a sharp reminder that the bloom is leaving the rose. To the man or woman who has had no marital success or has not quite made it to the top in career goals, the involution marks the need to relinquish ambition. To many it is a time to stop and count one's disappointments and losses, rather than achievements and gains. The odds are that unfulfilled wishes or needs are not going to be filled; sins of omission or commission will lack atonement or compensation. Hence the depression.

Formerly, the nature of the depression in involutional melancholia was quite specific. The outstanding features were severe depression, marked agitation, and one of two types of delusion, sometimes both. One type of delusion sprang from guilt. It held that all the ills of the world were attributable to the sufferer's previous sins, "I am the most unworthy person in the world. I have committed the unpardonable sin. Everything that happens in this world that's rotten is because of me." Obviously, such people are intensely suicidal. The second type of delusions are called delusions of *Nihilism* (nothingness). "The reason that I don't eat is that I have no insides." "I can't think because I have no mind." "I don't exist and soon nothing else will exist." Obviously, such delusions stem not from disorder of thought process, but from disorder of mood, severe depression. Currently, it is rare to see this fully developed illness because of the early use of antidepressant medication. What is generally seen is a man or woman in the involutional period who has many bodily complaints, who is eating and/or sleeping poorly, is mildly depressed, with some tinges of guilt, and with a general dampening of enthusiasm and questioning if it's all worthwhile.

There are two possible offenses which make involutional melancholia of particular interest to the corrections worker. The first of these is rarely commented on in textbooks, even though it is frequently seen. Not uncommonly one of the early signs of involutional melancholia, in men as well as women, is shoplifting. Such shoplifting has to be distinguished from compulsive shoplifting, from shoplifting as a purely antisocial form of behavior, or as a part of a general life style. This shoplifting represents a complete departure in the behavior pattern of those involved. They have the necessary funds in their possession to buy the articles which they attempt to pilfer. If apprehended, they are quite at a loss to explain even to themselves what has happened. In quite simplistic terms, they are repeating what many young children go through; namely, stealing as a symbolic act to repair a loss of affection. At times the articles stolen point directly to the actual underlying mechanism.

> A striking example of that is Mrs. L, forty-nine-years-old. Mrs. L was referred for help in presentence investigation following her second conviction in three months for shoplifting. These were the only convictions, indeed the only offenses, on her record. She lived in a good, middle class neighborhood,

her husband had a good job, and she had charge plates in her purse for each of the stores in which she had been apprehended. The police reports reveal that in each case the only articles stolen were baby clothing, one dress in each offense. On questioning, Mrs. L reported that in each instance she had been invited to a baby shower. Two of her close friends each had a pregnant daughter. Mrs. L was childless. With encouragement Mrs. L was able to talk of her feelings about the lonely life ahead for her. She was envious of her friends who had grandchildren to "keep them young." She was even afraid that her husband might leave her. Looking back it could be seen that the depression had been developing for about a year before her arrests. The invitation to the showers had crystalized her feelings. Her shoplifting expressed her wish to have a grandchild, her resentment of those friends who were about to have one, and her awareness that she would never have any grandchildren of her own.

Mrs. M had a somewhat similar story, at least as far as her age, social status, and childlessness were concerned. She was arrested after she was noticed slipping an extra can of soup into her bag at the supermarket without putting it through the checkout. Her life seemed to be quite uneventful and her future secure. However, questioning revealed early delusions of nihilism. "We won't have anything left. I know we're going to lose everything we have in the world. I will need that extra can of soup some day." She, too, had been in an undetected depression for almost a year.

The story of Mr. N can only be conjectured on the basis of media reports. For two or three days in 1974, each of the major television networks gave unusual prominence to the story of a second rank executive of a major motor car company arrested for shoplifting in a cigar store. Sixty years old, just short of the pinnacle of success, why should he steal a two-dollar lighter? Many assumptions could be made, but the most likely one is that Mr. N was in the still undetected stages of involutional melancholia, forced to admit the loss of his dream of going to the top.

The second type of offense committed by these people comes about through agitation, the feeling that "I am such a horrible person," the terrible feeling that this is a horrible world. The same mechanism takes over as has already been noted in psychosis with childbirth (see Chapter 3), where the sufferer attempts to kill herself and her loved ones who are going to be punished eternally for her guilt. She wishes to spare them that punishment. Here, however, the loved ones are apt to be no longer young children nor is the defendant necessarily a woman. The crimes are apt to be more violent.

A conviction for shoplifting in a middle-aged person should ring a bell in the corrections worker's head. This, of course, is particularly true if there has been no previous record and no obvious motive. The presentence investigation in these instances should focus on uncovering any evidence of depression in the immediate past. It is particularly helpful in this context to look for disturbances in appetite, sleep patterns, general feelings of well-being, in addition to the much more obvious feelings of depression. Sometimes a relative will be unable to clarify the situation any further than, "He (or she) has not seemed like the usual self these past few months," or, "She (or he) seemed somehow withdrawn and worried but I can't get her to talk about it." With these clues, it is usually not too difficult to elicit a fairly clear-cut picture of depression. A recommendation for treatment rather than due process might help arrest this depression at this point, and then reverse it.

The role of the corrections worker in cases of filicide, or even killing of a spouse, as a consequence of involutional melancholia is very similar to that described in Chapter 3 in relationship to psychosis due to childbirth. The age of the offender, who is now on the down-slope of life rather than the up-slope, makes the role of the worker more difficult. Every effort to improve socialization must be made. Here too, involvement in community enterprises which entail helping others can be of utmost benefit. Care must be taken to protect the offender from too eager representatives of the press and other news media. (To this day it is incomprehensible to me why so much was made of the case of Mr. N over the television.) Some of the stories are sensational and wide dissemination can badly hinder rehabilitation.

MANIC-DEPRESSIVE ILLNESS
(MANIC-DEPRESSIVE PSYCHOSIS) (296)

Manic-Depressive Illness (296) seems at first glance to embrace many different conditions. However, as in the various forms of schizophrenia, these various conditions have many common attributes. The first of these is that the condition occurs in discrete attacks, which run a limited course (although without treatment, a single attack may last for several years). In the interval between attacks there is nothing to suggest that the individual had ever been ill. Unlike schizophrenia, there is no tendency to show deterioration, regardless of the number of episodes. In this respect, this condition is analogous to the common cold. No matter how many times an individual has a cold, unless complications develop, no change can be found in the nose, the throat, or lungs after recovery from the attack. In general, people who suffer from this illness have personalities quite different from those who develop schizophrenia. In contrast to the withdrawn, solitary, daydreaming individuals so often described in the premorbid personality of the schizophrenic, those who develop manic-depressive illness are customarily outgoing and gregarious. They are doers rather than dreamers. The first attack of the illness is rarely seen before the early twenties, although on rare occasions it may occur in adolescence or even in childhood.

Three interesting developments emerge from recent studies of these conditions. The first is that the attacks themselves, especially the depression, are either accompanied by, or are due to, specific changes in the chemistry of certain areas of the brain, changes which are reversible by chemotherapy. The second is that hereditary factors play a large role in this condition, to the extent that it has almost become possible to predict that certain people have a tendency to develop or transmit the illness. The final development is that it now appears possible, by medication which will be discussed later, not only to treat an attack, but possibly to prevent any recurrence of further attacks.

Three groups of manic-depressive illnesses are recognized:

Manic-Depressive Illness, Manic Type (296.1); Manic-Depressive Illness, Depressed Type (296.2); and Manic-Depressive Illness, Circular Type (296.3). These may very easily be illustrated graphically. Figure 1 demonstrates the variation in mood in the average person. The mood oscillates mildly above and below a baseline normal for any particular individual. The oscillations may or may not be connected to an environmental circumstance. They may be *exogenous* (caused from without) or *endogenous* (caused from within).

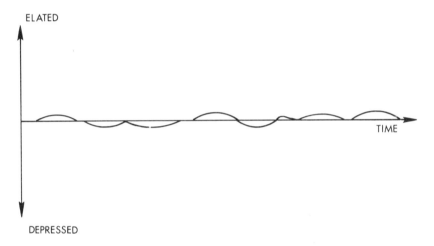

Figure 1. Normal State.

In its fully developed form, the manic phase of manic depressive illness is easily recognized. Figure 2a illustrates the swings above normal of the manic individual. The patient is highly excited, usuallly extremely elated and *euphoric* (full of feelings of joy), or may exhibit marked irritability. At times the excitement is so great that delusions of grandiosity may occur. Occasionally, there will be delusions of persecution and even rarely hallucinations. These disturbances in the content of thought are generally an extension of the exaggerated mood. The patient is markedly over-talkative. Speech is speeded up and seems to spew out of the individual's mouth as though it were under pressure and simply had to come out (this is called *pressure of*

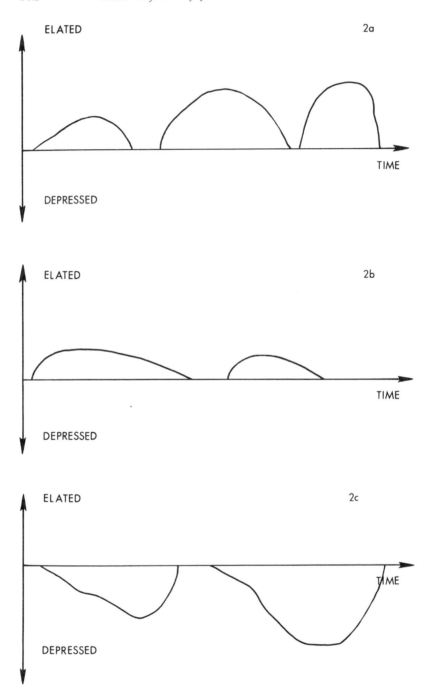

Figure 2.

speech). The speech content is characterized by what is called *flight of ideas*, that is, one idea follows another extremely rapidly. No constant topic is maintained. This can be differentiated from the looseness of associations seen in schizophrenia by the fact that the alert listener can always tell what the associations are. This is generally true even if hallucinations and delusions are present. They are public associations rather than private ones. Sometimes the association stems from the topic under discussion, sometimes it stems from the sound of the word, sometimes it is rhyming, sometimes it is punning. A typical example of flight of ideas might be:

> Here comes the doctor to see me, look at me, view me, pursue me, screw me. I'd like to screw you. Who are you, anyway? Anyway at all is fine with me. If you see me as I see you, we'll both be happy and untrue. I never told a lie in my life. Some people are terrible liars, but I'm not one of them, you can ask anybody. Anybody, everybody. Are you a buddy of mine? You can't be a buddy of mine and keep me in here when I want to be out there.

The cardinal signs of manic-depressive disorder, manic phase, are euphoric mood, pressure of speech with flight of ideas, and psychomotor excitement. A fully developed manic attack rarely develops suddenly. It is usually preceded by a period of slowly increasing activity. This build-up, which sometimes lasts for weeks, is referred to as the *hypomanic state* (*hypo* — under, less than; *manic* — to be mad). In this state, the individual is happier than usual, more active than usual, has more drive than usual, needs less sleep than usual, and not infrequently exhibits poorer judgment than usual. It is in the hypomanic state, Figure 2b, that much of the creative work of the world has been done. It is quite understandable why an individual in such a condition resists treatment. Indeed, it is debatable as to whether treatment of the hypomanic state is advisable in creative individuals. Unfortunately, the lack of judgment which frequently accompanies this hypomanic state will lead to such difficulties as squandering the family finances, writing bad checks, or performing other acts which bring the individual into conflict with the legal system. The first manic attack may occur at any age in life. First attacks are most common in the twenties.

An illustrative case of the hypomanic individual behaving in an antisocial fashion is that of Mr. O, a thirty-five-year-old businessman, head of a small but thriving industry, on his way back to his office on a Friday afternoon with the company payroll in cash. A pretty young girl is standing at a traffic light where he has stopped. She happens to be an aggressive sort of juvenile delinquent who makes fairly obvious advances to him. In his expansive mood, and with his poor judgment, he invites the girl into the car. One thing leads to another and they go off on a spree extending over several states and lasting until the money runs out.

He is faced on his return with a multiplicity of charges, ranging from conversion of company funds, contributing to the delinquency of a minor, all the way through to the Mann Act. A careful history, including a family history of manic-depressive illness, and a thorough psychiatric examination confirmed a diagnosis of hypomania. In this particular instance, the hypomanic phase changed almost immediately into a depression so severe as to require ECT. This, in turn, was again followed by a brief hypomanic phase before Mr. O stabilized. The course of the illness confirmed the diagnosis.

As the intensity of the manic swing increases, the situation becomes much more obvious to family and friends, and attempts are made toward hospitalization. Very often the individual becomes involved in highly aggressive, antisocial, acting-out behavior before treatment can be arranged, and the police are involved before medical professionals. Charges are usually dropped, and the individual is hospitalized. These people frequently begin to drink as they get high from their illness. Under those circumstances, they commonly get into bar-room brawls. It is not until they are sober that it is realized that the excitement is continuing and was not just due to the alcohol.

Mr. P presents an illustrative picture of this sort. Relatively young, a rather well built muscular male, he was building up to a manic attack. He got into a fight with his wife because of his hyper-irritability, left the apartment, and went to a movie.

He sat through only about half of one show and went to a bar where he proceeded to drink a great deal. He then went to the parking lot and after some difficulty he found his car, only to discover that it would not start because he had left the lights on and the battery was drained. This was a brand new car, but nevertheless he kicked the sides in because of his frustration and irritability. He was down to his last dime at that point and he used it to call his wife to tell her about his predicament. He wanted to ask her to come and get him. She recognized his voice on the phone and, still being very angry because of their quarrel, hung up on him. He had no choice but to spend a cold night in the car. In the morning he had to urinate and went to the movie theater, peeked through the glass doors, found the custodian and called to him. He explained his plight to the custodian. When the latter refused to let him in, he kicked in the plate glass door. He went to the toilet and in his own words, "When I got out I found every cop in the city around the place. It looked like a bubble gum convention." At that point he had no problem with transportation away from the movie theater. He was taken quickly to the nearest police station. In a relatively short period of time, it was determined that he was not drunk, but was in a manic phase and he was hospitalized.

The next illness to be considered is that of **Manic-Depressive Illness, Depressed Type (296.2)** (see Figure 2c). This is the opposite side of the coin. Rather than being over-talkative, over-active, and bubbly, the individual is underactive, shows poverty of ideas, and a definitely depressed mood. Such people rarely come within the purview of the probation officer, because the psychomotor retardation is so great that not only do they not commit crimes, they literally do nothing but sit. However, a mixed form is seen in which there is an agitated depression, with depressed mood and psychomotor over-activity. Then the picture is very similar to that already described in psychosis following childbirth and in involutional melancholia. People with agitated depression are more apt to commit suicide, because the increased motor activity allows the wish to be dead to be put into immediate action. If antisocial offenses are committed during an agitated depression, they take the same form as in the two conditions which the agitated depres-

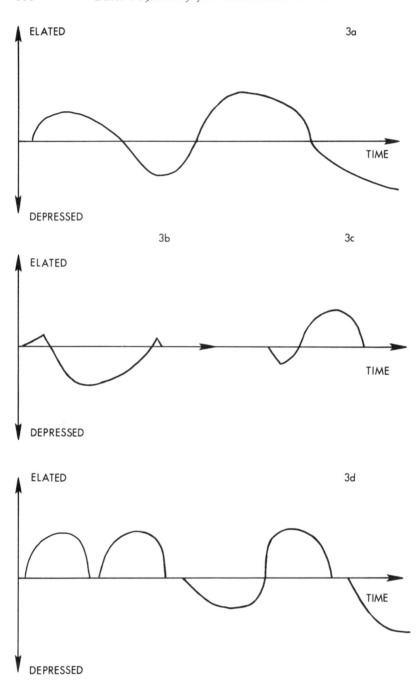

Figure 3.

sion resembles, and the handling of the offender is the same, except for specific preventive medication which will be discussed later on.

At least 50 percent of individuals who are subject to manic-depressive illness have it in the form of **Manic-Depressive Illness, Circular Type (296.3).** Figure 3 demonstrates vividly why the name manic-depressive illness is given to these two opposite conditions, namely mania and depression. Either phase may appear in the same individual in the circular type of manic-depressive illness. Figure 3a shows the picture of an individual with little, or no, normal intervals between mood swings. Figure 3b and c show forms of circular illness in which the predominant direction of the mood disorder is preceded (or followed) by a mini-disturbance in the opposite direction. Figure 3d demonstrates a case in which it is impossible to predict in which direction the mood will next fluctuate. It is of importance to note that the actual manifestations of a specific phase, for example the manic phase, are no different whether they occur in manic-depressive illness, manic type, or manic-depressive illness, circular type, manic phase. Those illnesses in which the swing is always in one direction, as in Figures 2a, b, and c, are referred to an unpolar illnesses; those in which both phases occur, as in Figure 3, are called bipolar illnesses. It should also be noted that no specificity exists either in regard to length of the interval between attacks, or whether this interval will increase or decrease with increasing age, or whether any attack will be the last.

It has been found that the salt of an ordinary metal called lithium, administered in doses which will maintain a definite level of lithium in the blood, flattens out the ups and downs of the manic-depressive's swings. Generally, it leaves the patient in a very mild hypomanic state in which he or she can be creative without being destructive. It should be emphasized that lithium is in no way a tranquilizer. It leaves no drowsiness, sleepiness, or feeling of being down. Under proper supervision, it can almost completely prevent the recurrence of these attacks. Since the frequency of these swings may vary from two to four manic episodes a year all the way to one every two to three years, the importance of such prevention can readily be seen. The ability to spot a manic attack quickly is a highly desirable asset for anyone who works in a jail or other detention facility. For the probation or parole officer, as in many other psychiatric conditions, one of the chief tasks will be to see that the individual continues to take the medication and continues to report to his physician to have blood levels monitored. This is extremely important because too low a blood level may lead to a recurrence of the condition, and too high a level can be severely toxic. The worker who is seeing a probationer or parolee on a regular basis is also in an ideal positon to pick up any incipient change in mood. In discussing schizophrenia it was noted that the worker's instinct when dealing with a bizarre individual was helpful in diagnosis. Similarly, in affective disorders a manic provokes a feeling of wanting to laugh *with* not *at;* a depressive patient stimulates a feeling of sadness in the worker. If such a mood swing is determined, the worker may then suggest an immediate check-up by the physician.

A final admonition is in order about managing the hypomanic person. The mood of joviality and happiness can quickly change to irritability and reactions of impulsivity and aggressiveness. This is best handled with a light touch. Instead of resorting to commands or force, which will only worsen the situation, the topic should be changed in a bantering way. It is quite easy to change the direction and nature of a manic's reaction.

PSYCHOTIC-DEPRESSIVE REACTION (298.0)

Although *DSM II* lists **Psychotic-Depressive Reaction (298.0)** under the heading of Other Psychosis, it is much more sensible to take it up under the affective disorders. In the instance of a psychotic-depressive reaction, the depressive reaction is quite similar to that in manic-depressive reaction, depressed type. It is distinguished from this latter condition by the fact that a genetic factor cannot be found and a precipitating cause can. It is rare for a patient with a psychotic-depressive reaction to be involved in antisocial behavior, at least when acutely depressed.

SCHIZO-AFFECTIVE DISORDERS (295.7)

DSM II lists the **Schizo-Affective Disorders (295.7)** under schizophrenia. It was felt advisable to describe them after the affective disorders had been discussed, because they are difficult to understand until something has been learned about both schizophrenia and the affective conditions. As the name implies, this illness has symptoms of both of the other two disorders. Like the manic-depressive states (or catatonic schizophrenia), it occurs in discrete attacks in which either excitement or depression is seen. Like schizophrenia, some disorder of thought process (paralogical thinking or looseness of associations) as well as *autistic* thinking with hallucinations and delusions also occur. In general it is believed that there is a progressive deterioration following each attack, but on occasion patients are seen in whom, despite rigorous testing, such deterioration can not be found. Since many of these patients respond well, both as an immediate therapeutic measure and in prevention of attacks, to administration of lithium, it may b that administration of this substance will serve as a so-called therapeutic test to differentiate schizo-affective disorders from catatonic schizophrenia. Those individuals who are in the excited phase of schizo-affective disorder may act in an antisocial way, sometimes quite impulsively. Ms. Q demonstrates such a case.

Ms. Q is a forty-seven-year-old female, referred for examination after she had practically disemboweled a young man, apparently without any provocation. Ms. Q occupied an apartment on the second floor of a home owned by a distant relative. On the day in question, as the son of this relative was coming home, he spotted a bunch of keys on the lawn. He called up, "Ms. Q are these yours?" She kind of grunted, and he walked upstairs with the keys. He knocked on the door, and as she opened it with one hand, she knifed him in the abdomen with a large butcher knife which she was holding in the other hand. Fortunately, he survived, but charges were pressed against her. She was taken to a mental hospital. Within a few weeks she was discharged as improved, returned to jail, and released on bond.

When examined for the court the following story emerged. She first came to the attention of the authorities fifteen years before the current offense. At that time, in her own home, she had been sitting on her boyfriend's lap. He got up to announce that his driver was there to take him to his job. She asked if he would take her to the state hospital the next day to visit her mother who was a patient there. He replied, "Of course, I always do when I have time," whereupon she picked up a pistol and shot him. She was obviously psychotic, and was taken to the state hospital. Her boyfriend refused to press charges, and after her apparent recovery she was released.

Between that episode and the offense which led to her current examination, Ms. Q was hospitalized twelve times in four different hospitals under the care of five different physicians. Diagnoses of schizophrenia, paranoid type; schizophrenia, catatonic type; and manic-depressive disorder, manic type had been made. Following her third hospitalization she had been discharged from her employment, and had been existing on her Social Security disability since that time. There were no other episodes of violence in her history.

When examined, Ms. Q gave an extremely interesting history. Her mother had died in a state hospital. One sister had committed suicide following a second admission to the state hospital. She described herself as having been an outgoing, gregarious person prior to her illness, a good worker with lots of friends. It is noted, however, that she had worked in three different cities before seeking permanent employment in her home town. She could recall no reason why she should have shot her boyfriend fifteen years ago, nor could she furnish any reason why she had knifed the young man, even though that event had taken place just four months before her examination. She did remember that she had been having difficulty for about three to four days prior to the offense. She had not been sleeping well. Strange things began to happen. The stove, the washing machine, and the refrigerator all began to talk to, and about, her. They began discussing her on the radio. Even after she had broken the radio by turning the dial rapidly in order to find a station where she was not being discussed, the conversation persisted. She could stop them from discussing her on television by turning the set off. She stated that she had recognized the young man when he called up to her apartment about the keys, but in the interval before he knocked on the door, she must have become confused and had mistaken him for an enemy, against whom she would have to protect herself. Asked if she thought she was insane at the time, her answer was, "When the stove and the refrigerator and the washing machine start talking to you, there's got to be something wrong. They can't talk."

Examination revealed an individual remarkably intact in every area for someone who had been subject to a disease process recurring thirteen times in fifteen years. She did have difficulty in remembering the details of each attack. Her ability to conceptualize and abstract was amazing. For example, her answer to "Explain the proverb, 'people who live in glass houses shouldn't throw stones' " was, "If you have a skeleton in your closet, and you are in the public eye, you should be extremely careful of accusing someone else of wrongdoing."

The one evidence of possible paralogical thinking was her plaintive statement that she could not understand why her relatives had made her move when she left the hospital. Asked what she would have done had she been in their place, her answer was, "Well, if I had known she was mentally ill, and didn't know what she was doing, I would have forgiven her." She was unable to comprehend the fear that this might happen again. Another point of interest in her story is that Ms. Q had never been on any medication other than the usual antipsychotic drugs. She objected to some of the side effects and took her medication only when she thought she needed it, rather than regularly. Once she became ill, she did not think of taking it. She had never had a trial on lithium.

The suggestion was made that if acquitted as not guilty by reason of insanity, she should be hospitalized, placed on lithium, and observed for a long enough period of time to see if this would prove to be an effective preventive.

PROSPECTIVE CHANGES IN DIAGNOSIS

At this juncture it is necessary to repeat that the current diagnoses of the affective disorders are being carefully studied. With the new edition of *DSM III* scheduled to come out in 1978 or 1979, these conditions will probably be called Major Mood

Disorders. They will be classified in a different way. The change in classification will be brought about due to the more recent findings of hereditary factors in these conditions, as well as increasing knowledge of disturbed biochemical functioning in the areas of the brain which have to do with mood. The new classification will still recognize the fact that manic swings occur and that they are associated with depressions. The diagnoses of neurotic and psychotic depressive reactions will probably be dropped. The mood disorders will be divided into major affective disorders and minor affective disorders. The affective disorders will then be divided into unipolar and bipolar. In unipolar mania or depression, no evidence of the opposite type of affect can be found no matter how careful the questioning. In addition, the hereditary factors differ from those seen in bipolar illness. Response to certain types of drug therapy may be different. The number of attacks any one individual may have is less frequent in unipolar depression, but the duration of individual untreated attacks is longer. Bipolar affective states include the alternating manic and depressive phases. Preventive measures with lithium alone are more successful in bipolar illness, while in unipolar illness lithium plus maintenance on antidepressants may be necessary to prevent recurrence. In addition, in unipolar depression psychotherapy may be of great benefit after the attack has stopped.

To summarize briefly, the depressive reactions of significance in corrections are involutional melancholia and agitated depression. Hypomanic reactions, full-blown manic reactions, and schizo-affective reactions of the manic type all may be linked to antisocial behavior. The corrections worker has an important role to play in the early recognition of the fact that such disturbance may underly antisocial behavior in particular individuals. In following up these individuals, equal attention must be given to the integration of the defendant into the community and helping to monitor the regular use of medication to prevent recurrence.

Chapter 7

PARANOID STATES

GENERAL CONSIDERATIONS

THE chief abnormalities in the **Paranoid States (297)** are delusions. These may be either delusions of grandeur or of persecution. These may occur either in sequence or simultaneously. The paranoid states may be contrasted to schizophrenia and to the affective disorders. In schizophrenia, the basic disorder is in the *thought process;* the majority of symptoms in that disorder stem from that abnormality. In the affective disorders, the essential disturbance is in the *mood;* all the symptoms of those disorders stem from the disturbance in mood. In the paranoid states, the essential disorder lies in the *content of thought;* any other functional disturbance, such as a disorder of mood, starts with the delusions.

Many writers feel that paranoid states are either less severe forms of paranoid schizophrenia or are more severe forms of paranoid personality disorders (see Chapter 11). It would seem, however, that there are definite differences among these conditions. Unlike paranoid schizophrenia, hallucinations are rare in the paranoid states. The age of onset is usually later in paranoid states than in paranoid schizophrenia, which itself has the oldest age of onset of all the schizophrenias. The delusional system is more tightly organized and much more logical in the paranoid states than in paranoid schizophrenia. Indeed, if the abnormal and irrational premises underlying the delusions of the paranoid states are accepted, the entire system built upon them would be credible. Finally, in contrast to schizophrenia, there is no deterioration in personality functioning no matter how long the condition lasts. Paranoid states are distinguished from paranoid personality in that definite delusions are present in the paranoid states and influence the individual's behavior. In the paranoid personality, specific delusions

113

are absent, but the entire attitude is one of suspicion.

The specific cause of the paranoid states is unknown. It has been proposed that paranoid states develop only in conjunction with repressed homosexuality. According to this hypothesis, the following schema explains what occurs. "I love him, but I am not allowed to love him. I do not love him, he loves me. I do not return his love. Therefore, he hates me and wants to harm me." It is true that this mechanism is seen in some paranoid people. It is equally true that paranoid states are seen in overt homosexuals, who have no reason to repress their feelings. In general it is felt that paranoid states develop in those people who were not able to develop a basic trust in others during childhood. There was no single, dependable, mothering person who was there at the time when the child was unable to minister to it's own needs. As a result, there would be times when lack of satisfaction of these basic needs, such as hunger, warmth, thirst, freedom from painful skin irritations, would be almost unendurable. Thus, the child did not develop a basic trust in the goodness of the environment. Another fertile soil for the development of paranoid states is the universal *fear of the stranger*. People transplanted to an alien culture, migrants, immigrants, particularly if there is also a language barrier, are more apt to develop paranoid states than those native to the particular area. Those groups more subject to severe discrimination also tend to have a higher incidence of paranoid states. This grows out of experential reality.

PARANOIA (297.0)

Paranoia (297.0) is one of the rarest of all mental illnesses. It is rarely seen by the corrections worker. When seen, it proves to be one of the most difficult, enigmatic, and baffling conditions encountered. Almost always, paranoia starts with a misinterpretation of a naturally occurring phenomenon. After a period of general suspiciousness, a specific event triggers the delusional system. For example, the phone of such a person will ring. When answered in adequate time, there is silence at the other end of the line. This is certainly an experience which is common to all of us. However, for the individual who is about to develop paranoia, it suddenly takes on extreme significance. Starting from the premise that possibly someone is bugging the telephone and wants to see if the bug is working, the patient elaborates an intricate system of delusions. Each delusion springs in logical order from the preceding one, until a network is built which may include in its web not only the police department of the entire city and state, but the FBI and the Interpol as well. They are all on the side of the enemy and are attempting to persecute the sufferer. Along with this, the paranoid develops a feeling of being unique, "I must be special if all this intricate network has been devised for me." Under the circumstances, it is not then uncommon to attempt to retaliate against one's enemies. The net result may very easily be antisocial behavior of a most drastic sort.

The striking thing about the situation in paranoia is the delusional system exists with almost complete isolation from the total personality. Even an in-depth evaluation may be completely negative unless the delusional system itself is explored. Such an individual may lead an apparently normal life for years, only to decide the net is closing too tightly and the persecution is becoming unbearable. Fortunately, most outbursts are verbal, but now and then some form of physical force is used to put an end to that persecution. At times it is only after such an act that it is learned that the supposed persecution had been going on for years. As a rule, family, neighbors, or friends will have heard the story before. Generally, they have either tried to argue with the paranoiac or just shrugged it off. The sufferer learns that others can not be persuaded to believe. From then on nothing more is said. In almost all those episodes reported in the press in which an individual killed two or three fellow employees, a supervisor, or an employer, apparently without provocation, it will be found that paranoia is present.

Chemotherapy may be helpful in paranoia. However, because of the patient's insistence that nothing is wrong, it is extremely difficult to get these people to take medication, or even to engage in psychotherapy. Very quickly both the medication and/or the attempt to help are woven into the persecutory network. If they are sentenced for an offense, their attitude is generally such that they serve maximum sentences. They will have proved to be recalcitrant and stubborn prisoners. It is rare for those paranoiacs acquitted as Not Guilty by Reason of Insanity to be released from a hospital as recovered. For this reason, as well as the rarity of the condition, they are seen infrequently by the community corrections worker. Wardens, guards, and others in penal institutions must be alert not to be included in the persecutory system, and hence fair game for retaliation. It is not good practice to agree with the delusions. On the other hand, it is extremely poor technique to attempt to argue point by point with these people. It further excites them, leads only to frustration, and it does nothing to remove the underlying ideas. Possibly the best advice in dealing with them is that given under the management of the person who suffered from schizophrenia of the paranoid type. There it was suggested that when delusional material is brought up it be ignored, and when other topics of conversation are discussed the listener enter in with interest and enthusiasm.

INVOLUTIONAL PARANOID STATES (297.1)

This is another one of those conditions which is not seen very frequently by the corrections worker. Since it is occasionally encountered it necessarily must be included. As might be judged from its name, this condition occurs in the involutional period. It is distinguished from Involutional Melancholia because delusion, rather than depression, is the outstanding symptom. It is distinguished from schizophrenia because there is no true disorder of thought process, and no deterioration goes on. The delusions in this condition are not as well systematized as they are in paranoia. This is another one of those situations in which there is relatively little the corrections worker can do; in most instances, the responsibility should not belong to Corrections.

This case, which is a good example of the involutional paranoid state, is complicated by another rare condition, namely, *folie a deux* (madness for two).

The protagonists, Ms. R and Ms. S, were unmarried sisters, thoroughly respectable citizens. Ms. R, forty-six, was a book-keeper. Ms. S, forty-four, was a school teacher. They had been quite frugal, saved their money, and owned their own home. In the boom just before the great depression of 1929, at the instigation of the older sister, Ms. R, the bookeeper, they had engaged in a practice which was quite common in those days. This was called pyramiding. A small down payment was made on a piece of property. This property was then used as collateral for down payment on another piece of property, and the pyramid was built as high as possible. They proceeded until they managed to stretch themselves so thin, that they had invested every penny they owned, including that obtained by mortgaging their own home. On paper they controlled somewhere between a quarter and a half million dollars' worth of real estate in their home town, a not inconsiderable figure in that period. At that point, the bubble burst and the depression of 1929 exploded in full force.

The Standard Oil Company had been bargaining with these women to lease a piece of property in order to establish a gas station thereon. The sisters were holding out for higher monthly rent than the company had offered. The depression struck, and they lost that property along with everything else that they owned. It was the older sister's firm conviction that the depression had been engineered by Mr. Morgan, who was at that time the head of Standard Oil of New York. He had done this, according to Ms. R, in order to get their property so the gas station could be built. She managed to sell this idea to her younger sister. With righteous indignation they purchased a revolver and took a train to New York City. On arrival there they headed to the nearest Travelers' Aid to ask how they could find Mr. Morgan. An alert worker asked why they wanted to see him. On being told that they had decided to kill him, they were steered to Bellevue Hospital where they were detained. When news of this detention reached their home community, the city fathers were sure that a mistake had been made. They descended en masse on the hospital, insisting that these were perfectly sane, respectable women, and that under no condition should they be considered mentally ill. They removed them from the hospital against medical advice and returned them to their home. Within twenty-four hours, they had purchased another gun and were again on their way to New York City with the same deed in mind.

Again they were intercepted, but this time there was no one to intercede for them. They were returned to a mental institution in their own community. Up to this point nobody in the corrections system had been involved. However, as happens so often in *folie a deux,* when Ms. R, the instigator died, Ms. S, recovered. At that time she was placed on trial, was found Not Guilty by Reason of Insanity, was deemed to have recovered and was placed on probation. It became the probation officer's duty to supervise her from then until her death. Other than the firm conviction that the state was responsible for her sister's death, she remained quite clear and presented no difficulty in management.

In the past, an involutional paranoid state might last until death. With newer methods of treatment, the danger of this happening is not nearly so great. As a result, the small number of these people who have been engaged in antisocial behavior find themselves rather quickly back out in the community and under the care of the corrections worker. For the most part, the same factors which were operative in bringing about an involutional melancholia are the factors which bring about the involutional paranoid state. The different clinical picture is due to the difference in the underlying personality structure of the individual who develops the illness. For this reason, on those rare occasions when the probation or parole officer's case load includes an individual of this sort, the approach will have to take into account the basic suspiciousness of that person. Possibly even more than in involutional melancholia, these people need help in socialization techniques, but they are also more apt to resist availing themselves of this help. The worker must be patient, must not bridle at the frequently expressed suspiciousness as to motivation, and must be persevering in the desire to help. As in any other form of paranoid illness, challenging the patient's delusional system or confronting the suspiciousness ·when true delusions are not present can only lead to disaster. It is only after a definite trust has been established that the slightest efforts can be made to hold up the mirror of reality. Even then, unless it is done gently, the fragile alliance may very well be shattered.

OTHER PARANOID STATES (297.9)

There remains one other condition to be considered under this heading of paranoid states, and that is **Other Paranoid States (297.9).** *DSM II,* interestingly enough, devotes less space to this condition than to any of the other conditions listed under paranoid states. In clinical practice, however, it is the most frequent paranoid disorder seen, other than paranoid schizophrenia. Other Paranoid States are relatively common. Symptomatically, they stand midway between Paranoid-Schizophrenia and Paranoia. Like the former, the delusions are not that well systematized; they are much more vague; they do tend to take on a mildly bizarre quality. Like the latter, there are no hallucinations. Also like the latter, no matter how long the condition lasts, the individual shows no sign of deterioration. People labeled as Other Paranoid States come into contact with the law when, because of their delusional system, they decide to take the law into their own hands, usually to protect themselves from, or to retaliate against, their imaginary persecutors. The delusions of Other Paranoid States are not as fixed as they are in true paranoia. It is sometimes possible for a worker who is able to remain in fairly close contact with such an individual to correct the misconceptions before they become deep-seated and elaborated. Some of the newer psychotropic medications are of benefit in altering the delusional system if the individual can be persuaded to take them.

There is a word of caution which should be introduced here. This applies when dealing with all those people who have been labeled paranoid. One should not automatically discount anything that such a patient has to say; there may be a great deal of veracity in it. One widely reported case was that of an individual who was kept in a hospital for years because of his claim that his wife and her lover had forced him to drink their blood. Someone finally got around to asking the wife how this strange idea ever got started, and she said it was not a strange idea at all, it was true; it was part of a custom of the country of their origin and proved that he had forgiven them. In an episode reported by a member of the staff at the Court Diagnostic and Treatment Center, a woman had been sent to the state hospital in which this staff member was an intern. The woman had been arrested on charges of speeding, reckless driving, and other traffic-related offenses. When arraigned she claimed diplomatic immunity, stating that she was an official representative of her country to the United Nations. Her clothing, her general appearance and demeanor, and her driver's license all failed to corroborate her story. It seemed to be bizarre enough so that it was decided that she needed hospital observation. What did emerge was that she did indeed work in the embassy of that nation and was a native of that country, even though she had no diplomatic immunity. The author has found that it pays, whenever possible, to attempt to get actual proof, or actual denial, of any rather bizarre statement that a patient makes unless it is so weird that it is obviously a part of the delusional system.

There is another interesting subdivison of paranoid states which is not found in *DSM II*. There is a definite question as to whether it belongs under paranoid states, which are psychoses, or under Personality Disorders, Paranoid Personality, a condition which is not psychotic. This subdivision involves an individual who is very suspicious, who does have mild delusions, but who reacts by filing a law suit against those who are perceived as persecutors rather than acting out against them. As a usual but not necessary rule, this is triggered by having originally been the defendant in a law suit. The number and insubstantial quality of suits filed bring the situation rather quickly to the attention of the authorities. The diagnostic term for such an individual is a **Litigious Paranoid.** The corrections officer does not come in contact with these people very often. If such a person does appear in the worker's case load, it is of paramount importance to record as fully as possible the exact nature of all contacts. There is an odds-on possibility that a suit might be instituted against the worker, and well-kept records will prove to be an invaluable protection against such a suit. There is also a possibility that the so-called jail-house lawyer might belong in this category, although, as far as can be determined, no specific study has been done which relates to this point.

ROLE OF THE WORKER

Taken as a whole, the various paranoid states do nothing to add to the joy of the correction worker's life nor does it seem that the worker has a great deal to offer such an individual. However, these people do exist and they must be dealt with when encountered. An open, empathic attitude is the most valuable. In one such case in this agency, an individual in a paranoid state was referred because of exhibitionism (the charge and the mental state bore no direct relationship). One worker in the agency was able to form a relationship with this man simply by listening to him. She did not argue with his delusions nor did she agree with him. During the time that she worked with him, the delusions did not change, but the intensity of his feelings about them lessened markedly, and his general adjustment in society seemed to improve a great deal. It would seem that this is about the most that can be expected of a corrections worker.

Chapter 8

NEUROSES

GENERAL CONSIDERATIONS

$\mathbf{M}$ANY attempts have been made to define the difference between neuroses and psychoses. Probably the most practical definition derives from the individual's perception of reality. In any neurotic state, with the possible exception of hysterical neurosis, which will be discussed later, there is no distortion of reality. External events are not misinterpreted. If the world appears frightening to the neurotic, there is still an awareness that the fear is internal and not caused by environmental factors. (If external events are really terrifying, the neurotic will experience fear to the same degree as anyone else. Indeed, some neurotic people react to terrifying environmental happenings with less anxiety than they generally experience.) In neurosis, the personality remains reasonably intact and does not exhibit disorganization. This is not to say that neurotic people are not sometimes as severely handicapped by their symptoms as are psychotic people. It is simply to say that the symptoms are of an entirely different nature. Furthermore, for the most part, neurotic persons are aware that their functioning is disturbed and, in general, troubled enough by this disturbance to seek help.

The core feature of all neurotic symptomatology is anxiety. This anxiety differs from the worry that is felt when a close relative is about to undergo major surgery, or the apprehension that occurs before taking an examination, or even the panic which sometimes takes over when someone yells "fire" in a crowded building. In those instances, the anxiety is based on immediate and perceivable reality. Indeed, there may be something abnormal if some degree of anxiety is not experienced under those circumstances. The anxiety of the neurotic person, in contrast, generally stems from situations in childhood, or in later life, in which experiences were unbearably painful at the time they occurred, and which could become painful again if they were recalled. In order to keep this recall from happening, various mechanisms are used to block out the recollection of the original anxiety. These defense mechanisms themselves may be symptom-producing.

Sometimes the anxiety itself is felt, but it is not felt in relationship to its original cause. Rather, it is experienced as a feeling of something about to happen which is frightening, but the exact nature of that something is unknown. This has been referred to as *free floating anxiety*. The anxiety may be displaced onto something that in itself is not anxiety producing for most people: crowds, open spaces, closed rooms, elevators, etc. This displaced anxiety is called a *phobia*. Anxiety and its defenses might also be viewed as learned behavior which then becomes automatic. While many types of neurotic reactions have been described, and while all sorts of neurotic individuals may be found in the worker's case load, only two are linked to antisocial behavior. Emphasis in this chapter will be placed on these conditions. They are **Hysterical Neurosis, Dissociative Type (300.14)**, and **Obsessive Compulsive Neurosis (300.3)**.

HYSTERICAL NEUROSIS, DISSOCIATIVE TYPE (300.14)

The **Hysterical Neurosis (300)** and the **Hysterical Personality (301.5)** (see Chapter 10) must be differentiated from the commonly used term, *having hysterics*. This term describes the loss of control frequently seen in an emotionally charged situation. It is manifested by prolonged and uncontrollable crying or laughing or a mixture of both. The hysterical neuroses are divided into two types — **Conversion Type (300.13)** and **Dissociative Type (300.14)**. The characteristic feature of hysterical neurosis of any type is that it is marked by a sudden, involuntary loss or disorder of one or another bodily function, including memory and state of consciousness. This loss is rooted in emotional disorder and comes on quite suddenly. Symptoms found in *conversion* hysteria include loss of bodily function such as sudden blindness, sudden deafness, loss of sensation in an arm or a leg, or paralysis of an extremity. Loss of memory and the altered state of consciousness are seen in *dissociative* hysteria. These latter changes range from such disorders as sleepwalking and excessive sleeptalking to functional amnesias, circumscribed loss of memory, and multiple personalities. It can be readily seen that it is important for the corrections worker to be aware of those conditions.

The classic case of a hysterical neurosis of the dissociative type is that situation which is so loved by fiction writers. An individual is found clasping a bloody knife, standing over someone who has been stabbed, and insisting, "I have no idea of who I am, how I got here, or what has happened." In these instances recall and reintegration of the forgotten or repressed memory may sometimes be brought about either by hypnosis or by so-called truth serum, that is, an injection of an intravenous sleeping medication. Neither of these methods is infallible. It has been demonstrated that the determined individual can maintain a cover story even under hypnosis or truth serum. Where it is feasible, it is better to allow memory to return slowly by removal of the individual from the scene of the traumatic or upsetting episode to a more neutral setting. There, with much encouragement and support, the true nature of what has gone on may be recovered and faced.

As a usual rule, such an hysterial or amnestic state develops after the commission of an act. It represents the offender's attempt to block the act from consciousness, because what has been done is so morally repugnant that the conscious memory rejects any possibility the individual might have performed this act or might be found guilty of such an act. The same mechanism is sometimes seen in an individual who has merely witnessed a particularly shocking act. Many times in blocking out that specific memory the mind blocks out other memories with it so no identifying personal data are available to the individual. Events are remembered only from the moment of regaining awareness of the surroundings. This capacity to retain somewhere within the personality a whole body of behavior which has been repressed and is not accessible to the conscious personality is called *dissociation*. Note the marked difference between this sort of dissociation and that dissociation referred to in schizophrenia where there was a dissociation between the mood and the content of thought. Here the dissociation is between behavior and the awareness of that behavior. The simplest example of this is sleepwalking. The individual who sleepwalks carries out a whole series of purposive acts without ever actually waking up and without any memory on awakening of what has transpired. The most complex form of this behavior is the *split personality* in which two, three, or more different personalities coexist within the same individual, many of them being unaware of the existence or the behavior of the others.

Regardless of whether the act of dissociation is manifested as a multiple personality or as an amnesia or forgetting, or even as sudden incomprehensible behavior, it is always the result of two opposing drives or desires. One is acceptable to the conscious personality; the other is not. In schizophrenia this results in ambivalence or blocking; in hysteria it results in dissociation. Dissociation occurs when a wish or a desire, morally repugnant to an individual's conscience, keeps on recurring and has to be kept from consciousness by a defense mechanism. The most commonly used mechanism is repression. Repeated environmental stimulation continues to evoke the wish, and repression becomes more and more difficult. The drive may get stronger or the repressing forces weaker. Some final incident serves as a trigger, and the repressed wish erupts in behavior. The behavior is so unacceptable to the personality that the entire event is blotted out — lost to memory or perceived as if in a dream, as though it happened to someone else. Dissociative hysteria generally occurs in a person with a known hysterical personality make-up, and after repeated stress.

Mr. T, a twenty-two-year-old male, was accused of having murdered his wife. He had burst into the shop where she was employed, and, in the presence of witnesses had fired at her twice at point blank range with a shotgun. He had left, driven several miles to a sporting goods store, bought another box of shotgun shells, driven to his parents' home and burst in saying, "I've shot my wife — call the police."

Mr. T had been involved in a poorly defined love-hate relationship with his mother since early childhood. He had been a sleepwalker since the age of three. The last episode of somnambulism had occurred about six months before the murder. He had a morbid fear of the dark and, until his marriage at the age of eighteen, had been unable to sleep without a light on in the room. His grade school career had been stormy. He had always been a show-off, the class clown. He had been put back in the middle of a grade, not because of learning problems but for "failure to adjust." As a result he had been teased unmercifully by his peers. In response he became rebellious, although never aggressive. As an escape he sniffed glue excessively until he entered high school. He loved the feeling of being free from his environment which the glue sniffing gave him. In high school, particularly after getting into vocational training, he blossomed. He never became what would be called gregarious or really outgoing, but he was comfortable and at ease with people. His wife was his first and only girl friend. He had met her his sophomore year in high school. They were married as seniors when she became pregnant.

Mr. T had idealized his wife and blinded himself to her obvious personality flaws. She had been under her father's thumb and was an extremely dependent person. She was quite petty and retaliated for small, sometimes unavoidable offenses. She had been brought up with marked sexual taboos. While she appeared excited during premarital sexual relations, she had never attained orgasm. Once they were married and the first child was born, she lost interest in sex completely. According to his story, she would literally submit to his advances while making remarks like, "Well, are you done? Then get off." She was an indifferent housekeeper. She worked for a while between pregnancies as a waitress. A second child was born two years after the first. Following this birth she went into a rather severe depression and ignored Mr. T completely. She would have almost nothing to do with him sexually. On those rare occasions when she did, he found himself suffering from premature ejaculation.

After about four months of this he suggested they should try to find help. She said she already had. He asked what she meant, and she replied that while she had been working she had had an affair. Through this she had discovered she was not cold, she could respond. The inference was that his failure to arouse her was responsible for their difficulties. He was stunned. The next day she took the children and left. Three weeks later she returned, after he had "gotten down on my hands and knees and begged her to come back." She insisted on working again, and now became open and flagrant in her affairs. She taunted him constantly on how much better than him other men were, not only in their love making, but in their physical endowments as well. His rigid repression of his hostile feelings broke down only once despite this provocation. On that occasion he struck her, only to beg forgiveness immediately. He had a desperate need to see her as his beautiful wife, whom he loved deeply and who loved him deeply.

Three weeks before the killing she confirmed she had been having affairs with his three closest friends. He had suspected this for a long time but was afraid to ask. At the time she told him this they were out riding. They passed the place where one of these friends worked. He stopped the car, got out, sucker-punched the man, and beat him up badly. He got back in the car quite calmly and said, "Let's go eat before the police come after me." Surprisingly, the assaulted man did not file a complaint. The next day his wife left him, leaving the children in his care.

He continued to entreat her to come back. His final effort to effect a reconciliation occurred on the anniversary of the oldest child's birth. His parents were having a special birthday party, and he decided to ask her to the birthday party. He left work during his lunch hour in order to send her a bouquet of flowers. He wrote a note which said, "Thank you for Freddie's life. We need you, miss you, and want you."

After work he picked the children up at their day nursery and drove them to his parent's home for the party. He went home, showered, and dressed. He called his wife at her work. She cut him off when she found out who it was. He drove there and went in to see her, only to discover she had given the flowers away, had torn up the card and thrown it away, and had dumped the vase in the waste paper basket. She was a receptionist and he was talking to her in the lobby of the place of employment. Fellow workers had come in to protect her while he was talking to her. At one point, he grabbed her rather roughly by the shoulders. As the workers started to move in toward him she motioned them off and dismissed them, implying that she could handle him herself. He felt belittled and humiliated by this. She picked the vase out of the waste basket and threw it across the room, shattering it. He walked out in a state of cmmplete confusion. He drove around for some time and found himself miles from the scene, not quite remembering how he had gotten there. In his mind he still saw her as the beautiful, desirable, lovable, "All-American girl" who was his wife. He continued to attempt to repress all his hostile negative feelings toward her.

He was an avid trap shooter. The past weekend he had been on the range and had shot two boxes of shells. Somehow he had kept the last two shells in his gun which he carried in his car. He explained this to himself as being protection if she came with her friends to try to get the children from him. After the final rebuff he decided there was only one thing he could do, kill himself. He found, by experiment, he could point the gun at himself and still reach the trigger. He drove back in the general direction of her place of employment, always pointing the gun at himself. He stopped in an adjacent parking lot, tried to pull the trigger, and froze. He drove to her building and again his hand froze on the trigger. He thought, "What's the point of doing it out here. The ambulance will come and take me away and she won't know what happened until she reads the paper. I must kill myself in front of her. Then she'll know." He was only vaguely aware of the hostile significance of this proposed act of killing himself in front of her and denied any implication that it would say to her, "See how you have made me feel." He insisted it was only in her presence that he would have strength enough to pull the trigger.

He entered her place of employment. She was sitting behind a waist high partition at a desk directly opposite the door. A fellow worker was standing there talking to her. According to him everything seemed strange. The carpeting felt a foot thick. There was an eerie silence. He thought, "Now I can do it." He heard the muffled sound of a gun. "It didn't sound like a shotgun on the range, but sort of muted and nuffled." He saw her half rise and turn with blood streaming from her elbow. He thought, "That *can't* be, I shot *myself.*" Another shot sounded and she fell to the floor, blood "spurting from her back like a fountain." He thought, "Now I can't kill myself, I have no shells left." For a moment he thought clearly, "I can't stop at the hardware store next door to get shells. The police will be here any minute." He drove to a store about four miles away to buy another box of shells. The whole act of buying shells was a nightmare and he began to believe that the clerk was deliberately slow in selling them to him so that the police could get there.

He went to his car in the parking lot, put one shell in the gun, and again he froze. He thought, "I can't let her father have the kids." (He had feuded bitterly with her father over the father's domination of the wife.) He actually said to the author in reporting this, "I can't let *their* father have the kids." He thought, "I must get to my father's house, lean on the horn, get him to come to the car so I can tell him about keeping the kids, and then shoot myself." He drove into his father's driveway, leaned on the horn and nothing happened. The horn would not blow. Leaving the gun in the car, he burst into the house and said, "I've just shot my wife. Call the police." and collapsed.

It is of more than passing interest that one of the first things he said to the police after having been given his rights was, "Her face wasn't damaged, was it?" (He still had to preserve his image of his "All-American girl.")

In this instance, there was no true amnesia. There was hysterical dissociation which occurred when his unconscious took over and aimed the gun at her instead of at him. Killing himself would serve several purposes. It would destroy the wicked wife which he kept buried inside himself. It would have partially satisfied his need to hurt her — "See how bad you made me feel. I'm killing myself because of you." But it was not enough. The strength of the hostile-destructive forces was greater than the strength of the repression, and dissociation took place.

The question is frequently asked, "What is the probability such an act would occur again?" Such a question has great practical significance, but cannot be answered with mathematical certainty. There are two variables which enter into the answer, the personality involved and the conflictual stresses to which that personality is subjected. These stresses are variables completely beyond society's control. It is possible by one thera-peutic means or another (there is no one therapy which holds the keys to the kingdom) to change the basic personality struc-ture so as to decrease the tendency to dissociate under stress. It is possible to provide an individual with means of handling unacceptable wishes other than to repress them. It is possible to learn to talk out rather than act out conflicts. In the case of Mr. T, the court did not acquit on the grounds of insanity, but did find him guilty of involuntary manslaughter. In the author's opinion, this was more than a crime of passion. It behooves the prison officials, or his parole officer when he is released, to become actively involved in assisting Mr. T to find help or there may be other sensational headlines.

Why is this presented as a case of hysterical dissociation and not as malingering or lying? It is felt to be hysterical dissocia-tion because the story as related by the defendant and the story, particularly the life history, as obtained by the clinic social worker were congruent. The sleepwalking and sleeptalking, the need as a child to escape his environment by glue sniffing, and the histrionic showing off in school all pointed to the sort of personality which is fertile soil for hysteria. The growing hos-tility was successfully repressed by the need to see her as loving, just as he had to see his mother as loving, until the final act broke down the ability to repress. In an example of this sort, the aid furnished by the corrections worker in terms of a pre-sentence, or where allowed by law, a pretrial history is just as important as the work done after the mills of the law have stopped grinding. The history furnished by means of the inves-tigation of the corrections officer can sometimes be most helpful in the detection of malingering. This holds true not only in terms of the description of the present offense, but in terms of the description of the childhood and earlier person-ality make-up of the offender. The history is particularly valu-able if the officer has held collateral interviews with relatives or friends.

It is possible for a single dissociative act to occur in an indi-vidual who has previously seemed stable and symptom-free, but is quite uncommon. People with hysterical neurosis of the dissociative type have been shown to be excitable, unstable, over-reacting, and histrionic prior to the time of the dissociation. They have shown evidence of behavior designed to attract attention, as well as to manipulate, throughout their past history. They are extremely immature and self-centered. As a usual rule they are completely dependent upon other people, both for emotional and physical sustenance. They dramatize almost every act which they perform. The simplest, most intimate behavior is made to appear as though before a wide audience. Females frequently act in a very seductive fashion. Usually a history of sleepwalking, sleeptalking, or other minor forms of dissociation will be present. The presence of such a history serves as an excellent corroborative evidence for a claim of dissociation. Stories obtained under hypnosis or "truth serum" frequently reveal the true facts and confirm or indicate the diagnosis of hysterical dissociation. These procedures, of course, may never be used without the permission of the defendant and, as noted earlier, are not infallible, nor are they admissible as evidence.

The case of Mr. U is also relevant as a case of feigned dissociation. This twenty-one-year-old man was examined on a charge of aggravated murder while committing a robbery. He was reported to have entered a hardware store and had asked to buy a box of shells. While the proprietor had his back to him, he had struck the proprietor many times over the head with a crowbar and had then stabbed him several times with a hunting knife. He yanked the man's wallet from his pocket, even though it had been attached by a chain. He then rifled the desk and cash drawer and departed as unostentatiously as possible from the rear of the store. He went to his house trailer and attempted to wash the blood from the knife. He hid the loot in the trailer. Later he went around town paying off bills.

He claimed to have only a patchy memory for what had happened. He said he recalled striking the man with a crowbar since it was handy, but stated he did not remember anything else about the event until sometime thereafter. When one of his friends said he had heard about this man's murder on the radio, he wondered to himself if it could possibly be he who was the murderer. As time progressed and as different people questioned him, more islands of memory would pop up in the middle of this story. It was learned that although it was a warm day in the summer, he was wearing gloves when he came into the store. He had removed them to write his name in acknowledging the purchases of shells which he had ordered but had put them back on again when the man turned around to get the shells. No prints were found on the murder weapon. It is also significant that he made an attempt to hide the knife and the money when he got home, and he washed the blood from his clothes and the knife.

The degree of attempted concealment serves as one of the tests which helps to assign responsibility in those cases in which it can not be determined whether the dissociation is real or malingered, or whether it occurred before or after the offense. In the case of Mr. T, he argued with his wife in front of witnesses; he shot her in the presence of a witness; even though he drove out of his way to buy shells it was not to escape ultimate detection, but enabled him to have the means to commit suicide; he drove directly to his parents' home, where he knew the police would obviously come, and stated, "I have killed my wife." Mr. U, on the contrary, evaded witnesses, tried to wash the blood off his garments, washed and hid the knife, at first denied his involvement to the police. Even if he had dissociated, the behavior of the dissociated personality demonstrated knowledge of wrongdoing, and Mr. U would have been responsible.

Hysterical dissociative behavior must also be differentiated from that occurring in epileptic twilight states. In epileptic fugue the behavior is generally more primitive and more loosely controlled. A past history of epileptic seizures will almost always be available. An electroencephalogram which demonstrates typical electrical seizure discharges in the brain waves is almost confirmatory of this differential diagnosis.

Hysterical dissociation does not always involve such lethal episodes. When it does, the offender is not apt to be free in the community until after prolonged incarceration with or without treatment. The corrections worker is more apt to be involved in those instances where dissociation accompanies a white collar crime. The probation worker must be aware of the manipulative, seductive and dramatic maneuvers of many of these individuals and be prepared to deal with them. If any indication of multiple personality is shown, this calls for instant referral for treatment. It must be remembered that dissociation, whether before, during, or after the commission of an offense, implies the offending behavior is not acceptable to the individual's conscious personality and hence does not represent a cop-out in the usually accepted meaning of that phrase. It may well be the individual's attempt to cop out from the demands of his own conscience. The officer's attitude should be that of acknowledging the good intentions of the offender and aiding in finding more acceptable ways of meeting needs. The officer will also be of help by identifying the seductive and manipulative maneuvers as they occur. It is quite helpful to use these instances as they occur in relationship to the officer, in order to demonstrate this is the way the individual deals with other people in the environment. It can be demonstrated how self-defeating this sort of behavior is. In many instances the person will have been well aware of both the behavior and its implications. Under those circumstances if the officer is convinced of the sincerity of the attempt to change, and does not believe this to be another con or manipulation, referral to psychotherapy may be of help. At all times the corrections worker must avoid being caught up in the manipulative web of these people.

OBSESSIVE—COMPULSIVE NEUROSIS (300.3)

In **Obsessive-Compulsive Neurosis (300.3)**, some form of ritualistic behavior is used to control anxiety. Obviously, if the ritualistic behavior is not antisocial, then, except incidentally, the sufferer does not come within the province of a corrections worker. An example from this group would be the individual whose compulsive hand washing guards against anxiety generated by the pressure of erotic thoughts, or guards against the guilt over childhood or adolescent masturbatory practices. At times however, rituals may be quite antisocial. Compulsive exhibitionism is an example of this type of ritual. Here exposure of the genitals is a compulsive act performed to ward off feelings of anxiety. As will be discussed under the antisocial sexual deviations (Chapter 11), the minority of exhibitionists are obsessive-compulsive neurotics. Other compulsions are seen frequently in fiction but much less commonly in the criminal system. These are acts such as kleptomania, the urge to steal things, or pyromania, the urge to set fires. The dynamics of behavior of this sort are extremely complex and are beyond a book of this sort. They do, however, occur as compulsive acts.

A description of the pattern involved as an aid in identifying such an offender, however, is certainly germane. The mechanics of a typical, antisocial, compulsive act goes something like this. The individual is aware of a vague feeling of anxiety. This is a familiar feeling which has been experienced before. Since from experience it is known to precede an antisocial act, a sincere attempt will be made to direct attention away from these feelings of anxiety by involvement in other tasks, by drinking, or by taking medication. However, the anxiety continues to grow more and more intense. As it does, the urge to perform the forbidden act begins to intrude on consciousness. The individual fights it for as long as possible. Control then gives way, sometimes suddenly and impulsively, or sometimes in a fashion planned to avoid detection. This is a situation in which definite evidence of planning to avoid detection, while indicative of knowledge that the act is wrong, is not necessarily indicative of nonneurotic causation. This is in marked contradistinction to the behavior that was discussed under the heading of hysterical dissociative reaction. There it was noted that any attempt at concealment tended to lessen the probability of neurotic causation. At any rate, in this sequence, whether impulsively or in a planned fashion, the compulsive act is eventually performed. Immediately, there is release of tension. This release is accompanied by a marked feeling of well being. Following this, at times almost immediately, at times following a somewhat longer period of comfort, intense feelings of guilt and remorse develop. These feelings are accompanied by repeated promises to the self never to perform this act again. The release engendered by the performance of the act lasts for varying lengths of time. Then the whole cycle begins to repeat itself: anxiety, struggle, awareness, struggle, action, relief, guilt, remorse, relative peace, anxiety.

Only rarely will an individual seek help with this sort of compulsion, no matter how upsetting it may be. This failure to try to get help is one of the chief reasons why a claim to such disability is so often disbelieved. This claim seems particularly paradoxical since, if apprehended, the person's reaction is almost invariably, "Thank goodness you've caught me. Now, possibly I may get some help." This paradox of not seeking treatment yet being relieved to be caught is apparently brought on by shame and embarrassment. Possibly a more compelling reason for concealment is a complete inability to believe anyone could understand such obviously bizarre and antisocial behavior if it were to be confessed openly in order to seek help. At times the individual feels no one will take his symptom seriously. At other times he fears the symptoms will perturb the listener as much as they do him, and immediate institutionalization will result. At times the obsessive-compulsive defense threatens to break down, and the resultant turmoil leads to a state almost indistinguishable from schizophrenia. The following case of an extremely severe obsessive-compulsive disorder illustrates this aspect.

> Mr. V, a thirty-three-year-old white male, married, father of two children, was arrested after having inflicted multiple stab wounds on a prostitute, within two minutes of the time they entered her apartment. When she managed to stagger to the kitchen and pick up a small paring knife to defend herself, he suddenly became calm, said, "I'm sorry," and walked out. Since he had been seen picking up the prostitute and his identity was known, he was quickly apprehended. When arrested he spontaneously confessed to beating a bar maid the previous week. This attempt had also terminated abruptly when she started to say a *Hail Mary*. He also confessed spontaneously to a two-year-old, unsolved murder. In that instance, the body of a young woman had been found in a lovers' lane, stabbed to death, with bite marks on her cheek. He was privy to facts that only the murderer could have

known, so there was no question that this was not a false confession.

He had been a model boy until the age of thirteen. While he was enlisting a young woman as a customer for his paper route, he had without any provocation stabbed her in the breast. At that time the dynamics of his problem were quite clear. He had been completely dominated by a mother with chronic heart disease who used her illness as a means of control. Any rebellious thoughts were said to be utterly sinful. As his sex drive began to emerge in adolescence, both parents treated it as though it were poisonous, sinful, and unthinkable. He had to repress his sexuality just as he had to repress the rebellion and the hostility toward his mother. The two fused and the act against the woman at the age of thirteen was symbolic of his feelings at that time. Intensive therapy was recommended for him then but was not carried out. At eighteen he had joined the service to get away from home. Overseas he was introduced to oral sex as well as to various sadomasochistic practices. While in the service, he went to see a psychiatrist to talk about his fears of homosexuality, and as a result was discharged from the service.

Following his discharge from the service he began to be obsessed with thoughts of killing a woman, dismembering her, and eating the body, starting with the breasts and genitals. He had married shortly after discharge and this obsession became so severe he feared he would harm his wife and children. It was almost impossible for him to get his thoughts off of this topic. He became confused and disorganized. It was necessary to hospitalize him. He was given electroconvulsive therapy and placed on medication. Following this he was relieved of his obsessive thoughts for the first time in years. For approximately nine months he got along quite well, so well he discontinued his medication without informing anyone or returning to his doctor. The obsessive thoughts began to return with maddening intensity. He started drinking, began to stay out of work and to seek out prostitutes for oral and sadistic gratification. The obsessive thoughts worsened in spite of this behavior. At this stage he murdered one of the girls he had picked up. He did not dismember her, but he had bitten her in the cheek just before stabbing her to death. He had had no sexual relations with her.

He confessed this murder to his priest but was not believed. He developed terrible pains in his chest and was hospitalized to be evaluated for a possible heart attack. He again consulted the psychiatrist. He did not tell him of the murder, but complained of a recurrence of the obsessive thoughts. Medication helped but did not remove them completely. He again became disorganized and had to be hospitalized. On release he felt better again, but the thoughts recurred. Now they included not only his wife and children, but even the childrens' girl friends and the babysitter. He was remodeling his house and he bought a circular saw ostensibly to help with this project. In fantasy he used it to cut up his victims. He daydreamed of putting the limbs and parts in the freezer, and eating them slowly one by one. There was scarcely a waking moment he was free from these thoughts. It was in this state the two final events occurred. To him it was a tremendous relief to be able to confess.

What is the corrections worker's role in relationship to offenders with obsessive-compulsive reaction? It is necessary to be aware that such a situation can exist before anything helpful can be accomplished. The worker must learn not to react with immediate scorn to the individual who commits antisocial acts and then says, "But I couldn't help what I did." This seems like such an obvious con that it is sometimes difficult to accept the possibility that it may not be one. If the worker is to have any sort of relationship at all with the offender, he must not even hint that he thinks it is an attempt to con until some definitive decision is made as to whether it is or is not. Prior to that time, in a presentence report, the probation officer can do a great deal to help those who have to make that decision by compiling an adequate social history. Among the details that are extremely helpful in that history are the answers to whether the individual has had ritualistic behaviors of other sorts in the past. There are as many rituals as there are those who carry them out. Common ones include having to dress in an inflexible order, having to check every gas jet or electric switch before leaving the house (sometimes several times), and having to count objects to a certain number and starting all over if one is missed, repeating the counting until the last number comes out at the last object. Any time one of these rituals is done improperly, or is not done at the usual time, anxiety results. (In the older literature these sorts of neurotic behaviors were called *anancasms*. The neurosis itself has been labeled *psychothenia*. The worker should be aware of these terms are they are still occasionally used.)

Other clues to obsessive-compulsive personalities include fussiness, rigidity, excessive cleanliness and neatness, perfectionism, and an insistence on everything being precisely in its place. Whenever possible these traits should be confirmed by collateral sources. Once the decision has been made that the individual is ill and probation with mandatory treatment has been agreed upon, the probation officer has another important function, namely that of liaison with the therapist. The therapist will not share the confidences of the offender, now a patient, but, since treatment is mandatory, the probation officer has a perfect right to expect regular reports from the therapist. These reports should cover whether the patient is (a) keeping his or her treatment appointments and (b) actually entering into treatment rather than just going through the motions to satisfy the court. In the latter instance, the probation officer can also be of help to the offender, not by being a punitive figure in a sense of pointing out, "If you don't cooperate you're going to go to jail," but rather of being supportive in the sense of, "Only by cooperating will you rid yourself of this scourge with which you have been whipped for so long." Corrections workers should be aware of their responsibility in those situations in which treatment has been made a mandatory part of probation. Not only is the probation officer obliged to keep up-to-date on the status of treatment, he is also expected to obtain court consent for any radical change in treatment plan. In a suit heard in 1976 in the United States Court of Appeals for the Fourth Circuit[1], both the psychiatrist and the probation officer were held liable for civil damages in the death of a young woman killed by the probationer. The latter had been changed

[1]Semler vs. Wadeson, Number 74-2345 and 2346 (Fourth Circuit, February 27, 1976).

from institutional care to day care with the permission of the court. When he was transferred from day care to twice-a-week group therapy, the court was not consulted. The probationer then killed the young woman, and both the psychiatrist and the probation officer were required to pay damages to her family.

Above all the worker must realize compulsions are among the most burdensome defenses against anxiety which an individual has. No matter how bizarre this behavior, it deserves a sympathetic ear and not scorn or contempt. Common sense injunctions to stop are of no help. Rarely, commanding an individual to go through the ritualistic routine repetitively will be of some help. Even more rarely, rewards for giving up routines for longer and longer period of time have been found to be helpful. These methods should not be attempted without backup from a skilled therapist, as complete disintegration sometimes results when these are attempted unskillfully. Obsessive-compulsive reactions are notoriously among the most difficult psychiatric conditions to treat, and the worker should encourage the offender to continue treatment even though little progress seems to be being made. By the same token, if a worker is attempting to help such an individual on his own, either because therapy is not available or the offender refuses to avail himself of it, the worker should not look for early success. Quite naturally these remarks are not to be taken to refer to an individual like Mr. V. Someone of this sort, with the sort of compulsions that Mr. V has, must be treated in an institution both for the safety of the community and for his own peace of mind.

OTHER NEUROSES

As has been stressed repeatedly, people who commit offenses may be psychotic or neurotic, but there may be no connection between the offense and the illness. Sometimes these people are assigned to the worker with the label neatly attached to them, and the worker should know what the labels imply. At other times, it may help the worker in understanding the noncriminal behavior of a client when there is awareness that such behavior does occur in people. For these reasons, the remaining categories of neuroses will be discussed very briefly. Probably the most common of all neuroses is the **Anxiety Neurosis (300.0).** Up until relatively recently, anxiety was the most common symptom seen by all physicians. In the last few years, it has been replaced by depression. In anxiety neurosis, attacks of fear, which may reach the status of panic, occur without any obvious precipitating stimulus. This fear may be experienced as a diffuse feeling of tension (worry, thoughts of some vague, approaching doom) or it may be felt as definite physiological symptoms (perspiration, goosebumps, rapid heartbeat, palpitation, tightness in the pit of the stomach, or rapid breathing).

At times the rapid breathing becomes so excessive as to produce what is called a *hyperventilation syndrome.* Because of the excessive overbreathing produced by the anxiety, too much carbon dioxide is blown off through the lungs. This lowers the acidity of the blood and brings on a whole new set of symptoms. The hands and feet begin to prickle and tingle, the muscles become stiff, and the individual may faint. As soon as this happens, the overbreathing stops and the system returns to normal. Then the fear of having another such attack induces anxiety, and a circular type of reaction is set up. Although reassurance does little to help the individual with anxiety neurosis, if the corrections worker can keep cool when confronted with such a situation, it can be a big help.

Phobic Neurosis (300.2) is also characterized by a display of fear. In this instance, however, the fear is of a specific object, situation, or place which, in actuality, is in no way threatening. The number of phobias is legion, and no attempt will be made to list them all. Some of the most common ones are fear of high places, fear of sharp objects, fear of closed places, and fear of open spaces. In these instances, the fear is actually caused by something of which the individual is unaware, and the fear is displaced to a neutral object. Those who suffer from anxiety neurosis sometimes develop phobias by association. For example, an anxiety attack occurs in a grocery store, and from that time on there is a phobia about going into grocery stores. The patient is completely unable to enter them. These people know the fears are completely illogical and it does no good to tell them so, or to try to laugh them out of it. Fortunately, since phobias appear to be learned behavior, people can be trained to unlearn them.

Depressive Neurosis (300.4) has already been referred to in Chapter 6 when the major affective disorders were discussed. Depressive neurosis, or reactive depression as it is more commonly called, is most frequently seen in reaction to a loss, whether great or small. It is of particular interest in corrections because the consequences of antisocial behavior may entail two significant losses, loss of freedom and loss of reputation. This will be discussed in greater length in Chapter 17 when indicators of potential suicide are discussed.

Neurasthenic Neurosis (300.5) or Neurasthenia is, because of its very nature, rarely seen by the corrections worker. The chief complaints in neurasthenia are chronic fatigue, exhaustion, lack of energy, and weakness. Almost everythng is too much effort. Such people may become drug addicts or alcoholics in an effort to alleviate these symptoms. Surprisingly, however, they are much more apt to turn to over-the-counter medications. Apparently, the brief relief afforded by uppers does not compensate for the intensive contrast in their symptoms when they come down. Obviously they rarely have the energy to engage in antisocial behavior.

Depersonalization Neurosis (300.6) is extremely uncommon. Depersonalization, or a feeling of unreality, not quite fitting in one's own body or surroundings, is not an unusual symptom as an accompaniment of other illnesses. It is seen commonly in schizophrenia and just as commonly at one stage of the common cold. When the head feels full and light, stimuli seem to come from far away, and everything takes on a strange, unreal quality. Feelings of depersonalization as the only manifestations of a neurotic reaction, however, are not usual. This must be differentiated from a hysterical dissociation, as well as schizophrenia.

Hypochondriacal Neurosis (300.7) is a very common condition, and certainly is frequently seen in any institutional setting. It has also been called *hypochondriasis*. This condition is manifested by constant preoccupation and worry about bodily parts and their functions. To a hypochondriac, a pain in the chest is instant heart disease, a spot on the skin is cancer. If a day passes without a bowel movement, constipation; if there should be two in one day, diarrhea. Unless there is some understanding of what is going on, these unfortunate people can be seen as nuisances, as frauds, or as attention seekers. Actually, the concern for the body protects against the intrusion of too painful thoughts, just as the obsessive-compulsive ritual does. Only too often a real illness is overlooked because they have "cried wolf" so often no one really listens any longer. Hypochondriasis should be differentiated from Conversion Hysteria, where there is a real loss of function which does not follow the lines of any known illness.

The corrections worker is not expected to be a psychologist or psychiatrist and is not expected to heal people suffering from these various illnesses, nor even to diagnose these conditions. It is hoped, however, it will be easier to be empathetic, and particularly easier not to assume the individual is feigning complaints, if a little is known about the conditions.

Chapter 9

PERSONALITY DISORDERS
(PART ONE)

GENERAL CONSIDERATIONS

ALTHOUGH there are four disorders listed under the general heading of **Personality Disorders and Certain Other Non-Psychotic Mental Disorders (301-304)**, only the **Personality Disorders (301)** and **Sexual Deviation (302)** will be considered in Part One of the book. The discussion of **Alcoholism (303)** and **Drug Dependence (304)** will be postponed to Part Three where they more logically belong. The greatest number of people with mental disorders seen by corrections workers are those with Personality Disorders (301). At the same time, there is no other category in which there is as much confusion in terms of conceptual clarity. At this point it might be wise to refer back to the manual from which these diagnoses are obtained, namely the *Diagnostic and Statistical Manual of Mental Disorders.* The word disorder should be underlined because there is even disagreement as to whether personality disorders represent mental illnesses or not. At one time, they were felt to be more the product of nature than nurture. It was believed the individual was born with certain defects and could not escape them no matter what life events occurred. That concept is no longer held. While the general heading in *DSM II* is that of Personality Disorder, the subheadings under it speak of specific types of *personality*. It would almost seem as though having that type of personality were, in and of itself, a disorder.

A very crude analogy might help make some sense of the relationship between the basic disorders in these individuals and antisocial behavior. A child may be born as a perfectly healthy, normal child. In the course of growth and development, a combination of factors such as malnutrition, vitamin deficiency, and inadequate maternal care may increase the vulnerability to injury. The child may break a leg. Through faulty healing because of the predisposing factors, the child may be left with one leg that is shorter than the other, or more crooked than the other. A limp will be the result. This shortened leg, or the limp which is a symptom thereof, cannot be called a disease or illness. At the same time it is not normal. Neither is it something with which the child was born. Yet, unless it is corrected, if it is possible to do so, it is going to distinctly influence the course of that individual's life.

This is also true of a personality disorder, which grows from various factors influencing the development of the child, although there may be some genetic factors involved. Unless the person receives some form of help (even if that help consists as in the above analogy in inserting a lift to raise the affected heel an inch to stop the limp), the individual, and at times society, is going to suffer permanently. Personality disorders are usually manifested by the time of adolescence, and become an integral part of the individual's personality by early adult life. The patterns are deeply ingrained, extremely maladaptive, and notoriously refractory to treatment. These aspects will be discussed as each of these conditions is described. It should be stressed again that it is the life-long nature of these maladaptations which distinguishes them from the various mental illnesses which have been discussed up to this point. These patterns are so deeply ingrained they have become a part of the character of the person involved. Indeed, some writers in this field do not refer to these conditions as personality disorders but as *character neuroses.*

As has been the rule throughout this book, only the sort of personality disorders which bring individuals into relatively frequent contact with courts and correction systems will be discussed extensively. Thus, the **Asthenic Personality (301.6)** will only be mentioned briefly. The **Paranoid Personality (301.0), Cyclothymic Personality (301.1), Schizoid Personality (301.2),** and **Obsessive-Compulsive Personality (301.4)** will be discussed only to differentiate them from the psychosis or neurosis of similar name. In general, this differentiation between the personality disorder and the psychosis is made on the basis that the personality disorders represent character traits of life-long standing and are not new conditions engrafted on the personality. Individuals with these disorders may decompensate under stress. If they do, then the illness which corresponds to the personality trait is the one most likely to develop.

EXPLOSIVE PERSONALITY
(EPILEPTOID PERSONALITY DISORDER) (301.3)

Semantic confusion is present at the very onset of the discussion of this condition. This is brought about by the use of the term *epileptoid*. There are two misnomers involved here. The first is the fact that the person with explosive personality does not necessarily suffer from a seizure disorder, does not-necessarily have a positive electroencephalogram, and does not necessarily have amnesia for an explosive outburst. The second is the fact, which was stressed in the chapter on organic brain disorders, that epileptics, as a group, have been much maligned by the implication they tend to be dangerous and explosive. As was pointed out in that chapter, only a small percentage of epileptics behave in this way. The majority are not subject to such explosive outbursts.

An individual with an explosive personality reacts to situational stress with major outbursts. Sometimes, these outbursts are confined to verbal abuse in which it almost appears that the individual is deliberately working up to a stage of rage. At other times the outbursts may be accompanied by physical assaultiveness, smashing furniture, kicking out windows, and similar maladaptive behavior patterns. Occasionally, individuals will smash their fists into a wall or through a pane of glass. In many ways, these outbursts resemble the temper tantrums of a spoiled child. Most characteristic is the fact they are so different from the individual's usual nonagressive, pleasant manner. These outbursts are generally unpredictable. At times seemingly minimal environmental stimulation will set them off; at other times the individual seems to stand a tremendous amount of stress before blowing up. These attacks are differentiated from any form of epileptic clouded state by the absence of positive electroencephalographic findings, the absence of familial history of seizure disorder, the absence of a past history of seizures, and the absence of the confusion and somnolence which are seen after epileptic seizures. At times, following these outbursts, an individual with an explosive personality will report an intense feeling of relaxation and calm, in some ways almost analogous to the relaxation which follows orgasm.

The worker should be familiar with other characteristics of the explosive personality. The outbursts occur most commonly in relationship to family or close friends rather than to the community at large. As in so many other instances, alcohol tends to act as a solvent, dissolving the tenuous control of these people. Hence, under the influence of alcohol, outbursts may occur away from the home. These outbursts may be differentiated from acute alcoholic intoxication or from pathological intoxication by the clear memory following the episode.

Included also under this heading (301.3) are those personalities diagnosed as *aggressive personality*. Many sociologists, criminologists, and psychiatrists feel it is individuals with aggressive personalities who commit the greatest number of assaultive crimes. These are people whose personalities may best be summed up by the words "chip on the shoulder." They are the people who muscle their way to the front of the line. They are the people who are quickest to take affront at an insulting remark, even though a moment before they may have made an equally offensive statement to another individual and have expected it to be overlooked. It is always difficult to know where to draw the line between normal competitive aggressiveness, hopefully directed to getting ahead in the world, and the degree of obnoxious aggressiveness which characterizes the aggressive personality.

Certain features in the childhood history of this personality disorder seem to stand out. There is generally a history of an abusive, alcoholic father, with frequent family fights and uproars. As young children, these people have a tendency to be more active than the children around them. Hence they are more prone to falls, bumps, bruises, broken bones, and even head injury. (This activity, however, is not great enough so the diagnosis of hyperkinetic or minimally brain damaged child can be made. (see Chapter 13.) Interestingly, they are generally compact, stocky, and muscular rather than lean and willowy in body build. This may be a genetic factor, but it would seem much more obvious that a lean, willowy type would not be able to get away with the aggressive sort of behavior which these people exhibit and which, at least in childhood, has to be backed up with the ability to use one's fists until the neighborhood is pretty much impressed. Sometimes the history may be obtained that they had reputations as bullies as children. At times, even cruelty to animals may be elicited.

In many ways, the aggressive personality resembles the chimpanzees described by Van Wyck-Goodall. Chimpanzees rarely fight each other, even in mating season. However, a constant struggle for dominance in the herd goes on. This struggle is conducted more by swagger and bluster than by actual use of force. The loudest animal arouses the most fear. Indeed, Van Wyck-Goodall cites one rather weak male chimpanzee who became the dominant chimp in the herd by dragging behind him two or three empty ten-gallon gasoline containers which by their clattering made more noise than any other chimp could make. Thus, the weaker chimp took the dominant position. So it is, very often, with the aggressive personality. This swagger and bluster conceal deep-seated feelings of inferiority and inadequacy. As in the chimp, if the bluff is called then there is no other way out but to fight. Hence, the explosive outburst.

One of the ways in which the aggressive personality is frequently manifested in an individual in America, in contrast to the apes in the forests of Africa, is by the aggressive use of the automobile. The arrest record of such a person is apt to be dotted with traffic offenses of all kinds. These offenses usually start in adolescence, frequently before the age at which a license can be legally obtained. This misuse of a car should not be surprising. If the basis for the aggressive personality is actually a feeling of inadequacy, then there is no other single outlet which gives one more a sense of power than having an unlimited supply of horsepower at the touch of a pedal. The automobile has almost become a symbol of *machismo* in this country. To drive faster, louder, and more recklessly is universally recognized as a symbol of dominance, just as is the swaggering of Van Wyck-Goodall's apes.

At times a real or fancied slight may cause such a person to retreat temporarily, brood over this blow to the pride, magnify it out of all proportions until there is a seething caldron of inner anger, an explosion waiting to be set off. Under these circumstances, a disparaging look, real or fancied, from a hapless passerby may cause displacement of that anger onto the innocent bystander with a resultant explosion, verbal or physical. It was said of John L. Sullivan, "the Irish strong boy," the first heavyweight champion of the modern era, that he would stride into a saloon, slam his fists on the bar, and declare, "I can lick any son-of-a-bitch in the house." With his reputation, proof was unnecessary. The explosive personality, given the proper circumstances may figuratively do the same thing. Unless he is in his own neighborhood with a known reputation this statement may have to be proved.

This would seem to be a good place to discuss the Episodic Dyscontrol Syndrome. It is difficult to know whether to place this syndrome under organic disorders or here under the explosive personality. It is not included in the official nomenclature of *DSM II*, but it is a term which the worker is going to run into with increasing frequency. Some people feel that the Episodic Dyscontrol Syndrome is due to an actual short circuit occurring in the brain. Normally when a stimulus is received, it is distributed through many channels before there is a response. Such elements as forethought, consideration of consequences, and matching stimulus against past experiences, all enter into the choice of response. In the episodic dyscontrol syndrome it is postulated that under certain circumstances no delay occurs between stimulus and response. The abrupt acts which occur seem to be based on the most primitive feelings: rage, fear, sex. These acts seem to demonstrate no long range concern for the consequences, neither to the object or the perpetrator of the behavior in question.

It almost appears that in this behavior there is a postive

disinhibition of any restraining force. Normally, within the nervous system there is a whole set of checks and balances in which certain behavior is inhibited because other centers are brought into play. In this syndrome it would seem as though this inhibition does not occur. Thus, brutally aggressive and destructive behavior may be seen. Viewed as a whole, the behavior, while bizarre, seems to have some sort of intention which, when carried out, fills a primitive need or serves to relieve tension. At no time, however, does there appear to be even a recognition that alternative behavior is possible. When the behavior is over it seems, even to the perpetrator, that meaningful action has taken place without any clear sense of "Why." There is always the feeling about such an episode that the perpetrator has not been fully aware of what is going on at the time. There may or may not be evidence of epilepsy, either in the history or in electroencephalographic tracings. Even when there is a positive history of epilepsy, the behavior in episodic dyscontrol differs from that seen before or following a seizure. There is no true confusion; the motor behavior is more goal directed; a specific need is gratified, a specific wish fulfilled. Like other forms of explosive behavior, it is more readily released by alcohol. Indeed it has been stated that alcohol is the universal solvent of inhibitions.

In spite of the fact that episodic dyscontrol syndrome occurs in those who show no evidence of epilepsy, many individuals with this condition respond dramatically to one of the medications used to control epilepsy, Dilantin® Sodium®. Paradoxically, in some of those instances where epilepsy and episodic dyscontrol are present in the same person, Dilantin controls the seizures but not the explosive action. Indeed instances have been reported where as the number of epileptic seizures decreases, the amount of acting out behavior increases.

Monroe, who coined the term episodic dyscontrol syndrome, differentiates this behavior from that of the antisocial personality. In his view the antisocial personality considers the consequences of the behavior, and discards delay in favor of immediate gratification. The individual with episodic dyscontrol does not take time to consider. Once the behavior is past and the individuals look back on it, they feel as though it were not in keeping with their character. The act itself is not denied, as in the malingerer, nor repressed as in the hysteric, nor rationalized as in the antisocial character. Rather it is admitted, but seen in such a way that it leaves its perpetrator in a state of remorse, shock, and bewilderment. "I must have done it, but I don't know how I could have done something like that." Thus, it becomes extremely difficult to know whether to class this syndrome as an organic syndrome or as a special sort of epileptoid personality.

People with explosive and aggressive personalities or with episodic dyscontrol syndrome are frequently on the probation or parole officer's caseload. How should they be dealt with? First, forewarned is forearmed. Understanding the nature of the reaction and its general unpredictability allows the officer to be constantly on guard, particularly if the parolee or probationer has been drinking. It is important dynamically that the officer remembers always to be completely within the law's boundaries. In this way, the corrections worker does not have to become one of Goodall's chimps and outswagger and outroar the aggressive personality. The officer must remain calm, cool, but always self-assured, not giving way to the aggressiveness of the other, but at the same time not demeaning, threatening, or belittling. While the probation or the parole officer is not meant to be a therapist, getting beyond this shell of bluster and into the empty, inadequate, inner core of the individual's personality may lead the way toward effecting a profound personality change.

Awareness of the fact that another human being is suffering underneath (and may be assuming a facade to assuage that suffering) can be extremely reassuring. This is particularly true if this knowledge is expressed in deeds and not in words. Helping an explosive personality define an area in which to excel, to display confidence, and to feel adequate is a very effective technique. This is particularly true vocationally. The corrections worker can join forces with the vocational counselor to help steer the explosive personality towards a trade or vocation in which success is possible. Efforts should then be directed to helping the individual avoid antagonizing trainers and employers. The core of self-respect placed there by the correction worker's attitude can be greatly enhanced in reality by a job which affords real self-respect.

At times, professional help may be effective. This may take the form of medication, either to be taken constantly to dampen irritability or to be taken as needed when the individual becomes aware the destructive impulses are about to erupt in anger. The second form of professional help is that of psychotherapy. Under the present system of delivery of health care this is an extremely difficult resource to find. At times the offender will be aware of the tremendous need for help and will submit to voluntary hospitalization. There, a combination of medication, therapeutic environment, and psychotherapy may be necessary for several weeks. This can be followed after discharge with further therapy by the therapist and support by the probation or parole officer. At times, seeing the client's spouse conjointly with the client may be very effective in teaching a better understanding of the situation. In this way it may become possible for the spouse to spot oncoming rage, to learn to avoid known irritants which may precipitate it, or to simply get out of the way until the rage is dissipated. This may be a very necessary stopgap while other measures are being taken. To repeat, the core attitude in coping with and helping the explosive personality is to avoid any expression of fear while conveying the firmness of authority without flaunting or theatening its use.

THE ANTISOCIAL PERSONALITY (301.7)

Antisocial Personality (301.7) is the latest in a long series of names given to a specific type of personality disorder recognized through the ages. Earlier terms which have been used to describe this particular disorder have included such things as "moral insanity," "constitutional psychopathic inferiority," "psychopathic personality" and "sociopathic personality." *DSM II* describes the antisocial personality as, "Individuals who are basically unsocialized and whose behavior pattern brings them repeatedly into conflict with society. They are incapable of significant loyalty to individuals, groups, or social values. They are grossly selfish, callous, irresponsible, impulsive, and unable to feel guilt or learn from experience and punishment. Frustration tolerance is low. They tend to blame others or offer plausible rationalizations for their behavior. A mere history of repeated legal or social offenses is not sufficient to justify this diagnosis."

The term sociopathic personality was used in *DSM I*, published in 1952. At that time it included three specific personality types: the asocial, the antisocial, and the dyssocial. This latter term, dyssocial, is currently classified under the heading number **Social Maladjustment without Manifest Psychiatric Disorder 316** and is classified as **Dyssocial Behavior 316.3.** This term is used to describe those people who are the products of their culture. In this respect, it is analogous to cultural-familial mental retardation, referred to in Chapter 2. This is not, in any way, to infer that dyssocial individuals are mentally retarded. It is simply to say they are the product of their family mores. For a person brought up in certain areas of Appalachia, there is nothing wrong with the manufacturing and selling of bootleg whiskey. Indeed, not only is it not wrong, sometimes family tradition and pride are involved in it. Similarly, although this tendency would seem to be lessening at the present time, it is not at all uncommon for a male brought up in this culture to be involved sexually with females ten, twelve, and fourteen years old with a complete lack of awareness that there is anything wrong in this behavior.

Individuals transplanted from these areas to large northern urban areas frequently find themselves in conflict with the law, not out of any specific attempt to break the law but because their culture teaches such behavior is perfectly legitimate. In the urban ghettos of large cities, many children are raised to believe that shoplifting, mugging, breaking and entering are perfectly legitimate ways of acquiring extra money; the only sin is to be caught. Such people cannot be called antisocial, they are truly dyssocial. Indeed the term "the Fagin syndrome" has been applied not uncommonly to young children brought up in this manner. This syndrome is named after the character in Dickens' *Oliver Twist* who shelters youngsters and teaches them to pick pockets in order to pay for the care which he gives them. A true dyssocial individual then should not be confused with an antisocial individual.

The term *asocial* is really no longer in use. This term was reserved for those individuals who grew up unable to distinguish right from wrong, unable to comprehend what society's rules are because those rules were never taught. It is now fairly well agreed that it would almost be necessary to grow up on a desert island without any sort of social input in order to reach maturity without a knowledge of what society's expectations are, whether one chooses to live up to those expectations or not. The term asocial has been dropped, therefore, and these people are now included in the definition of antisocial personality.

Possibly the best approach to the description of the antisocial personality is to analyze phrase by phrase the definition quoted from *DSM II*. Why are these individuals "basically unsocialized"? At one time it was believed that they were born unsocializable. This is no longer felt to be true. The influence of genetic patterns is still very much in question, and the nature versus nurture dispute may never be settled. Of all the explanations advanced for the development of this condition, there are three which seem to be fairly widely accepted. In an individual case, any one of the three might be applicable.

The first of these proposes that these individuals develop in this way because of insufficient mothering during the first years of life. It might have been that at a very early age they were placed in an institution where they were brought up with no *one* person responsible for seeing they got not only the physical but also the emotional nurturance necessary for proper development. It might have been they were born to mothers who were rejecting, neglectful, alcoholic, or drug dependent, who, for whatever cause, failed to give the child any affection and stimulation during the first three basic formative years of life. As a result of not having one significant mothering figure to please, these people learned only to please themselves. They did not form even a rudimentary conscience. Their behavior is limited only by what external limits are set. It is never limited from within.

The second theory holds that, while the mother was basically completely rejecting of the child, she felt so much guilt about her rejection she overcompensated for it. Hence, she overindulged and overprotected the child. In this way the child was never made responsible for his or her own behavior and never made to face the consequences. These people learn to view the world as designed to gratify all their needs. They feel entitled to take forever without giving. There are an amazing number of parents who consistently attempt to aid a child in avoiding responsibility for behavior. Every juvenile court worker knows parents who scream, "Take this child. I can't stand him any longer. He's a dirty little thing! I want him put where he can't steal any more." The next day they are in court with an attorney demanding his release.

The third theory holds attempts *are* made to teach the child to use proper discipline, but either one of two things happens. Either discipline is inconsistent, so the child never learns what is expected, or the delay between the child's faulty behavior and the punishment is so long the child makes no connection between that behavior and the results which follow from it. This is particularly apt to happen in a home where the mother is so fearful of losing the child's love, or feels so unsure of herself, that misbehavior is followed by, "You just wait until your father gets home, I'm going to tell him and he'll certainly take care of it." At this point, the child has lost either way. If the father does "take care of it," either the time interval between the offending behavior and the punishment is so great no learning takes place or else there is no consistency in the mother's reporting to the father and the child learns to get away with almost anything.

There is a fourth hypothesis which does not state the child is unsocialized, but maintains socialization and motivation do occur but in the wrong direction. According to this theory, the child responds to the unspoken wishes of the parents rather than to the spoken prohibitions, and actually gains love by breaking rules.

W exhibits this mechanism beautifully. This fifteen-year-old boy lived with his mother and stepfather. When he visited his father on weekends he was allowed to ride the father's motorbike which he enjoyed tremendously. When he returned home from the weekend he would comment on what a good time he had had and what a great sport his father was to let him ride his bike. The stepfather, who was extremely jealous of the father, had shown no interest whatsoever in motorcycles. Now he bought a bigger, stronger, faster motorcycle than the father. He warned the boy not to use it under any circumstances. He then proceeded time after time to leave the keys in plain view where it would be impossible for the boy not to get the double message. Finally, at the mother's prodding, he hid the keys but retained the motorcycle. The boy was eventually brought into court for theft of a neighbor's bike which he had used for joyriding. The stepfather professed shock at this behavior.

The story of X also demonstrates the same mechanisms. She is a thirteen-year-old pregnant girl. For months, each time she left the home, she would hear her mother say, "I don't know what's getting into young people in their behavior today. They never had this kind of freedom when I was a girl. I sure know what I would have done with it. Now you be sure you don't let a boy take advantage of you." The pregnancy was inevitable.

These last two cases illustrate what are called *Super-Ego Lacunae,* holes placed in the conscience. Where this mechanism is at work in antisocial behavior, the antisocial pattern will usually be limited to one form of behavior and not generalized as it is in antisocial personality.

"Incapacity for significant loyalty" is a prominent trait of antisocial personalities. They are often described as being "with a group but not part of it." A careful study of the history will generally reveal, in addition to the factors covered in the preceding paragraphs, an early life replete with constant changes in environment. To use a very hackneyed phase, they have been shuffled from pillar to post. It is not at all unusual that an individual diagnosed as having an antisocial personality has attended ten to twelve schools during the first three or four grades. He or she will have lived with a bewildering succession of aunts, uncles, friends, strangers, agencies, and institutions. There is no opportunity to put down roots, no opportunity to really form loyalties to a group. These people learn at an early age it is painful to form relationships, because relationships always break up. You must be loyal to yourself because no one else will be loyal to you. At the same time, many of them are capable of inducing an almost unbelievable feeling of loyalty in others. Not uncommonly, the male with an antisocial personality disorder may be simultaneously, or serially, married to two, three, or four women, each of whom is devoted to him, even though each may know of the presence of the others and of their claim upon his attention. This does not imply such a male is necessarily charismatic, as would appear to have been the case with Charles Manson. The theory has been advanced that having lacked the proper mothering in infancy, they appeal to the maternal side of certain women. It may also be they act as a challenge to women, a challenge to effect changes no one else has been able to accomplish. What is probably the most plausible reason is that many psychopathic personalities have a tremendous amount of charm which tends to conceal their negative qualities.

"Brings them repeatedly into conflict with society" is the trait of the antisocial personality which is so frequently described as "being unable to learn from experience." This does not in any way indicate these people lack intelligence; indeed, many of them are of superior intelligence. Rather it would appear to be due to a marked difficulty in grasping cause and effect relationships, particularly as these apply to themselves. It is possibly for this reason that it is so difficult to apply operant conditioning techniques utilizing positive reinforcement in the treatment of these people. Reinforcement is required for a much longer period of time than with the ordinary subject.

The exact mechanism underlying this inability to profit from experience is unknown. It has been speculated the lack of anxiety has something to do with it. (This lack of anxiety will be commented on at greater length in a different context.) This theory may have some validity. Ingenious experiments have been performed in which adrenaline has been administered to these people just before the learning sequence trial has begun. Adrenaline simulates the naturally occurring signs of anxiety, such as rapid heart beat, increased respiration, dryness of the mouth, fluttery feeling in the pit of the stomach, and so forth. Learning is much more effective following this artificial production of anxiety than without it. Whatever the cause, this particular trait of inability to learn from experience is widely accepted as one of the pathognomonic signs of the antisocial personality.

"They are grossly selfish" is another phrase which is used to describe this disorder and ties in with another part of the definition, "frustration tolerance is low." The antisocial personality is characterized by an, "I want what I want, when I want it" attitude. There is an almost complete inability to delay gratification of need. For this reason, in addition to selfishness, impulsivity is a prime factor in the personality make up. From this trait, "I want what I want, when I want it," can be traced the callousness and indifference to the needs, wants, and feelings of others. When what is uppermost in one's mind is one's own needs, the implied attitude exhibited by behavior is the equivalent of "to hell with you." Another adjective which has been used to describe this attitude of wanting immediate gratification is that they are *hedonistic* (searching after pleasure).

"They tend to blame others or offer plausible rationalizations for their behavior." A great deal of discussion has been generated by this aspect of the personality of the antisocial individual. On the one hand there are those who claim that because of the lack of feeling of guilt, or responsibility for behavior, there is every reason for projecting the blame onto others. The majority of those who work with these individuals tend to feel the projection of blame is a deliberate attempt to con. This attempt, however, is more pervasive than it seems on the surface, because it would seem to be an attempt to con not only the listener but the offender as well. The antisocial personality is frequently successful in both aspects of this behavior, and hence repeats the same behavior over and over without learning from experience, as has just been pointed out.

The following illustration is informative not only of this point of believing the con one's self but of the general pattern of the antisocial personality.

Mr. Y was referred to this agency for evaluation on charges of gross sexual imposition. A thirty-year-old male, he had a confirmed history of having been sentenced for detaining a woman against her wishes and for grand larceny. In addition to this, correspondence from the police department in his home community indicated that he was well known to them; he had been arrested there many times for being a peeping tom. His last arrest there was on a charge of disorderly conduct. Mr. Y protested the absurdity of the current charges. (He had pled guilty to them, but insisted the only reason he entered this plea was so he could be placed on probation and not lose any time from his job. At the same time he indicated he was having difficulty keeping his appointments because he was dickering for two different and more prestigious jobs.)

Mr. Y was the fourth of four children. His mother had been deserted by his father shortly after his birth. There was some question as to whether or not the mother had been a prostitute. (To hear Mr. Y talk about her, she was an angel.) Because of her inability to support her children, he had been moved back and forth — in the local orphan asylum, to foster homes, back to his mother, back out to the community, to a relative, back to his mother, etc. He stated it was a tradition in his family that whenever anyone felt that they were old enough to be on their own they could simply so announce it and leave. He states he did this when he was thirteen and has been on his own ever since. It was pointed out to him that the arrest record in his home town showed many offenses after the age of thirteen. He insisted he had left there for good at that time and stated flatly that the record was absolutely impossible, he could not have been there. It might be noted he stated the same thing about all the rest of his record, which will be described, even though this record was based on FBI information and had fingerprint as well as photographic authentication.

As noted, he denied he had ever had any previous offenses. He amended this to state, "Yes, I have been arrested for grand larceny. The problem was I was asleep, under the influence of drugs in the back seat of my car while friends used the car to knock off a business place, and then deserted me alone in the back seat."

He spoke about how after he left home at the age of thirteen he was hitchhiking. He was picked up by a man who was quite impressed by him and said, "If you ever want a job come to see me." Although he had bragged he was completely on his own since leaving home, in telling his story he stated that he hitchhiked to the home of an aunt in the town where this man lived. After living with the aunt for a while he decided he should not burden her with his presence without paying her, so he looked the man up. The man gave him a job in his hardware store. This was the largest hardware store in the community. According to him, at the age of thirteen he became the best salesman in the whole store. He stated he even figured for a contractor the exact amount of material down to the last nail he would need for building a house, and this without any floor plan. The gratified owner made him second in charge of the store. He wanted to teach him about stock market manipulations, but he was eager to be on his own so he left and went to college.

He claimed while at college, in Dade County, Miami, he became a narcotics addict, but he conquered that habit *cold turkey* by getting himself drunk over a long weekend. A friend helped him to kick the habit by restraining him from going out to get drugs. He then stayed more or less drunk for four or five weeks until the habit had been kicked completely. He insisted, however, the narcotics habit had now been replaced by alcohol. He used the rationalization it was better for him to drink a fifth of rum a day then to use narcotics, on the grounds that (1) it was not against the law and (2) it was cheaper. Therefore, he did not have to indulge in illegal activity to uphold his habit.

Returning to the question of the larceny for which he was arrested and sentenced to serve two years in the penitentiary, he insisted he only served six months. He stated, indeed, he was the first person ever to be granted furlough from a state penitentiary. (He had told a coworker he was the first person ever to be granted probation, but changed this when I read the word furlough directly from the file.) He explained furlough to mean he was released on condition he go directly to a job or to an educational situation and he had done this.

When confronted with the dates, which showed a year's gap between his leaving the institution and his entering the university, he stated he had not been able to get his credits together in time to go to school He stated he had spent that year in the following manner: for three months he was a deputy sheriff in a local jail and for six months he was an aide in a local halfway house for alcoholic offenders. These dates could be easily checked. They were and were found to be false; he had never worked for either of these institutions.

He was currently married to a woman who was eight years his senior, whom he stated was tremendously in love with him and believed in him in spite of all the harassment and persecution to which the law subjected him. In spite of the fact he was continuing to drink a fifth of whiskey a day, and that due to his position he was on the road which meant he was absent from home most of the week, she loved him unreservedly. He portrayed these periods of being away from home as being a steady bash, with both liquor and women, and stated on many occasions he did not even do the work he was supposed to do. He professed to be extremely ashamed of his behavior, but there was nothing in his manner which corresponded to his words.

According to him, the current charge was completely false. Whereas the complainant and the police report both stated he had forced his way into her car and attempted to molest her, his story was they both had been in an afterhours carry-out and had struck up a conversation. He had followed her into the parking lot of her apartment, continued to converse from his car to her car, and then had driven off to return home. He professed complete surprise at the charges of detaining a woman against her wishes and gross sexual imposition.

He readily admitted to past offenses for which he had not been charged, such as pimping, stealing betting tickets and then selling them, and conversion. He also insisted that in a few hours he would be getting his master's degree from a local university. Confronted with his transcript which showed very clearly he still had not been granted a bachelor's degree, and none of the courses he was taking were at the master's level, he explained this by the fact they were still trying to reconcile records of previous courses which he had taken while in the correctional institution.

As he was leaving the interview he turned and said, "Oh yes, I remember what that other charge might have been of detaining a woman. I've often wondered what happened to that. That was when I was quite young and three or four of us tried to break into an empty house. When we got in, a woman started to attack us with a broom. She must have been trying to put the house in order for tenants. We went out through a window taking out sash and all. We were never apprehended and I often wondered what the outcome of that was." When the author pointed out to him that under the United States law nobody can be sentenced in absentia and certainly no one serves a jail sentence if absent, he pointedly passed this over. At all times Mr. Y appeared to believe his own rationalizations and wanted to persuade himself they were true just as much as he wanted to persuade the examiner they were true.

"A mere history of repeated legal or social offenses is not sufficient to justify this diagnosis." It is extremely important to point out that many recidivists are not antisocial personalities. It should be stressed the majority of recidivists do not fit this diagnosis. Rather, these are people who have made crime a way of life, a life style which fits them and to which they are committed. In examining this group, it is not uncommon at all to hear the statement, "Well, maybe I will serve ten years for this offense, but just wait until I get out. I'll make up for it then. I'll pull a job that will leave me on easy street and nobody will catch me." Never would the antisocial personality be guilty of such a statement. His attitude is always, "I didn't do it. If I did do it, it was not my fault, it was somebody else's. If and when I am free from this sentence, you will never see me do anything of this sort again."

The lack of anxiety has been mentioned. This too is a cardinal feature of the antisocial personality. This lack of anxiety does not apply where acute situational stress is concerned. The antisocial personality frequently shows a high degree of anxiety immediately after having been arrested for a serious offense or while undergoing examination in connection with that arrest. Tension while awaiting trial can mount to high levels. The first few days in prison after being sentenced may produce anxiety almost at the panic level. Even a temporary or minipsychosis may be produced. Once the acute stress is removed, the psychosis clears. Subsequent behavior is that of the model prisoner, with the goal of making as much "good time" as possible in order to facilitate early release.

The anxiety which accompanies this sort of situational stress must be differentiated from the all-pervading anxiety which so many people show. This particular type of anxiety of the antisocial personality stands in marked contrast to the life history, in which there is no evidence of any of the common fears of childhood, where there is no evidence of any anxiety before, after, or during commission of the act from which the apprehension or sentence resulted, and there is no evidence of the common tension anxiety from which so many people suffer. This lack of anxiety is a positive attribute for the male antisocial personality who finds himself in the military service during a time of war. Such a male generally makes the world's worst peace-time soldier. He cannot stand the military regulations, he cannot bear to be in a situation where he is not allowed to do what he wants, when he wants. He goes AWOL, is subject to frequent court martials, is constantly engaged in disciplinary infractions. Usually under such circumstances he either is given a bad conduct discharge, a dishonorable discharge, or an unfit for the requirements of the service discharge. In wartime, however, if he lands in a combat unit, his behavior is entirely different. There, the lack of anxiety, the failure to foresee consequences, the impulsivity, may all very well lead him to a Congressional Medal of Honor. This has happened not uncommonly in our nation's history.

To sum up the traits of the antisocial personality in somewhat different language: The cardinal points are the inability to form deep relationships with other people, the lack of conscience or remorse, the failure to learn from experience, the impulsivity, the inability to delay gratification, the callousness to the feelings and rights of others, and the freedom from anxiety other than situation anxiety.

In marked contrast to the situation which has been delineated in regard to other psychiatric diagnoses, it is almost impossible to list specific offenses as being more prone to be committed by the antisocial personality. *Polymorphous perverse* sexuality is frequently present, but not in all such individuals. (This implies the ability to engage in any perversion and will be taken up in greater detail in Chapter 11 of this book.) Other offenses range from confidence games to murder.

There are only a few optimistic notes which might be mentioned. There is general agreement that the best time to attempt to involve such an individual in treatment is the period between late adolescence and early adult life. There is also general consensus that with advancing age the signs of antisocial personality tend to "wear out." Most offenses have been committed before the defendant is thirty-five years of age. As a general rule, although there are always exceptions, the antisocial personality does not commit any more transgressions of the law much beyond the age of forty-five. No satisfactory answers have been found as to the reasons for this change of behavior with age. If we could answer the question as to why these people do seem to burn out and apply this knowledge in terms of treatment and rehabilitation, a great deal of prevention could be done. Possibly more than with any other sort of disturbance, the signs of the antisocial personality are already present at a very early age.

As far as the probation or parole officer's contact with these individuals is concerned, the only universally applicable comment is, "Keep your guard up at all times." In practically no other situation is it so necessary to check and double check every statement which is made, to doubt every assertion set forth, and to keep as close tabs as possible on the offender. Elopement from one jurisdiction to a safer community is common. Other offenses may be committed almost under the unsuspecting eyes of the probation officer. Since there is such a great difficulty in forming relationships, any attempt to put the corrections officer-offender relationship on the sort of footing which attempts to control the offender by means of the relationship is doomed to failure.

It is pointed out by many observers that many antisocial personalities never come in contact with the law. A special term has been coined for these people, namely *Compensated Antisocial Personality*. They are frequently seen in high offices in large corporations where they have fought their way up the ladder, ruthlessly displacing anyone who would stand in their path. It is quite possible that some people in political life who obtain high office belong to this special group. At times in the past it has seemed that their machinations outside the law have been of such magnitude that confrontation might pull down the whole fabric of society.

Chapter 10

PERSONALITY DISORDERS (PART TWO)

PASSIVE-AGGRESSIVE PERSONALITY (301.81)

WHAT is meant when the label **Passive-Aggressive Personality** is used? The very name of the personality disorder appears to be contradictory. Passivity and aggression are usually thought of as the opposite ends of a continuum of behavior. In *DSM I* this heading was actually broken into three divisions: (1) passive-aggressive personality (aggressive type); (2) passive-aggressive personality (passive-dependent type); and (3) passive-aggressive personality (passive-aggressive type). Number 1 is now included under explosive personality. Number 2 is no longer used at all, although it would certainly seem to fit a great number of people. Presumably they are currently labeled as either schizoid personality or inadequate personality (q.v.). Since they do not really seem to belong in either group and since they present a special problem to the corrections worker they will be discussed independently.

The only type of Passive-Aggressive Personality still so labelled is the passive-aggressive type. How is it possible to aggress by passivity? Two episodes emerging in the story of an individual recently seen in presentence status will illustrate this point very well, while at the same time demonstrating how far back in the life of the individual these personality traits extend.

Z was a twenty-two-year-old male seen prior to sentencing on a charge of gross sexual imposition. His life history revealed placement in foster homes and institutions from very early childhood. A vivid memory of one of these placements, when he was five or six years of age, is of being hit over the head with a frying pan by an angry foster mother. She had been trying to question him about an incident in which he had been involved. No matter what tactic she used, he simply remained absolutely mute. The aggression inherent in this

165

passive mutism so infuriated her that she lost control and struck him with the frying pan. Fifteen years later, in the second year of a three year hitch in the Navy, he had reacted in the same way to a petty officer who was trying to question him as to the reasons why he had fallen asleep on duty and was not properly dressed in uniform. Again, no matter what the questions, he remained absolutely silent, until the petty officer could stand it no longer and struck him.

Two years later, when questioned about this latter episode, he was still unable to understand why the petty officer got angry, and why the charges against the petty officer were dropped. He felt it was quite unreasonable that at a captain's mast he was found guilty on all charges. He was asked what he thought the outcome should have been. It develops this had been a typical passive-aggressive maneuver. He had expected to be given thirty days in correctional detention and then an honorable discharge. He had wanted to get out of the service. He still feels hurt that he was given an immediate discharge under other than honorable conditions.

It *is* possible then to aggress in a passive manner. Foot dragging is another pattern used in a hostile aggressive way. Further examples of the sort of behavior which characterizes the passive-aggressive personality are never quite finishing a task; being late for appointments; excessive use of the term "sir" or "officer" with a slightly provocative tone. Possibly the outstanding example of passive-aggression in history is the famous passive resistance movement of Mahatma Gandhi followers in India.

There is some confusion as to whether aggression in a chronically passive individual should be included in this category. Not infrequently, extremely violent behavior is seen in an individual who, throughout all his life, has repressed all hostility, anger, and aggression, and who then, when the head of steam has built up inside to an intolerable level, suddenly blows in a completely uncontrollable fashion. This is not passive-aggressive behavior in the strict sense of that term. Such an individual should generally be classified under the heading of explosive personality. If there has been a history of sleepwalking, amnesia, or other hysterical symptoms in the past, then a diagnosis of hysterical dissociation would be more fitting.

As in so many of the diagnostic categories that have been discussed, the passive-aggressive personality is generally not related in any causal fashion to the offense. Thus, this particular personality disorder may be seen with any sort of offense. (Z who was cited as an example happened to be a sexual offender.) There is, however, one sort of crime which in a sense flows from the personality structure. This is theft, particularly when the victim is the employer of the offender. The mechanism of this behavior is as follows: A passive-aggressive male (or female) is employed at a job in which he feels he is being underpaid, where he feels his talents are not fully appreciated, and where he feels he does not have enough responsibility. Instead of asking directly for a raise or for more responsibility or opportunity, or instead of looking for another job, he steals from his employer because in his mind he deserves the money.

The probation or parole officer who becomes aware of the passive-aggressive traits of a probationer or parolee is in position to be of considerable help. Undoubtedly it is true that it is difficult to change the characterological traits of a lifetime. The corrections worker, however, seeing the individual repeatedly in a mandatory relationship, can begin to demonstrate exactly how these habitual reaction patterns displayed to others are self-defeating and can only antagonize others. This can be done by pointing out how habitual tardiness for appointments, or failure to keep them, disregard of probation or parole conditions, and obsequious politeness irritate the worker. Once recognition of the passive-aggressive nature of this behavior has been acknowledged, the worker can steer the individual to the proper source for help. These people may improve greatly with group therapy, particularly in a behaviorally oriented, assertive training group, a T.A. group, or a gestalt group. Effecting a beneficial personality change apparently will have no direct effect on antisocial behavior, but if this aspect of personality function is improved, more appropriate social behavior may follow, and there will be an indirect effect on criminal activity. The corrections worker can strengthen greater adherence to the rules of society in the client by recognition and reinforcement of the improved personality functioning.

Passive-Aggressive Personality, Passive-Dependent Type

This section on the passive-agressive personality is brought to a close by a discussion of the second type listed in *DSM I* under this heading, the passive-dependent personality. These people are best described by the popular expression "clinging vine." They seem to be unable to stand on their own feet. They constantly need support from outside sources, whether other individuals or agencies. They can be differentiated from schizoid personalities in that they are not loners or turned inward, do have a wide range of emotional responses, and do not have a rich fantasy life. They are distinguished from the inadequate personality in that, given the proper support, they can function quite successfully at work and in society. What they are quite unable to do is to act independently. If a job is found, they work well. If a blind date is arranged, they are good company. If someone plans a break in, they are good lookouts or participants. Completely on their own, they are helpless. Occasionally, a basically passive-dependent personality hides behind a facade of rugged individualism and independence. These people will not lean, even in situations in which dependence is acceptable, for example serious illness, disabling fractures, the death of a close relative. This latter group who hide their dependence not uncommonly suffer from digestive tract disorders, particularly ulcers.

As in the passive-aggressive personality, passive-aggressive type, so too in the passive-dependent type, there is little causal relationship between the antisocial behavior and the disorder. Since they are so dependent, however, they are easily influenced by others, and then they may participate in various burglaries, thefts, or confidence schemes. Only very rarely are they involved in violent offenses. By their very dependency however, they turn out to be special problems for corrections officers when they have been involved in crime. In prison they can usually be dominated and led by more independent individuals. They sometimes become pawns in a struggle for power and indirectly incite a great deal of unrest. At times this may necessitate their being placed on a security range, not only for their own protection, but also to remove a source of irritation.

In the status of probationer or parolee, they may suck the unsuspecting corrections worker dry. Without being quite aware of what is happening, the worker may find that not only has the suggestion been made that the parolee go to X company to look for a job, but the worker has been sucked into calling the company, arranging the interview, and even driving the offender there. It cannot be emphasized sufficiently that this sort of response can never be really helpful. On the other hand, before long the corrections worker will find himself dreading contacts with such an individual, whether by phone or in person. Anger will mount as the exploitation continues, and unless care is exercised the client will be busted without much provocation. On the other hand, doing things for a dependent person is really no help. It simply fosters dependency. The most helpful procedure after having assayed the personality structure is to continue to insist that the individual do the indicated tasks without further help from the officer.

INADEQUATE PERSONALITY (301.82)

The characteristics of the **Inadequate Personality (301.82)** are well summarized by that label itself. Probably there is no other diagnostic category in which the very label seems to instill such negative feelings in the user of that label. It becomes extremely difficult to avoid automatic value judgments as to behavior and automatic pessimism as to eventual outcome once this diagnosis has been made. The inadequate personality is apt to have been unofficially titled *sad sack* or *born loser* by his peer group long before coming into contact with an agency or a diagnostician. The diagnosis itself frequently seems to be one of desperation. There is no other pigeon hole in which this person can be neatly stuffed, yet obviously there is something wrong. It becomes frustrating not to be able to identify what that something is. The intelligence of such an individual may fall anywhere along a scale from borderline mentally retarded to superior intelligence. Physical strength may vary from weak and languid to extremely strong. (It is not uncommon for males with this personality structure to take up weight lifting as a compensatory mechanism. This should in no way imply that all weight lifters are compensating for inadequate personalities) Stamina is reported to be lacking, but this is not-universal. *DSM II* stresses the word *ineffectual* in its definition and this is probably the most descriptive term which can be found.

There is probably a good reason why these people have never developed social skills in their progress from infancy to adulthood. If so, it has nothing to do with cultural levels. They do not show the same features as do those with mental retardation due to cultural and environmental deprivation. They come from all classes of society. If there has been a specific disturbance in parent-child relationships which is causative it has yet to be identified. It would be very tempting to insist this must be a congenital condition. Exhaustive studies, however, have failed to demonstrate a genetic factor, and there is no evidence which would suggest a causative physical problem during pregnancy or early infancy.

These people can be differentiated from passive-dependent personalities by the fact they do not cling. Indeed, one of the ways in which this social inadequacy is frequently manifested is by ineptly timed assertion of independence. It is possible careful psychological testing will reveal some people so diagnosed should in actuality be diagnosed as schizophrenia, simple type. The true inadequate personality, however, has no disorder in thought process, is not a loner by choice, and does not show any signs of deterioration with passing time.

A characteristic history will reveal repeated job changes with rare promotions. Sometimes they quit a job when success would appear to be within their grasp. More often they are fired for incompetency, even though physically and mentally they should be capable of performing the required tasks. Personal relationships tend to be just as temporary, and it is not unusual to find five, six or seven marriages, whether legal or common-law, entered into over the course of years.

As might be expected, these people are not very successful criminals. They are apt to be known to the welfare agencies far more than to corrections. There is however a tendency to behave impulsively and immaturely in ways which may at times lead to aggressive, even serious, offenses. As in any diagnostic category, any sort of offense may be committed. Quite often, the inadequate personality seen by the corrections worker is either alcoholic or drug dependent. Naturally the presence of either of these two conditions worsens the prognosis.

This brings us full circle to the opening paragraph of this section. The diagnosis once made, particularly if complicated by drugs or alcohol, tends to become a self-fulfilling prophecy. The corrections worker (and many psychiatrists as well) subsequently throws in the towel and makes no effort. Incarceration is not the answer. It adds no skills; it complicates integration into society. There are occasions, admittedly rare, when the social experience of being treated as a worthwhile human being can have a profound effect on the career of such a person. The worker in attempting to enter into a relationship with an inadequate personality runs the very definite risk of being let down. The risk of fostering dependence and being sucked dry is not present as it is with the passive-dependent personality. The odds of being blamed for the individual's misfortunes are miniscule, as compared to the paranoid personality. The chances of being shut out completely do not begin to approximate those encountered in dealing with the schizoid personality. The possibility of being exploited is almost nil compared to the antisocial personality; of being attacked, minimal compared to the aggressive personality, and of being seduced zero as compared to the hysterical personality. Yet once this value judgment, the diagnosis of inadequate personality, is made, it is the rare worker who will attempt to mobilize all the means at his or her command to help these people.

HYSTERICAL PERSONALITY
(HISTRIONIC PERSONALITY DISORDER) (301.5)

It was noted in Chapter 8 that hysterical neurosis was frequently associated with a hysterical personality. The two however may exist independently.[1] It is hard to quote exact statistics about any of the personality disorders, largely because the borderline between the various conditons are so poorly demarcated. (The points at which personality traits become personality disorders are also quite imprecise, a fact which must have been obvious on reading these last two chapters.) What statistics are available tend to show the greatest number of people with hysterical personality *do not* develop a hysterical neurosis. The same statistics indicate about 90 percent of hysterical personality disorders occur in women.

The outstanding characteristic of the hysterical personality is the need to be center stage, to be the focal point of all eyes, the only source of conversation. Such women do not come into a room; they make an entrance. They do not tell a story; they enact a drama. Not only are they immature, superficial, and shallow in their emotional reactions, they are also extremely vain and self-centered, with little awareness of the feelings of others.

The single event which in my experience best seemed to epitomize this last aspect of a woman with a hysterical personality disorder follows.

> Mrs. A.A., a twenty-nine-year-old married female, pulled up in front of her home at two o'clock in the morning with her boyfriend. A violent argument broke out when he, first jestingly and then in earnest, as he saw her getting more upset, refused to kiss her goodnight. She literally charged into the house, burst into the bedroom, and awakened her husband with the imperious demand that he get out of bed, pursue and beat up the boyfriend, because he had dared to treat her in this fashion.

These women are said to be quite seductive sexually but basically frigid. They tend to be manipulative and, as seen in the example above, quite disturbed when thwarted. Physical complaints may be legion and usually have no organic founda-

---

[1]This situation is further complicated by a suggestion that these conditions be divided into three groups: hysterical personality, hysteria, and *Briquet's syndrome*. This has little practical significance to the corrections worker except to indicate that the term *Briquet's syndrome* is connected with hysterical personality.

tion. In the past the diagnosis could sometimes be made on examination of the surface of the abdomen. This was frequently referred to as a road map, because of the large number of crisscrossing operative scars. The past tense is used advisedly because such futile operations are much less common today. More common now is a similar picture of scars on the under surface of the wrist and forearms. Impulsive and manipulative suicidal gestures are an extremely frequent occurrence in hysterical personalities. The word "gesture" was not chosen because it sounded good. It *is* possible for an hysterical personality to commit suicide, but when it happens it is more apt to be by mistake than intention. Hubby is due home at five; wife turns on the gas jets at 4:45 PM. The draw bridge is up today, or his car will not start, or the rail crossing is blocked, or he unaccustomedly stops in for a beer. He gets home at six instead of five and by then it is too late.

This is of practical significance for the corrections worker. If such a client calls in a thick voice to announce that she has swallowed a bottle of tranquilizers, the call deserves a response. That response should be to dispatch the proper crew — emergency squad, fire unit, police department, life rescue squad — not to answer the call personally. If contacted by the emergency room, the proper statement is to have them use their own judgment as to admission, but in the worker's opinion the person is better off treated adequately and released immediately. The less attention paid beyond the essential, the quicker the behavior will be abandoned.

In what ways do those with hysterical personalities come in contact with the corrections worker? Manipulative attempts are sometimes extremely close to confidence rackets, and the margins blur. Frequent police contacts due to overdoses lead to suspicion of drug involvement. One study reported the hysterical personality to be found in a high percentage of female felons, female relatives of male felons, and wives of known antisocial males. Immature, impulsive, self-centered behavior frequently precipitates arguments, which, particularly if alcohol is involved, can readily turn into brawls. The hysterical personality, once she has lost control, is very apt to resist arrest and another charge is added.

As might be gathered from the above discussion, dealing with a behavioral pattern as complex and deeply ingrained as this is not a simple task. This is one area where the corrections officer should make no attempt to be the leader of the rehabilitative team, if one exists. Even without assuming leadership there are two major areas which must be kept in mind when dealing with these people. One is to be constantly aware of attempts to seduce and manipulate and to handle these attempts gently but firmly and effectively. The other is to keep a constant check with other agencies involved, lest the hysterical personality play one off against the other, divide, and rule.

PARANOID PERSONALITY (301.0)

CYCLOTHYMIC PERSONALITY (301.1)

SCHIZOID PERSONALITY (301.2)

OBSESSIVE-COMPULSIVE PERSONALITY (301.4)

These four personality types are lumped together at this point not because they have that much in common with each other, but because their characteristics can be inferred from the major illnesses after which they are named. People with these personality disorders are probably involved less frequently in the criminal justice system (with the possible exception of the schizoid personality) than are those with any of the other personality patterns we have discussed to this point.

The **Paranoid Personality (301.1)** is the descriptive term applied to those people whose usual reaction is one of suspicion, resentment, and hostility. They use the psychological mechanisms of denial and projection and hence tend to blame all their difficulties on others. These mechanisms are normal in a young child. "That D on my report card is because the teacher doesn't like me." "See what you made me do." There is no evidence to suggest these are unhealthy mechanisms in children, nor that their excessive use leads to development of a paranoid personality. Certainly, if these mechanisms are encouraged in childhood or even silently accepted, it is easy to see how they can become an integral part of the character. On the other hand, when dealing with a fully developed adult paranoid personality it is a technical mistake to attempt to set the record straight and to make the individual assume responsibility, rather than allowing him to put the blame on others. The best stance is to listen attentively, neither agree nor disagree, and focus on the feelings. It is generally agreed that paranoid personalities rarely develop paranoid psychosis, that is they do not actually break with reality. Such a break may occur under two conditions: (1) acutely under stress, in which case the psychosis is generally short lived and self-limited; (2) in the aging process, when these people in addition to becoming querulous old men or women may become actively delusional as their cognitive functions fail.

Cyclothymic Personalities (301.1) are those who correspond in personality type to manic depressives. They are subject to periodic mood swings without external cause. These swings do not reach the depth of true depression or the heights of mania or hypomania. When antisocial behavior occurs it generally bears no direct relationship to the personality. However, the probation or parole officer working with a cyclothymic personality over any period of time should be able to spot the change in mood quite quickly. It scarcely needs saying that supervision must be much more intense during an upswing because it is then the cyclothymic personality has the increased drive and energy which can lead to effective action on dormant plans.

The **Schizoid Personality (301.2)** is such a common personality disorder that we have probably all come into contact with several of these people through the course of life. These are the people who are loners. They are extremely shy and timid; at times they try to hide these qualities behind a jovial mask, which never completely does hide them. Their peers consider them to be eccentric. They do a great deal of daydreaming or fantasizing but are well able to differentiate between fantasy and reality. They tend to be oversensitive, but have trouble expressing hostility when hurt. Indeed, it is difficult for them to show any feelings, so that they commonly display what appears to be detachment. It is extremely difficult for them to form relationships, and if anyone treatens to become close, the schizoid personality tends to panic and run. As with the other personality disorders, these traits have been present throughout life. If these people do become psychotic, they develop schizophrenia.

Bizarre major offenses have been committed on rare occasions by schizoid personalities, but the majority of those personalities who are in conflict with the law stumble over problems with their sexuality. Two cases will illustrate this.

> A.B., a sixteen-year-old black male was arrested for exhibitionism. A high school junior, he was on the baseball team but had no contact with his teammates off the field. One of five children, he seldom interacted with his siblings, who all thought him peculiar. His mother stated he had seemed different from early childhood, always preferring to be alone, doing a lot of daydreaming, saying little. As far as she knew, he had no close friends. The only constructive activity on his part she was aware of was baseball, about which he seemed passionately enthusiastic.

> On the morning of the offense, he had been out soliciting funds for uniforms for the baseball team. A teenage white girl whom he vaguely recognized as being a classmate answered his ring at her doorbell. She had apparently just arisen and was dressed in a nightgown and rather sheer robe. She closed the door to get some money, and when she came back he had his cannister close to his groin, his zipper open, and his penis in full display next to the cannister. She ran to awaken her brother who apprehended A.B. just three doors down the street. He insisted to the brother, and later to the police, that it was an accident, his zipper was faulty. He told the writer, in a tone of voice and body set which suggested he was talking about someone else, it was not an accident. He was stimulated emotionally and hoped that, if she knew him, she would not be alarmed by his behavior and, indeed, might even ask him to come in the house.

> Mr. A.C., a forty-three-year-old white male, was arrested for

exposing himself to two teenage girls on a Saturday evening in a public park. The girls had been walking down a path when he stepped out from behind a bush with his penis exposed. This was the third complaint the police had had of a similar occurrence in that park in the past month, always on a Saturday evening. He had said nothing to the girls on any of the occasions. He had made no attempt to harm them. Mr. A.C. was perfectly willing to talk. There was a mildly paranoid tone to his complaint, since he did project the blame for his behavior on to the *do-gooders*. However, the picture he painted was of a typical schizoid personality. His mother and two sisters were living, all within two to three miles of him. He had seen none of them in twelve years. There had been no quarrel. He had never gone to visit them and they had tired of coming to visit him. In spite of the fact that he had been employed steadily for years in a well-paying, routine, factory job, he lived in what could only be described as a shack at the edge of a city dump at the end of an unpaved road.

Until about three months prior to his arrest, his routine had been the same. He would go to work in the morning, stop for one beer by himself on the way home, pick up a few groceries, and retire to his shack. He read paperback novels by the light of a kerosene lamp until bedtime and then went to sleep. He aparently banked the greater part of his money. Every Saturday evening he took a bath (his only one of the week), changed his clothing (the only change of the week), and went to a local house of prostitution. There, he chose a different girl each week, paid his money, satisfied himself sexually, and went home. There was no report of any deviant sexual practices with these women. Three months before his arrest, the county administration had changed hands. Every house of prostitution in the country had closed down until the heat was off. Even the taxi drivers were unable to take Mr. A.C. to a rendezvous. *He* was totally unable to approach a girl on the street and could not trust one who approached *him*. As he said, "The do-gooders did me in." The closing of the houses of prostitution took away his only sexual outlet. His schizoid personality boxed him in. His behavior was designed, like that of the previous case, to say, "Do you want me?"

The **Obsessive-Compulsive Personality (301.4)** furnishes the basis from which an Obsessive-Compulsive Neurosis (Chapter 8) develops. Repetitive thoughts and compulsive behavior serve as defenses against anxiety in the compulsive neurotic. The obsessive-compulsive personality is marked by constant straining to find perfection. (Only by being perfect can these people satisfy the tremendous inner feeling of guilt.) Their dress tends to be impeccable (at least on the outside; they may wear the same underwear for weeks). This exterior also serves to say, "Everything must be all right inside." The standards for themselves and those around them are extremely high and very rigid (only in this way can they protect themselves against the terrible thoughts beneath). They are meticulous in everything they do. They tend to collect things almost to the point of hoarding.

Such people make marvelous bookeepers, tabulators, surveyors, any occupation which demands conscientiousness and scrupulous accuracy. Their families, however, can be driven to distraction by the constant insistence on, "A place for everything and everything in its place." (Extreme disorder reminds them that something is in disorder inside themselves.) It is rare for obsessive-compulsive personalities to become involved in crime. When the deeply repressed inaccessible thoughts break through, they do so in the form of severe neurotic symptomatology and even frank psychosis, rather than in antisocial behavior. Indeed, it is questioned whether the obsessive-compulsive personality who disintegrates to the point where the repressed forbidden actions break through to consciousness ever carries these forbidden wishes out. Mr. V, cited in Chapter 8, was certainly an exception to this rule. There is another school of thought which insists that this behavior must be schizophrenic.

THE BORDERLINE SYNDROME

Like the Episodic Dyscontrol Syndrome, which was discussed in Chapter 9, the borderline syndrome is not officially recognized as such by *DSM II*. Care must be taken not to confuse the borderline syndrome with borderline mental retardation. The intelligence of those who exhibit this condition of borderline syndrome may vary from borderline mental retardation to superior intelligence. It is being described under the personality disorders because there is general agreement it does not represent an illness engrafted on the personality, as is the case with the organic conditions, the psychoses, and the neuroses. Rather, individuals who exhibit a borderline syndrome seem to have never progressed beyond a very early and primitive stage of personality development.

The first attempt to define this group was made in 1935. Since that time at least twenty-one different labels have been applied to these people. The borderline syndrome seemed to have become the accepted one during the past three to five years. Even the exact meaning of the term *borderline* itself has been somewhat hazy. In one sense it means that these people occupy the borderline between neurosis and psychosis, between reality and unreality, between integration and disintegration. Recently this has been expanded to mean that they stand at the border, probably crossroads is a better term, where normals, personality disorders, neuroses, and psychoses join. Most characteristic is a movement backward and forward, into and out of, one or another of these territories. This feature of the condition has been referred to as a *stable instability.*

Because of this baffling array of symptoms, it is very hard to describe the clinical picture of borderline patients. They come into contact with corrections because they "act out" their problems, rather than either thinking them through or talking about them. According to some authorities, this is because acting out is the family method of communication. It is generally held that parents of borderline patients are themselves borderline. These people seem to be capable of feeling only two emotions. The most frightening of these is anger, which is deep-seated and diffuse and tends to focus on anyone in the environment. The other emotion is depression. This is not in reaction to any specific occurrence, but rather to a deep feeling of loneliness, of an awareness of an inability to commit themselves to others in a world where this sort of interaction takes place. As a result, they frequently appear to be what has been called "as if" people. They act *as if* they were college students, mothers, or criminals, and yet they give no evidence of any consistent self-identity; they do not know who they are themselves. They do not often show pleasure, nor are they often emotionally flat.

Strangely, they are usually quite adaptable and generally get along well for a period of time wherever they are, be it at school, work, or prison. And yet this always breaks down in some inappropriate behavior. They tend to go on binges. They eat too much, drink too much, use drugs excessively, or pursue sex avidly, for a period of time. They then turn away as if satiated and even become ascetic. Generally, they are in excellent contact with reality, but under varying degrees of distress they can have mini-psychoses, lasting from moments to days. When they do interact with others, they tend to swing between superficial transient relationships and intense dependent ones in which they become extremely manipulative and demanding. These last two paragraphs seem to be quite explanatory of the term stable instability.

In spite of the fact that the borderline syndrome does not find recognition in *DSM II*, it is a diagnosis which is being made with increasing frequency. The definite statement was made in 1970 at a meeting of the American Psychiatric Association, "The number of borderline patients are increasing at a higher rate than that of any other diagnostic category." Whether this is due to an increasing number of people in this category or to an increased recognition of the syndrome itself is difficult to say. It is my considered opinion, particularly in adolescents seen at the Child Study Institute (the Juvenile Detention Home for Lucas County, Ohio) and at the Adolescent Unit of the Toledo Mental Health Center, that the increase is in the number of borderline patients rather than an increasing use of this diagnosis.

These people represent an extremely difficult problem in management, whether by the psychiatrist or the corrections worker. They do best when strict limits are imposed. This would imply very specific conditions of probation, reinforced by a suspended sentence. Indeed, for a while they settle down very well in either a hospital or jail. However, in either of these settings for longer than two or three months they become very dependent and may badly regress. They easily become pansexual, and homosexuality or lesbianism become the common way of life for them in an institution. It is important the corrections worker keep two of the descriptive features of people with this syndrome constantly in mind when working with them.

The first of these features is the anger which they display. It is of the utmost importance this be recognized as a reaction to inner emptiness and loneliness and not seen as directed against the worker, even though it may be focused on the worker. Here is one place where limit-setting may defuse a potentially bad situation. "It's all right if you want to say to me, 'I think you're a son of a bitch,' but you may not say 'You son of a bitch, you.' " The second point which must be kept in mind is the matter of *stable instability*. At almost no point in a relationship with a person with borderline syndrome may the worker relax and feel, "Well, at least XYZ is doing well." Two days later, XYZ will have given the statement the lie. The author has no suggestions as to how to avoid having such an attitude of expectant watching keep from being a self-fulfilling prophecy.

THE CORRECTIONS WORKER AND
THE PERSONALITY DISORDERS

As each of the personality disorders was discussed, some attempts were made to indicate how the corrections worker might best deal with the specific problems involved. This chapter will be concluded with some generalizations which apply to all of these conditions, including the borderline syndrome. All of these diagnoses refer to deeply ingrained character traits. Under certain circumstances, some of these traits are quite desirable. It was pointed out that the obsessive-compulsive personality, with the need for perfectionism and compulsion and the attention to small details, makes an excellent bookkeeper. It might be pointed out with equal truthfulness that these same traits make for an ideal counterfeiter.

This then is one area in which the corrections worker might operate helpfully; the area of helping the individual to use character traits in socially acceptable ways. This would mean, for example, helping the obsessive-compulsive personality to become a bookkeeper rather than a counterfeiter or helping the hysterical personality, if the talent exists, to become an entertainer rather than a con artist.

It is admittedly a herculean task to change the character traits of a lifetime, particularly if the individual does not want to change. This is another area in which the corrections worker has an unparalleled opportunity because of the mandatory relationship. This opportunity lies in motivating the individual to want to change, and then identifying the mental health resources which may offer some chance that change can be brought about. It seems to have become a fairly well-accepted fact, both in corrections and in psychiatry, that people do not change in prisons regardless of therapy. (Some few voices dissent from this.) The reason given is that when incarcerated the motive to enter therapy is not to change, but to pile up good time, to make the record look better when parole is being considered. These same factors do not operate outside institutional walls. Both probation and parole are for definite periods of time. They may be revoked, but they are generally not shortened for good behavior.

In some instances, in some jurisdictions, and for some offenses, treatment is made a mandatory condition of probation. When this is the case in an individual with a personality disorder, it places a special burden on the probation officer. The fact of mandatory treatment does not relieve the worker of the responsibility of seeing the probationer, nor of working in other areas of rehabilitation. It does add the burden of frequent checks with the therapist to insure that appointments are being kept and the probationer is doing more than going through the motions of cooperating. The worker may share behavioral observations with the therapist, and in turn may receive instructions as to how to reinforce the therapeutic process. The worker must also keep in mind the matter of his own responsibility as discussed in Chapter 8.

Finally, this group of people (those with personality disorders) are probably the most irritating and least rewarding of all those with whom the correction worker deals. They also make up a fairly large share of the caseload, certainly the largest share of that caseload to which a psychiatric diagnosis can be applied. It may be of small comfort to be aware the large majority of these people do not want to be as they are. The greatest part of their antisocial, upsetting, seemingly senseless, and at times dangerous behavior grows out of deep inner-feelings of alienation, loneliness, discontent, inferiority, inadequacy, and nothingness. This is a feeling that is all the more painful since it is so diffuse as to be almost unrecognized by those experiencing it. This is not to suggest that the community should not be protected against them because they are unaware of the well-springs of their own behavior. It is probably easier for the corrections worker to cope with the feelings of dissatisfaction which occur when no change takes place, when behavior worsens, when actions seem to have personal motivation, if the deep roots of this acting out are kept in mind. The satisfaction is multiplied immeasureably when one of these people turns the corner and the worker feels, "I helped bring that about."

Chapter 11

SEXUAL DEVIATIONS
(PART ONE)

GENERAL CONSIDERATIONS

IT is extremely difficult to determine what sexual behavior should be included in a discussion of sexual deviations. From the viewpoint of corrections, it is not the sexual deviation which is of primary importance, but the offense which occurs as a result of that deviation. For example, a male offender was referred to this agency (Court Diagnostic and Treatment Center) for evaluation on presentence status following having pled guilty to a series of armed robberies. During the course of the evaluation, it was discovered he had an extremely bizarre sexual deviation in which, among other things, he would insert a broom handle into his rectum and manipulate it until he bled. The dynamics of this deviation were fascinating but had no causal connection with the offenses for which he was being evaluated. Hence there is no need to discuss this sort of anal erotic behavior. Such behavior occurring in connection with a highly sadistic murder, however, might be extremely significant.

From a slightly different point of view, there is a question as to the inclusion of a discussion of homosexuality. According to the results of a survey conducted in 1974 among the members of the American Psychiatric Association, homosexuality is no longer to be considered a sexual deviation. Yet, in the majority of states, homosexual acts, even between consenting adults, are illegal. In 1976, the Supreme Court of the United States upheld the decision of a state court to this effect. Even in those states in which such behavior is no longer considered illegal, arrests are still being made for soliciting, or sexual importuning of one male by another. (It is interesting that in our culture the law is mute about female homosexuality [lesbianism] unless the cus-

184

tody of children is involved, while a tremendous turmoil continues to rage around male homosexuality.)

Oral-genital sexuality is no longer considered a sexual deviation. Most sex manuals and educational films are explicit in their approval of these sexual activities in foreplay. At the same time, laws in many states prohibit any form of oral-genital contact, even between husband and wife. To a large extent, it would appear the law as to what is legal or illegal is somewhat at odds with the value judgments of the community as to what is moral and immoral. Is this behavior to be considered a deviation, and if so, should it be included?

From the viewpoint of the corrections worker who has to deal with sexual offenders, it appears the most important question is, "What does the presence of this particular sexual deviation imply as far as behavior which might be harmful or dangerous to others is concerned?" The answer to this question in many instances depends more on the individual manifestations of the deviation than on the nature of the deviation itself. A discussion of **Fetishism (302.1)** will serve to elucidate this statement.

Fetishism is a form of sexual deviation in which a part of the sexual object stands for the whole. In its socialized form, with which we are all familiar, some men are particularly stimulated by breasts, others by buttocks, still others by thighs. The fetish may be an object of wearing apparel, a shoe, a purse, a bra, a pair of panties. True fetishists are not only stimulated by the object, they are impotent in its absence. Many fetishists use a woman's panties as an accessory in masturbation. Truly, this would appear to be a harmless means of sexual gratification. If, instead of purchasing the panties from a store, they were borrowed from a sister, it would be annoying. The sister would probably consider this a real nuisance. If stolen from a neighboring laundromat, the deviation becomes more serious. If it is necessary as a part of the fetishistic act for the panties to be stolen by breaking into an apartment, the police are certainly going to be involved. And, if the only way the individual can gain orgiastic satisfaction is by using panties which he has removed from a woman's thighs, that act would be considered dangerous. That is particularly true if the woman does not know him, is unaware all he wants is her panties and not her, and resists vigorously.

This question of what topics to include in these chapters on sexual deviation is further complicated by the fact that many apparently nonsexual offenses, such as kleptomania (compulsive stealing) and pyromania (compulsive firesetting), may have their origins in faulty psychosexual development. Many psychiatrists interested in the dynamics of antisocial behavior consider breaking and entering, particularly in young adolescents, to be symbolic of rape, which *is* a forcible breaking and entering. At the same time, rape itself, which would appear to be the most blatantly sexual of all offenses, is considered by many writers to be primarily an act of aggression and not a sexual act. Prostitution is an offense which, while studied by psychiatrists, is not considered a deviation.

Fortunately, some positive general statements about sexual deviation can be made. There are many widely held myths about sexual offenders which must be dispelled. The great majority of sexual offenses are of a nuisance rather than of a dangerous variety. The great majority of sexual offenders do not progress from one deviation to another. The exhibitionist will probably never commit other sexual offenses than indecent exposure. The fetishist will probably never turn into a Jack the Ripper. Mentally retarded individuals do not commit more sex offenses than those of normal or superior intelligence. Homosexuals are not perverts waiting to pounce on innocent individuals. The bushes are not full of lurking strangers about to molest little children.

The attainment of normal adult heterosexuality is not an easy achievement for many people. It is generally held deviations result from failure properly to fulfill the requirements of each stage of development from birth to adulthood when heterosexuality should be attained. This failure may be the result of biological factors, of faulty education, of faulty parenting, of failure to have proper models with whom to identify, and so on. In a book of this scope, it is impossible to explore all of them in detail. Where a theoretical formulation of the development of a particular deviation will be of help to the worker, not only in understanding the deviation, but also in helping the offender, it will be included.

GENDER IDENTITY

Problems in development of gender identity contribute to the genesis of many sexual deviations. A discussion of this development follows, since it so well illustrates the complexity of the developmental faults.

Gender identity is that concept which enables a boy to think, "I am a male," or a girl, "I am a female." Surprisingly, it does not depend completely on the possession of either male or female sex glands or external genitals. As in so many other areas which have been discussed, the question of gender identity is a mixture of biological, social, and psychological factors. It was mentioned in Chapter 2, in the section on the XYY syndrome, that the Y chromosome in the nucleus of human cells is necessary to produce an anatomical male. It has been known for some time that during the first three fetal months, the sexual glands, or *gonads* (the testes in the male, the ovaries in the female), are still undifferentiated. If the Y chromosome is present, then during the fourth month, these glands develop as testicles and secrete male sex hormones (androgens); in the absence of a Y chromosome they become ovaries and secrete female sex hormones (estrogens). It has been learned recently, if development is progressing normally, this flooding of sex hormones influences the central nervous system as well as the reproductive system. The brain in the male becomes, as it were, masculinized at this time. This leads in later life to the development of masculine patterns, both in sexual and general behavior, even though there is less difference in masculine and feminine behavior in the human species than in any other. It has been shown the increase in aggressiveness and competitiveness in the male over the female is partly the result of the *androgenization* of the brain in the male during the fourth month of pregnancy. This is not to be interpreted as a value judgment as to the worth of these characteristics.

In the past, both estrogens and androgens have been administered in the first four months of pregnancy in an attempt to prevent miscarriages in women who are known to have a high risk of miscarrying. The male children of mothers in whom estrogens were used for these purposes are found to be less aggressive, less combative, and less inclined to engage in contact sports than their male siblings carried through pregnancy without the use of estrogens. Similarly, the female children of mothers given male sex hormones during the first four months, may, in adolescence, develop a specific syndrome characterized by virilization (deep voice, flat chest, masculine distribution of hair on the extremities) and increased sex drive. This latter characteristic is probably attributable to the fact that small quantities of male sex hormones circulating in the blood stream increase the female sex drive.

Biological factors then definitely enter into this question of sexual identity. The most important single factor in the formation of this identity, however, is the attitude of the parents. Naturally, presented with a boy the parents will raise him as a boy; with a girl, they will raise her as a girl. Occasionally, however, cases do occur in which the sex of the child is misidentified at birth. A combination of undescended testicles and *hypospadiasis* (the urethral opening is on the undersurface of the penis rather than at the head) may on examination be mistaken for female genitalia. *Pseudohermaphroditism* may cause the external genitalia of the female to resemble those of a boy. There are other causes for honest mistakes in diagnosis. It has been demonstrated if such a child is raised for the first three years as a member of the sex opposite to the true anatomical and chromosomal sex, that child will continue throughout life to regard himself/herself as a member of the assigned sex.

In other instances there is no possible doubt of the anatomical sex of the child, but the parents, or probably more frequently a parent, will treat the child as though that child were a member of the opposite sex. The fifth consecutive girl in a family may well be named Jacqueline or Henrietta, shortened to Jack or Henry. Her early toys may well be model racing cars, boxing gloves, or tiny footballs. Many mothers desperately want a girl to be the firstborn, and when a boy arrives never really accept that fact. Certainly, this has a definite effect on the formation of gender identity.

Although this basic gender identity is formed in the first three years of life and remains throughout life, males seem to develop more doubts and problems about their masculinity than females do about their femininity. This may be due to the fact that for almost everyone, the first period of life is spent in much closer contact with the mother than with the father. During the first nine months the relationship between mother and child may be so close that is is referred to as *symbiosis* (a mutually dependent relationship). While it is necessary for the child to *individuate* in order to become a person, this task is more difficult in the boy than in the girl, who does not have to put so great a distance between herself and her mother because they do not have to be that different. This difficulty may in a large part be responsible for the overwhelming disparity in the prevalence of all sexual deviations in males as opposed to females. (For example, it is rare to see a female exposing herself publicly for other than commercial reasons.) Fathers are more apt to be distant and threatening figures in a family, and it may be more difficult for a boy to identify with such a figure than for a girl to identify with a warm, supporting mother. The opposite may, of course, also be true. It may be the father who is warm and the mother distant. Doubts about masculinity are present to a greater or lesser degree in almost all males at one time or another.

The presentation of the sexual deviations in these chapters will attempt to proceed from those which create the least physical and psychological trauma to the victim to those which are the most dangerous. In many instances, the so-called nuisance offenses may present as dangerous under the proper circumstances.

TRANSVESTISM (302.3)

TRANSVESTISM (302.3) consists of a desire to dress in the clothing of the opposite sex. This behavior may range all the way from wearing only one article to complete cross-dressing. As an offense, it falls in the category of an offense against public decency, although it is a little difficult to understand why it is presently so considered. It is almost exculsively a male offense, probably because we are so conditioned to seeing women in masculine-like attire no attention is paid to this phenomenon.

Transvestism may be looked on as one extreme on a continuum running from transvestism through homosexuality to transsexualism. (Transsexualism consists of a life long pattern of thinking of oneself as belonging to the opposite sex, behaving as though one belonged to the opposite sex, and ultimately desiring surgical intervention to appear and function as much as possible as a member of the opposite sex.) Transvestism must be differentiated from *dressing in drag*, which implies a homosexual's attempt to appear as much like a woman as possible. Most transvestites are overtly heterosexual; many of them are married and have children. In a high percentage of these latter instances, the wives are quite cooperative, even buying female clothing for their husbands. (It would appear the male transvestite is more potent when dressed in female clothes, and that may be why the wife is so willing to buy the clothing for him.) In most instances, the clothing is worn only in the privacy of the home. Occasionally, a transvestite fully attired in woman's clothing will walk outdoors at two or three o'clock in the morning. However, exhibitionistic transvestites have been reported, who do enjoy showing themselves in public areas. Professional female impersonators may belong in this group. It may be that writers who describe exhibitionistic transvestites are really talking about the homosexual in drag.

Almost all transvestites give a history of a mother who wanted a girl. These mothers would not allow their son's hair to be cut until it was time to go to school and insisted on dressing him as a girl until that time. Some writers feel the transvestic tendencies become fixed when sexual excitement is first associated with dressing in female attire. In this respect, it is comparable to fetishism.

As noted, transvestism can under no circumstances be considered other than a nuisance offense. It is rare for a transvestite to commit any other sexual offense. There is even a question as to whether transvestism should be treated. This is particularly true if the behavior is not disturbing to the spouse. The probation counselor's role (it is very rare for a transvestite to receive custodial sentencing and hence parole), is first and foremost to evaluate the situation in the marriage. If this is stable, routine reporting plus the strengthening of the resolve to stay off the streets while cross-dressed is all that is necessary. If the marriage is shaky, then the couple should be encouraged to seek conjoint therapy.

HOMOSEXUALITY

Homosexuality is still an offense in most states, even though the act between two consenting adults has been decriminalized in others. It is, therefore, necessary to consider it among the sexual deviations even though it is no longer so considered by the American Psychiatric Association. (It is classed as a "sexual orientation disturbance, to be treated only if the individual is in conflict and desires a change.") As a usual rule, the term homosexuality, as such, does not appear in the statutes; the statutes are concerned with *sodomy* and *unnatural acts*. Until now, homosexuality as an offense has been confined to males.

Statistics as to the incidence of homosexuality in either sex are largely educated guesses. All of the reported studies, of which those of Kinsey in 1948 and 1953 are the best known, have had built-in methodological defects. For this reason, they can be used only as estimates. According to Kinsey's figures, 10 percent of American males and between 2 and 6 percent of American females have been more or less exclusively homosexual throughout their lives. Thirty-seven percent of men beyond adolescence have had some homosexual experience to the point of orgasm; 38 percent of the women in the study were aware of having been homosexually aroused, 13 percent to the point of orgasm.

There are a great many theories as to the cause of homosexuality. The following attempt to organize these theories is admittedly over-simplified and dogmatic. It is written in the interest of clarity and should not be interpreted as the final word on the subject nor as being complete in all details. The statements made refer in general only to male homosexuals. While lesbianism is historically as well known as male homosexuality, it is only within the last two decades any attempts have been made to study it intensively. For this reason, the situation regarding the cause of lesbianism is less clear even than for male homosexuality.

This attempt to organize these theories derives from the saying that, "Some men are born great, some achieve greatness, and some have greatness thrust upon them." That can be paraphrased to read: Some people are born homosexual, some become homosexual because of their interaction with the environment (particularly their family) in their early developmental years, and some are made homosexual by seduction by an adult in adolescence. If this formulation is valid, it has important implications for those who wish help in changing their sex object preference. Currently, there is a growing public opinion, reflected in court decisions and legislation, which states no one has the right to involuntarily change the sexual orientation of any adult.

It is important to keep in mind the distinction between homosexual behavior and homosexuality. Homosexual peer group play is generally accepted as a normal stage in adolescent development. This may range from adolescents' *"goosing"* one another, or of rubbing each others' genitals while *"horsing around,"* through mutual masturbation to a relatively brief, but intense, affectionate and/or sexual affair. After adolescence, homosexual behavior may occur under conditions of prolonged, enforced separation from members of the opposite sex, as in the military service or in penal institutions. In the latter instance, the homosexual act may be the result of intimidation, coercion, or even force. Still other isolated acts of homosexuality may occur without being indicative of a basic homosexual orientation.

Another distinction that must be made is between *latent* and *overt* homosexuality. In the latent homosexual, the homosexual tendencies are more or less unconscious. That is, the individual is unaware he possesses such tendencies. (It has been claimed some homosexual tendencies are present in everyone.) At times these tendencies are kept unconscious only at the risk of distorted behavior. One very common example of this is the individual who over-reacts to a homosexual. "That dirty fag propositioned me, and I let him have it right in the face. I hope I broke the bastard's nose." This tremendous abhorrence of those who are overtly homosexual serves only to hide one's own latent tendencies from oneself. The defenses of latent homosexuals not infrequently break down under the influence of alcohol. When drunk they may initiate homosexual behavior, only when sober to be appalled at their own actions. (It must be clearly kept in mind that, in those states where homosexual behavior is prohibited, "I was drunk and didn't know what I was doing," is a frequent assertion of the *cruising* homosexual when arrested. (This phrase will be described later.)

The distinction between latent and overt homosexuality must also be differentiated from the distinction between the *closet* homosexual and the homosexual who has *come out*. The latent homosexual is truly unaware he is homosexual. He may successfully repress this knowledge all his life, or he may slowly become aware of his homosexual preference and engage in overt homosexual behavior. This overt behavior may still be kept secret from the world, except for his partners who are frequently anonymous. In that case he is a *closet* homosexual. He may acknowledge his homosexuality openly. Then he is said to have *come out*. This dissemination of the fact of homosexuality is usually limited to the gay world. With the current emphasis on the rights of the individual, homosexuals are more frequently proclaiming their status to society at large.

In spite of the fact the most important item in the development of gender identity is parental assignment of sex role, there are many boys who without discernible cues from the environment display feminine mannerisms from the moment they are able to respond. As they develop, they prefer to play with girls rather than with boys. They shun rough games and sports. They walk and talk in a girlish way. This is in spite of the fact that their parents wanted a boy, treat him as a boy, and do everything in their power to make him more *manly*. These children are not confused about their gender identity. They are well aware that they are boys. They are also aware that they do not want to be. They are removed only a short distance from the transsexuals on the already mentioned continuum of transvestism, homosexuality, transsexuals. These are the born homosexuals.

This does not mean effeminate males are necessarily homosexuals, any more than rugged, athletic *"he-men"* are necessarily heterosexual. It simply says there is a group of males who not only have effeminate mannerisms but who also are interested primarily in males as sexual objects throughout life. The statement some males are born homosexual would seem to be supported by the biological data as to the effect of sexual hormones on the developing embryo. However, until recently, the final proof was lacking, namely a demonstration of the difference between homosexuals and heterosexuals in sex hormones circulating in the blood or the presence of the broken down products of these hormones excreted in the urine. With the use of newer techniques, it has been demonstrated there is a difference in ratios of various fractions of circulating hormones in certain homosexuals. The ratios of these hormones found in some homosexual males is almost identical with that found in the heterosexual female. These findings are still to be confirmed by other investigators.

The second group of homosexuals was stated to be those who achieve homosexuality in their reactions to their environment during the critical developmental years of early childhood. It has been difficult to make other than theoretical statements about these individuals, since no one person has had the opportunity to study development of a significant number of homosexuals in depth. One attempt to circumvent this problem of too few subjects was made by Bieber and those associated with him in the study. A number of psychoanalysts pooled their findings in 106 people who were under treatment because they wished to change their sexual object preference from homosexual to heterosexual. The most frequent common features found in the developmental history of these people were the presence of a close-binding, intimate (CBI) mother and a cold, distant, rejecting father. Under these circumstances, it is much easier for a boy to identify with his mother.

A second theory identifies the mother as being dominating, punitive, and symbolically castrating. According to this theory, the boys fears the mother and, by extension, all women. Such men are said to fantisize the vagina having teeth that will bite off the penis. (Almost all theories hold that some fear of women plays a role in homosexuality.)

The most widely held theory about developmental homosexuality is based on Freud's original formulations. This theory holds that, in normal development, the boy becomes sexually attracted to his mother at some time during the fourth to sixth year of life. At the same time he fears (in fantasy) his father's jealousy of this rival. This fear is that his father will castrate him should he find out about the desire for the mother. The normal solution of this dilemma is to give up the mother as a love object, identify with the father, love the mother through him, and then have a woman of his own later in life. If the father is rejecting, punitive, or distant, then the boy cannot identify with the father and must renounce not only his mother but all women. If the mother is CBI, then he is also in more danger of identifying with her. These, then, are some of the ways homosexuality is achieved.

It was mentioned that homosexual play is usual in adolescents. For the individual who has done a good job of solving the problem of the family drama (this is the well-known Oedipal conflict), this adolescent homosexuality is just another stage in the progress towards heterosexuality. For those who have been unable to resolve the Oedipal conflict, this adolescent homosexual play may confirm their homosexuality. If those people who have had difficulty in solving the Oedipal conflict do not by chance become involved in adolescent homosexuality they may become unconscious (latent) homosexuals.

One other possible pathway to male homosexuality remains. This is the path frequented by those referred to as having homosexuality thrust upon them. Here, too, a special predisposition is necessary. This is not necessarily an incomplete resolution of the Oedipal complex. This is more apt to happen in the adolescent who realistically feels unloved and unwanted in his own home, who usually has few if any close friends among his peers, and who is then seduced homosexually by a male adult. For such a youngster, the important thing is the warmth and affection which he has never experienced in the past. In an attempt to achieve this feeling of acceptance, he continues to repeat the homosexual experience. Interestingly, in these instances, when adulthood is reached the preferred sexual objects of such a male are adolescent boys. It is almost as though he were forced to duplicate the entire experience throughout life. (When an adolescent female in the same circumstances, that is craving warmth and affection, is seduced by an older male, the experience predisposes her to promiscuity. As yet, little is known of the reaction of an adolescent girl who is the subject of homosexual seduction by an older woman.)

A clear distinction must be made between the behavior of this type of seduced adolescent male and the behavior of the exploitative male adolescent. Many male adolescents have sexual relationships with adult males strictly for financial gain. It is not at all uncommon then for the adolescent to blackmail the adult. Another fairly frequent practice is to lure the adult to an area where he can be jumped by the adolescent's friends, beaten *to teach him a lesson,* and then rolled. The adolescent remains secure in the knowledge he will not be reported to the authorities because of the resultant embarrassment and humiliation to the victim, not to mention the risk he runs of being accused of contributing to the delinquency of a minor. These assumptions of the adolescent are generally correct. Such adolescents are generally firmly heterosexual in their basic orientation. They do have severe character defects.

It must be stressed again that this brief review of the causes of homosexuality does not cover all the theories of homosexuality. (For example, the long held view that all people are basically bisexual has not even been mentioned.) It has reduced the theories offered to the most basic terms. It affords a simple framework on which to construct a larger knowledge.

The nature of the type of homosexual behavior does not bear any relationship to the cause (with the possible exception of the forced choice of an adolescent object by those who have had homosexuality thrust upon them). There are many popular myths and misconceptions about homosexuality which should be dispelled. All homosexual males do not look and act like *queens,* nor all lesbians like *butches.* The most masculine-appearing men may be homosexual, the most masculine-appearing women heterosexual. There is no correspondence between the role taken in the relationship, i.e. dominant or submissive, and the role taken in sexual behavior, i.e. active or passive. Homosexuals are not by nature more promiscuous than are heterosexuals. It is quite true that hit and run homosexual activity is much more common than the same sort of heterosexual behavior. (The latter is certainly increasing as public attitudes toward promiscuity change and contraception is more widely used.)

Similarly, the amount of homosexual *cruising,* i.e. moving from one spot to another looking for a one night stand, would certainly lessen if it were not for all the factors which presently make secrecy and anonymity essential. These factors include public revulsion, fear of blackmail, police harassment, fear of loss of job. (There are some exceptions to this. Certain males seem to be almost compulsive in this cruising activity and some have been known to achieve eight to ten relationships in a day.) Even in the face of these factors, there are many stable relationships carried on over a number of years. Many writers are of the opinion that more stable relationships would be the case if public and legal attitudes toward homosexuality changed, and if, as in heterosexual marriages, some form of divorce preceded dissolution of the relationship.

In any urban area, specific places become known as gay territory. Many bars have an almost exclusively homosexual clientele. (Almost all the heterosexuals present are there either as voyeurs or dabblers in homosexual behavior.) Many of these bars have suggestive names, "The Open Closet," "The Come On Out Club," "The Gayety." Many feature female impersonators, run beauty contests, and affairs of like ilk. Others are conservative and decorous. Turkish baths, public toilets, certain streets, and particular areas of specific parks may become almost exclusively homosexual hangouts. Arrests for loitering are not uncommon in these areas. Another police device is to make the first approach, go to a secluded spot, not uncommonly the defendant's car, lead the talk vaguely to sexual matters, and as soon as any bodily contact is made, e.g. the defendant places a hand on the officer's thigh, an arrest is made for soliciting or importuning. Not uncommonly, if such a case comes to trial it is thrown out of court because of the behavior of the officer. As a general rule, the defendant will plead guilty in the hope of keeping his name out of the papers. Under the influence of the Gay Liberation Movement and The Mannichean Society, more and more such cases are being brought to trial.

The role of the corrections worker in these matters of homosexuality will be included in greater detail when their role in relationship to sexual offenses in general is discussed at the end of these two chapters. Here, one thing will be stressed. That is the danger of suicide in the case of the middle aged homosexual, on presentence status following his first arrest, and terribly ashamed and afraid of what revelation might do to his career. (It has been my customary experience that, unless the individual involved is a public figure and subject to a news story, the media do not feature such stories.) This possiblity of suicide, however, must be on the correction worker's mind when doing a presentence examination, and it should be gentle, supportive, and reassuring. The following is an example from one of my earlier cases in this field; I have encountered many since.

> Mr. A.D. was a forty-seven-year-old, single, white male. He had never been interested in women and had no known homosexual interests. He was a research chemist in a large industrial firm and had a steady work record. He was a devout Christian and attended church twice weekly. His chief hobby was Civil War history, and he had a large collection of memorabilia of this period. He was devoted to his nieces and nephews. One of the latter had just turned sixteen and was on

summer vacation between his junior and senior years in high school The uncle asked to take him on a four-week trip around the famous battle fields of the Civil War. They had a fabulous trip. Everything had gone without incident until the last night. On the way home the uncle induced the nephew to engage in mutual masturbation. (There had been no previous solicitation.) The nephew felt troubled by this and about two weeks later reported it to his mother, the chemist's sister.

It so happened that there had been a falling out over their mother's estate. The sister did not feel she had received her fair share. She reported the episode to the police. The uncle was charged and pled guilty. Under then existent Ohio law, it was mandatory for him to undergo examination by three psychiatrists. I happened to be one of them. In our unanimous opinion, this man was a latent homosexual. We believed this urge had broken through under the stress of the daily close contact for a month with a desirable sex object, and that up until that time it had been well sublimated in work and hobbies. Indeed it may even never have reached consciousness in the past. It was also our unanimous opinion that incarceration had nothing to offer this man, that he was not dangerous to the community, that he was not in need of treatment, and that the only purpose of probation would be to reinforce his own wish to never be in a similar situation again.

Unfortunately, at that time it was the practice of psychiatrists to dismiss the defendant while they discussed their findings and recommendations. All he was told was that a report would be sent to the court. His trial was scheduled for a Tuesday morning. When he did not show up, those who were sent to look for him found him hanging from a rope in his garage. He had hung himself Monday night.

A very few words about types of treatment. For those who are "born homosexual" it would appear that little can be done. Certainly, past efforts with hormonal treatment have been useless. It may be that some day specific hormonal changes can be identified and such treatment could be successful if initiated early enough in life. There are also some preliminary reports that suggest behavior modification techniques may be successful if used in early adolescence. These involve many techniques other than the usual positive reinforcement or aversive conditioning. They may include training in changing gait, mannerisms, and speech patterns from feminine to masculine, as well as self-assertiveness training. Positive results have been reported in a few cases with these methods.

For those who "achieve homosexuality," depth therapy, usually psychoanalytic, is generally recommended. Bieber and his group claim a large proportion of success in these cases.

For those who have homosexuality "thrust upon them," the outlook is much more favorable. Individual psychotherapy directed toward the basic feelings of loneliness and rejection and more acceptable ways of satisfying these feelings is the usual method employed. In these individuals, group therapy has also proved highly successful, both in completely homosexual groups or in groups with differing sexual orientations. Currently, the entire question of the ethics of attempting to force sex orientation change are being widely discussed. While these questions do have tremendous moral connotations, and are certainly significant from that point of view, they would appear at present to be largely academic. It is generally agreed that the greatest single factor bearing on successful treatment is the degree of motivation for treatment.

LESBIANISM

This imprecise knowledge about the origin of male homosexuality is clear and definite in comparison to our knowledge of the causation of Lesbianism. This gets its name from the ancient Greek poetess, Sappho, who lived about 600 BC on the Island of Lesbos, about which it was written, "Oh burning isle of Lesbos, where Sappho loved and sang." While the incidence of lesbianism is generally placed at about one-half that of male homosexuality, it may be much higher. There is increasing awareness that many married women may be basically homosexual and may have homosexual experiences throughout their marriages. While society, as presently constituted, actively denounces homosexuality, it practically ignores lesbianism. Almost everyone who writes on this subject mentions girls may be tomboys with no questions asked, while boys who are girlish are called sissies and their masculinity questioned. Women may walk arm in arm, may even kiss each other on the lips in public, may live together for years, and no eyebrows are raised. Men indulging in similar behavior have serious questions asked (at least by gossips) about the nature of their relationship. It is also assumed a thirty-nine-year-old childless, still unmarried woman is that way through no choice of her own; a man in similar circumstances is thought of either as a hermit, a Don Juan, or gay. Sometimes the last two are synonymous in that Don Juanism may be a cover for either overt or unconscious homosexuality.

Similarly, it is very difficult to explain lesbianism on the basis of any of the theories advanced about the male homosexual. Attempts to utilize classic Freudian analytic theory have always seemed to require some of the historical facts to be distorted or rationalized to fit the theory, or else the theoretical speculations have to be strung so thin that they no longer can stand logical scrutiny. A new theory is that the movement toward women's liberation has made more women knowledgeable as to the opportunities available to them. Indeed, in some instances this theory has suggested homosexual behavior is politically (in the sense of male versus female) determined. It has been postulated a fear of males must underlie female homosexuality just as a fear of females is said to be a basis for male homosexuality.

As far as overt behavior is concerned, it ranges from kissing and fondling, caressing the breasts, through *tribadism* (mutual approximation and friction of the genitalia) and mutual masturbation, to cunnilingus. The use of an artificial penis (or *dildo*) in interfemale relationships is far less frequent in reality than in the general imagination. One of the behavioral differences between female and male homosexuals is that once a female pattern has been set it continues to be repeated, in contrast to male behavior where a variety of sexual activity is constantly sought. It should be noted that bisexuality (or at least the appearance thereof) is much simpler in females than in males. A female may simulate her role in heterosexual relations. Many homosexual males are completely impotent with women. For this reason, while no accurate statistics are available, it is beginning to be generally believed there are more female bisexuals than males. Whether the primary orientation of these females is primarily homosexual is not known. It has been suggested that the *swinging* represents a way of compensating for unsatisfactory marital sexual relations. A married woman may have a close female friend without arousing suspicion. Her husband would strongly question such a close relationship with a male.

Changing sexual attitudes have also made it more common for women to attend gay bars. I personally am not aware of exclusively female gay bars, although they may exist. The homosexual woman is more comfortable in the presence of the homosexual male than in the presence of the heterosexual. Less is expected of her. I am not aware of female homosexuals being arrested for deviant sexual practices unless these are in public.

Possibly the question currently asked most frequently about the female homosexual is whether her behavior has any effect on her children. Can a homosexual mother raise normal children, or will she inevitably warp their sexual development? This question has not been answered definitely to anyone's satisfaction. From the legal point of view there are mothers known to be lesbian who have been awarded custody of their children. Similarly, this same reason (lesbianism) has been used to deny a woman custody. The same factors seem to be of significance as have been utilized in determining if the male homosexual may have visitation and companionship rights with his children. The important factor is: Is the homosexual behavior or attitude flaunted by the parent? In one classic case, a father was denied companionship rights to his son after it had been demonstrated that the son had been required to march in a Gay Liberation parade while carrying a sign. Another case in point involved the rights of two homosexual women to retain custody of their children if they were to live together. Each had custody but was told the children would be removed if they cohabited.

Only two verifiable statements may be made about the treatment of the female homosexual. Studies as to treatment methods are extremely few in number and are contradictory as to methodology to be employed. Hopefully, this will be remedied in the future, although, with the changing attitudes toward both male and female homosexuality, the probability grows that fewer and fewer people will come for treatment for sexual orientation disturbance. The women's liberation movement is making a definite impact on sexual role stereotypes. No one can predict with any certainty what effect this impact, as well as the more permissive attitudes toward homosexuality, will have on young children, now and in the future.

VOYEURISM (302.5)

Voyeurism (302.5) is the need to observe members of the opposite sex while they are undressing, nude, or are engaging in some form of sexual activity. Voyeurism must have existed long before the exploits of Lady Godiva and Peeping Tom stamped it indelibly on the mores of mankind as an offense. As in so many other sexual deviations, the need to peep is almost entirely a masculine preoccupation. From the theoretical viewpoint, it is rather difficult to determine why this should be. Most of the common explanations for voyeurism might be considered to apply to females as well as males. One explanation holds voyeurism is the result of an unsatisfied desire of early childhood to know what went on behind the closed door of the parents' bedroom. The transition to voyeurism is the result of parents' unwillingness to answer the curious child's questions about sex. This leaves the child with a constant need to know. According to this theory, this sexual curiosity is the forerunner of all curiosity. The famous scientist is simply satisfying this curiosity in an acceptable way.

The second theory holds voyeurism, like its opposite, exhibitionism, is a regression to the normal childhood developmental stage of show and look: the boy and girl looking at each others' genitals and finding pleasure and excitement in that experience. This theory holds that stress in later life may cause a regression to this childhood stage. As might be expected, voyeurism and exhibitionism (the need to show) are considered two sides of the same coin and frequently coexist.

Certainly, whatever the theoretical cause, some degree of voyeurism is present in most of us, at least in most males. The striptease, the girlie magazines, and the blue movies could not flourish if it were not for these voyeuristic tendencies. An extremely interesting way of looking at voyeurism has recently been proposed in Scandinavia. This is to the effect that the voyeur is not immediately excited by the scene he sees. The scene is imprinted on his mind to be taken home and rerun as a film or video tape. Then it serves as a stimulus for masturbatory activity, and the *film* can be run over and over again. In support of this thesis, it is pointed out arrests for voyeurism have diminished to the vanishing point since pornography has become legal in those nations. It is no longer necessary for the voyeur to imprint a scene on his brain cells; he can buy it in the store, take it home with him, and use it whenever desirable.

Voyeurism belongs in the category of nuisance offenses. It is very rare for a voyeur to do more than peep, and if he is about to be detected, he will run. There are, however, a small percentage of voyeurs who progress to relatively serious sex crimes, including rape and rather brutal murders. In a history of a large number of these individuals, nonsexual offenses particularly breaking and entering will be present. As was noted in the general discussion on sexual deviations, breaking and entering can be considered symbolic of rape.

Although as a general rule voyeurism is a nuisance offense, it is naturally frightening to see a face peeping in a window when the intentions of the peeper are unknown. In actuality, the voyeur is in far more danger of being harmed by being shot, breaking a leg climbing a fence, or breaking a neck running into a wire in the dark, than any danger he poses to the person peeped at. In two of the voyeurs who have been seen by me, the nuisance aspect of their peeping was extremely traumatic psychologically to the victims. One of these males was a teenager; the other a man in his mid-twenties. In each instance, merely looking through a window at a woman undressing, or a couple making love, was not enough. Each was under a compulsion to climb through the window of a sleeping woman and pull the bedding from her, hoping to see her naked. Naturally, the woman awakened frightened. This initial reaction of fright was sufficient to have the peeper leave the house without uttering a word. The incident was even more frightening to the victim in the case of the older man who was always nude himself and was generally partially intoxicated. He gained a good deal of newspaper notoriety as "the peeled peeper" or the "nude dude." Each was caught and in each instance the real motive was to frighten the victim. The older man was just as much an exhibitionist as a voyeur. In each of these two instances, the psychological motivation was much more complex than in either of the theories advanced. In each instance there was a real hostility toward women in general. With such individuals, there is a realistic fear that at a later date this form of voyeurism might go on to more active types of sexual assaults.

As with exhibitionism, voyeurism is frequently a compulsion, and no amount of incarceration, without treatment, will help to control it. There is not too much the corrections officer *per se* can do for the voyeur. Certainly, his attitude should not be punitive but understanding. He is, however, an officer of the justice system, and all his efforts should be directed to helping reinforce the prohibitions of the law, while strengthening the need to seek help and to continue with that help until the problem is solved.

EXHIBITIONISM (302.4)

It is necessary to differentiate the sexual deviation **Exhibitionism (302.4)** from the associated offense, indecent exposure. Exhibitionism is a specific sexual deviation in which there is a need to expose the genitalia as a sexual end in itself. It would appear that it is confined entirely to males. Indecent exposure is the offense which results when the genitals are exposed in public. Women have been arrested for indecent exposure when they appear nude in a burlesque theater or go-go-bar. Sometimes the offense is named lewd and lascivious behavior or an offense against public decency. Possibly, the presence or absence of a G-string or pasties makes the difference. In men, indecent exposure may be the result of drunkenness, of many of the deteriorating conditions which have been discussed (schizophrenia, epileptic deterioration, organic brain syndromes or various sorts), or of exhibitionism. Indecent exposure is the most common sexual offense, and exhibitionism is the most common sexual deviation (if homosexuality is no longer considered a deviation).

Because of the compulsive nature of the behavior, indecent exposure has the highest recidivism rate of all sexual offenses. The actual rates of recidivism vary in different studies, but most studies agree the rate is higher for second offenders than for first and is still higher after the third offense. Exhibitionists are also apt to have nonsexual offenses in their records. Age of onset seems to have twin peaks, one at fifteen and one by the mid-twenties. Exhibitionists as such are rarely subject to other sexual deviations with the possible exception of voyeurism. Occasionally, on examination, the masturbatory fantasies of some exhibitionists are found to be extremely brutal and sadistic. When this is the case, the possibility of later and more traumatic sexual behavior must be considered. The thesis has been advanced that when an act is done in fantasy it is rarely carried out in reality. This is a dangerous assumption. In the author's experience, many aggressive acts have been carried out many times in fantasy prior to being acted on in reality. In one such exhibitionist, the aggression was eventually turned against himself and he committed suicide. The probation officer should ask routinely about the nature of masturbation fantasies when doing a presentence report on exhibitionists.

Exhibitionism is generally thought of as a nontraumatizing offense. However, if the objects of the exhibition are children, psychological trauma may result. It has been stated repeatedly the aim of the exhibitionist is to shock, and unless he gets some reaction from his victim, the act is not satisfactory. Like most generalizations about human sexuality, there are many exceptions. For most exhibitionists, the mere act of exposing the genitalia is an end in itself regardless of the effect on the viewer. Another generalization which is not true is that all exhibitionism is accompanied by or followed by masturbation. This belief may have arisen from observations of the behavior of deteriorated schizophrenics on the back wards of mental hospitals in bygone years. In these individuals, the exposure was incidental to the masturbation, rather than the masturbation being an integral part of the exposure.

There are many reasons for exhibitionism. Undoubtedly, some exhibitionists are fixated at the "look and show" level of sexual development which was discussed in voyeurism. In the cases I have seen, these people are in the minority. A far more important factor is doubt about masculinity. The following example is chosen because this element is so obvious.

Mr. A.E. sought professional help after being arrested for indecent exposure. Although this was his first arrest, he had exposed himself many times before. The pattern was always the same. He would be in his car and stopped at a stop light. Just as the light changed he would raise himself in his seat to expose his erect penis to a woman or women. He would almost wave it at them and then drive on. Only one sort of woman was so honored. She must have grey hair.

Mr. A.E. was twenty-six years of age, married, a successful automobile mechanic, the father of two children. He was the only boy in a family of four children. His father was a rather distant man, busily occupied with two jobs. He taught automobile repair at a vocational high school and worked in a local garage afternoons and evenings and through the summer. Mr. A.E.'s mother was a rigid, perfectionistic, belittling woman. At no time, from boyhood to the time of his arrest, did she ever give him any praise. Her constant refrain was, "You'll never be the man your father is." Mr. A.E. had gone to the school where his father taught, but had carefully avoided automobile repair. He had learned printing. He was drafted in to the Army immediately after his graduation from high school. In one of those ironic twists so common in the military service, he had been assigned to a motor pool, sent to truck repair school, and then back to the pool. By the time the war was over he had risen to the rank of Staff Sargeant, in large measure because of his excellence as a mechanic. When he got home and showed his stripes, his mother remarked, "You wouldn't have gotten that far if they hadn't known who your father was."

Mr. A.E. married shortly after his return from the service. From time to time his wife would chide him about not earning enough money. Once in a while she let him know he was not the world's greatest lover. One day after such an episode, he exposed himself. From then on a pattern developed in which, following a putdown by his wife, he would expose himself. The meaning of his behavior was self-evident. By exposing himself to older women he was in effect saying to his mother (and his wife), "Look at me, I'm just as good a man as my father ever was."

The reason for all exhibitionistic behavior is not so obvious. In some instances exposure is a response to stress, particularly if failure is involved. It is almost as though there is a need to regress to a childhood reaction. In those instances, where an expression of shock from the victim is a necessity for the offender, there is a combination of unconscious hatred of women and the need to assert masculine dominance. Exhibitionists are generally described as timid, nonassertive people. In agreement with other observers, I have often noted that most exhibitionists have an ambivalent feeling about the mother and are rather distant from the father.

The most common explanation given for his behavior by the exhibitionist himself is he was using this as a means of introduction to a woman. In most cases this is either "rationalization" (a mechanism in which unconscious irrational behavior is made to appear plausible) or an obvious con. To now, I have yet to meet an exhibitionist who actually attracted a woman successfully in this way. There are instances, however, in withdrawn, inadequate individuals, at times schizoid, in which this explanation is a true one. The cases of A.B. and A.C. cited in Chapter 10 exemplify this.

Many times exhibitionism seems to be as much impulsive as compulsive. In most individuals who exhibit themselves the final diagnosis would appear to be sexual deviation, exhibitionism. There are rare individuals in whom exhibitionism is just one of a multiplicity of deviant sexual behaviors. This ability to engage in all forms of sexual deviation is referred to as *polymorphous perverse* sexuality. In some instances, exhibitionism is a manifestation of *pedophilia* (sexual desire for children), which will be discussed in detail in the next chapter. Under those circumstances, exhibitionism is not an end in itself but serves as a prelude to sexual behavior with the child.

If indecent exposure is the result of an underlying deteriorating condition, then the psychiatric condition must be treated where possible. If it is incident to alcoholism, then that must be corrected. Where the indecent exposure is the result of exhibitionism, then treatment of the exhibitionism is in order. It is important to differentiate between the indecent exposure happening as an incidental aspect of acute intoxication and the exhibitionism occurring in an individual who is intoxicated.

Both group and individual therapy have been used successfully in the treatment of exhibitionism. The number of exhibitionists who express relief over being apprehended is amazing. The sincerity of these expressions can be determined by the motivation to continue treatment. Therapy in a group of fellow exhibitionists usually gets off to a good start, because it is a relief to know that this particular impulse is shared by others and does not imply being *crazy*. One of the most recent techniques employed is based on behavioral modification. This consists of making the individual expose himself to a woman, who, as a member of the treatment team, completely ignores the act. Success has been reported with as few as one such exposure. A colleague has frequently told of a spontaneous cure of one of his patients who exposed himself to the office nurse while waiting to see him. Her response was to say, "Who do you think you're going to impress with that little thing?" He was reported never to have exposed himself again. If done deliberately, such treatment would seem to be a little cruel, since, as noted, the exhibitionist is very apt to suffer from doubts about his own masculinity. Individual psychotherapy leading back to the childhood roots of the behavior has also been reported as successful.

As in voyeurism, incarceration does little to stop the exhibitionist from continuation of his behavior after confinement. The recidivism rate in first offenders is reported to be between 10 and 20 percent. Certainly, the remaining 80 percent of nonrecidivists do not all undergo treatment. The presentence report of the probation officer may be of tremendous help in deciding which offenders should be candidates for treatment and those who will probably do well on probation. In this regard, it is extremely important that collateral interviews be done with the spouse or members of the family. (It is quite interesting that a majority of exhibitionists are married, and although they may blame the problem on the temporary unavailability of their wives as sexual partners, this is rarely found to be the case.) It is a general rule that a careful presentence report, if accompanied by a collateral interview, will serve to pinpoint the areas of stress most likely to precipitate a return to the show-and-tell period of childhood. A prolonged period of probation, with joint efforts by the probation officer, the probationer, and the probationer's spouse to avoid or alleviate these periods of stress, will frequently be all that is necessary for a successful outcome. Group treatment is indicated where doubts about masculinity and feelings of inadequacy appear to be the cause. Individual psychotherapy is certainly indicated where any aggressive components are seen, and then the probation officer may well ask for psychiatric examination to confirm his fears. Most important in any successful work with the exhibitionist is the avoidance of belittlement, embarrassment, and shaming, unless done deliberately as a behavior modification technique.

Chapter 12

SEXUAL DEVIATIONS
(PART TWO)

GENERAL CONSIDERATIONS

U P to this point, the sexual deviations which have been considered may or may not be offenses. If they are, they are generally nuisance offenses and become traumatizing ones only under special circumstances. This Chapter will discuss those deviations which are universally offenses, and generally result in trauma to the victim. At one extreme are those offenses in which the trauma is more apt to be psychological than physical, i.e. pedophilia and incest; at the other extreme are such offenses as sexual mutilation and lust murder. There are multiple theories as to the causes of these conditions. Many of these theories are highly speculative. As in Chapter 11, theoretical speculations will be included only when they seem to have some practical value.

PEDOPHILIA (302.2)

Pedophilia (302.2) literally means "love of children." The offense corresponding to the sexual deviation, pedophilia, is *child molestation.* Mohr, Turner, and Gerry in their book *Pedophilia and Exhibitionism,* give the best operational definition of this condition that I have come across. They refer to it as, *"The expressed desire for immature sexual gratification with a prepubertal child.* According to the sex of the child, we can distinguish between *heterosexual pedophilia* and *homosexual pedophilia,* and in cases where there is no differentiation in the sex of the object, we use the term *undifferentiated pedophilia."*[1] It is important to recognize that a significant factor in

---

[1] Italics in the original.

determining whether the offense of child molestation has occurred is not only the age of the victim but also the age of the
offender. Thus, a fifteen-year-old boy, even if he has sexual
relations with a twelve-year-old girl, would not be considered
to have committed child molestation. It is usually conceded
that at least a five year gap should attain, while Mohr et al. feel
a seven to ten year gap would be preferable.

There are several myths about pedophilia which should be
dispelled immediately before any further discussion of the subject. The first is the myth of the stranger. There are a small
proportion of children who are molested by strangers, but by
far the largest percentage of offenders are males known to the
victims. (The pedophile is almost universally male. In my entire forensic practicer I can remember examining only two females with this deviation. Interestingly, in these cases, the
female is almost never charged with child molestation, but
rather with contributing to the delinquency of a minor. In each
instance, the female was well known to the boy.) If the results
of various studies are combined, only about 12 percent of offenders were complete strangers to the children. As might be
expected from this, the majority of offenses take place in the
vicinity of the victim's home, if not in the home itself. The
final myth which needs debunking is that the aim of the pedophile is coitus. The definition offered speaks of "immature
gratification." Thus, in cases of heterosexual pedophilia the
most common forms of sexual expression are caressing, fondling, and at times oral-genital contact.

This last statement may not be made so positively in homosexual pedophilia. In that condition orgasm *is* sought by the
offender, and all forms of homosexual practices may be utilized. Anal intercourse with a child, however, is rare. Mohr et al.
report that orgiastic satisfaction is also a goal in undifferentiated pedophilia. As a usual rule, violence per se is not present
in pedophilia. The pedophile utilizes his acquaintance with
the victims to attain what measure of gratification he wishes: to
touch or be touched; to show or fondle; to kiss or be kissed
(whether orally or genitally); etc. When force is used, it is generally, although not invariably, by strangers. Generally,

although also not invariably, it involves anal intercourse with a pubescent boy, rather than penetration of an immature girl. When the latter takes place in pedophilia, the offender, with few exceptions, is either intoxicated or psychotic.

The intelligence of pedophiles is not different in any marked degree from that of the general public. This may range from moderately mentally retarded to superior intelligence. According to Mohr et al., the age of incidence of pedophilia has three peaks: the late teens, the mid to late thirties, and from fifty-five on.

Pedophilia in teenagers tends to develop in withdrawn, socially immature, sometimes mildly mentally retarded males, whose behavior in regard to little girls represents a fumbling sort of sexual curiosity which, because of their general inadequacy, they are unable to gratify with girls of a more suitable age. The prediction of recidivism in this group is uncertain. It would appear to depend as much on their future social maturation as on any other factor.

Mr. A.F. is an eighteen-year-old young man referred to the Court Diagnostic and Treatment Center after he had been seen caressing an eight-year-old girl in a field adjacent to a school that was quite close to where they were currently living. "They" is used advisably because the girl in question was the daughter of the offender's mother's boyfriend. The boyfriend had three children by a previous marriage. For about five months these four shared a trailer with A.F., his mother, and his nineteen-year-old sister. A.F. had an I.Q. of 55. He was repeating the tenth grade in a special class. On rare occasions he had been the childrens' babysitter. He had never actually dated. On two or three occasions he had gone to a drive-in with an eighteen-year-old girl whom he had met through his family. She had arranged these outings. She weighed over two hundred pounds. The client had kissed her on one or two occasions and he admitted it had stimulated him sexually.

The police report was meager and there was no presentence investigation available at the time A.F. was seen. According to his story they had been playing with a basketball at the school playground. She went into the field to chase the ball.

She then beckoned him to come over. when he did, she lay down and asked him to kiss her between the legs. He states he did so but stopped after a moment because it seemed silly. He heard nothing more about it until he went to the municipal courthouse to report on a totally unrelated case and was placed under arrest for child molestation.

The second age group (mid to late thirties) contains more married men than single ones. Neighborhood children are frequently the victims. Not uncommonly, the victim may be a stepchild or in-law, or less frequently, a natural child (see Incest later in this chapter). Generally, the incident occurs when the offender is drunk, unemployed (in contrast to just not having gone to work), and/or has had a serious disagreement with his wife.

Mr. A.G. was examined at the Court Diagnostic and Treatment Center at the request of the court. He was a thirty-seven-year-old, married, black, unemployed male who had been arrested for child molestation. Walking down the street, staggering might be a better word, he had spotted the twelve-year-old, mentally retarded, younger brother of a friend of his sitting on a porch. He beckoned the youngster across the street, and, on the pretense of wanting to show him something, lured him into the basement of a vacant home. With some force, he sodomized the boy twice. After A.G. had passed out, the boy returned home and complained to his mother. Hospital examination revealed tears in the boy's anus, and the mother went to the police. Mr. A.G. was found asleep in the basement where he had taken the boy. He professed to remember nothing about the episode, then insisted that the boy was lying. A.G. had an extensive record of nonsexual crimes. He was of average intelligence, unemployed, and was separated from his wife at the time of the offense.

Males in the older age group (from fifty-five on) almost unfailingly have suffered a recent loss of their wives, by death or divorce. They are lonely and may have some degree of organic deterioration. Usually, there will have been no previous offenses, either sexual or otherwise in their history; recidivism rate in this group is minimal.

A fourth group mentioned by Mohr et al. and well known to

all who write on this subject, as well as those who work in forensic settings, are the chronic child molesters. Sometimes these people are sexually polymorphous perverse, that is, capable of any form of sexual gratification or deviation, with no preference for any one particular model. Sometimes they are sexual opportunists who take advantage of any form of sexual gratification available. Others are true psychopathic offenders with long prison records for other offenses, who are sexually fixated on children. At times, pedophilia may be obviously learned behavior.

Mr. A.H. was a thirty-seven-year-old white male, single, the product of a rural environment. Intelligence testing revealed him to have an IQ of 67 (mildly mentally retarded) with native potential as a high borderline retardate. He had attended a two-room country school where he was not passed but assigned from one grade to the next, but never achieved much beyond a second grade level. When he was thirteen, while on noon break, some of the other boys played a practical joke on him and locked him in the outhouse with two little girls. When the children did not show up for the afternoon class, a search was instituted. Mr. A.H. was found with the girls. The principal was so angry he had him committed to one of the state institutions for the feeble minded. (It is assumed that his family, who were also familosocial retardates, were willing to have one less mouth to feed; at least they did not protest.) He remained at the institution until he was twenty-one years of age. He was sodomized and fellated shortly after his arrival.

Soon after his discharge he had an acute psychotic break and was sent to the area mental hospital. Within one month of admission he ran away and was discharged from the hospital books. Within two months he had kidnapped and sodomized a little boy. He was tried, found not guilty by reason of insanity, and sent to the state hospital for the criminally insane. Several years later, under a Federal Court ruling, the hospital was surveyed for those who had recovered and could be discharged, or if unrecovered were deemed untreatable. He was held to belong to the latter category, and was sent to a less restrictive facility; in this case it was the state hospital from which he had previously run away. He promptly ran away again. This time he made his way to one of the southern states where he succeeded in maintaining himself as a woodcutter for a year.

He got homesick around Christmas and came home. He got drunk and was again involved with a ten-year-old boy. Since the Federal Court order prohibited it, he was not returned to the state hospital for the criminally insane, but instead was sent back to the local mental hospital. Again he escaped and this time went to New York City. He got along well for a few months, mooching food and sleeping in the parks. With the onset of winter, he had himself admitted to the psychiatric unit at Bellevue Hospital, was transferred to one of the New York State hospitals, and then, under the Interstate Compact, went back again to his local state hospital. He immediately ran away and returned home. Since he seemed to be making a good adjustment there, he was allowed to remain.

He worked on a neighbor's farm as a hired-hand for a few months. One Saturday morning he got dressed, went into town, and after the liquor store opened he bought a bottle of rum. He took it to the park and drank most of it. He spotted two boys fishing and managed to persuade the ten-year-old to go with him. The eleven-year-old boy ran, but by the time he had notified anyone, A.H. and the boy had disappeared. They were found twelve hours later in an abandoned shanty, where A.H. had kept the boy a prisoner and had sodomized him twice.

He was returned to the state hospital for the criminally insane for examination for competency to stand trial. Apparently, in an effort to do what they thought best socially, they declared him incompetent and returned him to court for disposition at an appropriate facility. The local state hospital refused to take him back saying, rightly, they could not hold him and would not be responsible for his behavior. Two institutions for the mentally retarded refused to admit him on the grounds that his IQ was too high. The judge, in desperation, referred him to this clinic for a second determination as to his competency to stand trial. There was no question that he filled all the criteria for competency. Indeed, he went further and, while insisting that he knew what he did was wrong and that he could refrain from doing it if he had not been drinking, insisted that the state had made him the way he was and owed him treatment. Incidentally, he had had heterosexual relations only once, that being with a grown woman who was also a patient at the state hospital; she had been the aggressor. He thought it was kind of "pleasant", but he would "never have the nerve to ask a woman to do something like that on my own."

This case is cited along with others to demonstrate that simply making a diagnosis of pedophilia does not in any way illustrate the complexity of the situation. In this instance, Mr. A.H. might respond to some form of behavior therapy, possibly even of an aversive nature. This is all but forbidden by the laws of the state, out of fear that in the wrong hands it would lead to mind control. He might find some relief from his sexual needs from antihormonal therapy. This is experimental in this country and cannot be given without the individual's consent, although it has been used with some success abroad, notably in Scandanavian countries. Since he is institutionalized for a crime, he cannot legally give informed consent.

Corrections workers rarely have much contact with the victims in cases of child molestation. It is important their situation be discussed. The belief that the child is universally damaged psychologically is one of the common assumptions underlying the revulsion this act arouses. Neither this, nor the companion assumption that the child is always an unwilling victim, is necessarily true. Certainly, a pubescent male who has been forcibly assaulted, as in the victims of A.G. and A.H., will have suffered severe psychological, and possible physical, trauma and should receive psychiatric first aid. Where force has not been used, the degree of psychological damage depends on two factors. The first is the way the incident is handled immediately after its occurrence. Intense emotional reactions on the part of the parents, repeated questioning by police, unpleasant appearances and cross-examination in courtrooms may all be as traumatic or even more traumatic than the offense itself. The second and more important factor is the emotional health of the child and the family at the time the offense occurs. Repeated studies have shown that children who are emotionally stable at the time of the offense, and who come from families who themselves are stable, have few lasting undesirable effects from sexual episodes in childhood where force had not been used. When such effects do occur in these children, they are apt to be subtle and not severely disabling. More serious after-effects occur in those instances where the child has felt unloved and unwanted prior to the victimization. Some of these effects have already been discussed in Chapter 11 in the section on homosexuality. Where disorganized and chaotic conditions exist in the child's home at the time of the offense, the resultant effects may be much more drastic. Many of these children may become life long schizophrenics.

It is equally important to note that in some cases the child is the victim only in the legal sense. The child may have submitted willingly or passively or may even have initiated the sexual activity. This in no way minimizes the role of the offender, who theoretically should possess sufficient judgment to withstand the blandishments of the child. To cite my own experience, approximately 70 to 80 percent of those adults accused of child molestation assert the child made the first advances. Many of them protested it was only after repeated overtures on the part of the child that they succumbed. It has commonly been my experience, in those circumstances where I have had the opportunity to examine the child, the adult is right roughly 40 to 50 percent of the time. It is impossible to arrive at accurate statistics, but in my overall estimation, the "victim" has actually initiated the behavior about 25 percent of the time.

This aggressiveness on the part of the child has been commented on by others. It is generally conceded these seductive children (both girls and boys) are beyond average physical attractiveness and charm, and they come from disorganized homes in which they get little attention. The following case represents a rather extreme example of such a situation.

Mr. A.I. is a seventy-eight-year-old white male examined by a panel of three psychiatrists after having been found guilty of child molestation. He was a self-employed tailor who maintained a three-room apartment above his tailor shop. He was a Greek immigrant who spoke barely intelligible English. Fortunately, one of the examining psychiatrists was of Greek origin and could communicate with him adequately. Mr. A.I. had been a widower for three years. He had employed one of the neighborhood girls to come in once a week to clean his apartment. She had moved about six months before his arrest and had suggested one of her girlfriends would be glad to work for him. Mr. A.I. had accepted this offer without inquiring about the girlfriend's age. Mary, the new cleaning girl, was a pretty, vivacious, eleven-year-old. When she stopped in the shop each week for her money, she would always carry on a conversation with Mr. A.I. After several weeks she began to suggest he ought to come up and visit her while she was working, so he could tell her exactly what he wanted done.

After about three such visits he went up to his apartment one day to find her working in nothing but a pair of shorts. He suggested she put on her clothes, but instead she came over and sat on his lap and put her hand on his genital area.

There was no coital activity at that time, but mutual caressing, touching, and fondling went on for several weeks. At that time she began to ask for an increase in pay, and when he refused, she threatened to tell her mother. He panicked and for one week did give her more money. The next week, however, he told her that she was fired, and he was going to get another girl to do his cleaning. She informed her mother she had been molested, and charges were filed. It was the impression of the panel of psychiatrists that Mr. A.I. was telling the truth, and that he was guilty of an understandable error of judgment. A recommendation for probation was made and accepted by the court.

Fortuitously, about six months later I actually had the opportunity to examine Mary. She had been referred to the juvenile court for forging checks. Intelligence testing revealed mild mental retardation, but this was not apparent on casual conversation. Only eleven-years-old, she appeared fourteen or fifteen. She was physically attractive, charming, and appealing. Her family history revealed a pattern of abandonment, rejection, and neglect. Her father had long since left the family. One older sister had a long juvenile court record and had committed suicide. A thirteen-year-old brother was also involved in the check forging offense. Blame for the entire difficulty was placed on him, although there was a general suspicion that the mother had actually masterminded the forgery. Both children denied this. (The brother later admitted it to his social worker while at the rehabilitation center.) When talking with Mary in connection with the forgery, confirmation was received of her role in the involvement with A.I. Here, too, there was the definite suggestion the mother might have masterminded the situation.

In follow up, it might be noted all attempts on the part of the juvenile court worker to help Mary were futile. Her intense loyalty to her mother, who constantly exploited and rejected her, nullified all attempts at therapeutic intervention. Two years later, an action of the mother placed Mary in a double-bind situation, and it was necessary to admit her to the adolescent unit of the local mental health center, where a diagnosis of schizophrenia was made.

Role of the Corrections Worker in Pedophilia

In cases of pedophilia, one of the most important tasks of the corrections worker is to make recommendations to the court as to the probation of the offender. One of the most reliable aids on making such a recommendation is the likelihood of recidivism. The following figures have been taken from Mohr et al. They estimate that in heterosexual pedophilia, "The reconviction rate for first offenders would be between 5 and 8 percent." ". . . for previous sexual offenders, the repeater rate should lie around 20 percent, and for previous sexual and nonsexual offenders, around 30 percent. For homosexual pedophilia, the best estimate would be about twice these figures."

It is extremely difficult to make specific predictions from general statistics. Obviously from the above, a homosexual pedophile, particularly one who has previously committed nonsexual offenses as well, is a poor risk for probation. As to the remainder, it has been my general experience that adolescent child molesters tend to fall into two classes. The largest of these is made up of relatively withdrawn, bashful, emotionally immature youngsters. Their approach to a child is based on a combination of unsatisfied sexual curiosity and an inability to make a satisfactory sexual approach to their peers. Dissatisfaction about these factors may be augmented by the conversation of their peers or by pornographic material. This adolescent group responds to a combination of probation, with socialization and sexual education. (It might be pointed out that since the expected recidivism rate is less than 8 percent, this response might occur without the suggested rehabilitation plan.) The second group of adolescents consists of those in whom the offense seems to be highly impulsive and accompanied by force. Such adolescents should have a period of psychiatric observation to determine whether there is a more serious personality problem, or even a psychosis, underlying the offense. Certainly, a second offense in an adolescent should always indicate a thorough clinical evaluation.

In the middle age group, the presentence evaluation should include a thorough work-up for any factors which might be operative. Psychoses and/or organic conditions are rare in this group. Serious personality disorders may exist in about 25 percent. The conditions which emerge most frequently in the presentence evaluation are problem drinking and marital difficulties; not uncommonly they coexist. If the offender in this group does not have a serious personality disorder and this is his first offense, the probation officer may feel fairly comfortable in recommending probation. The worker should then attempt to secure help for both the marital and drinking problems.

In the so-called senile group, recidivism is extremely rare unless definite organic psychosis due to arteriosclerosis or senility is present. The case of Mr. F. described in Chapter 4 delineates the role of the probation officer quite fully.

The disposition of the chronic pedophile poses a difficult problem. In those states which have so-called *sexual psychopath* laws, these individuals are usually sent either to special institutions for the sex offender or to the state hospital for the criminally insane. They are extremely refractory to standard treatment modalities. The use of experimental treatment is sharply curtailed in this country because of possible interference in the offender's civil rights. Recent Federal Court rulings have held such offenders cannot be detained indefinitely in such institutions, unless it can be demonstrated that (1) they are treatable and (2) an active treatment plan can be implemented. Thus, they are either transferred to less restrictive facilities from which they escape (see case of A.H.) or else they are sent to penal institutions to serve the remainder of their sentence. In either instance, the great majority of such offenders return to the streets. In that case they will usually be in the custody of a parole officer.

Reports of attempts at outpatient treatment with this type of offender are conflicting, but generally discouraging. Group therapy, in a group of sexual offenders, seems to hold more promise than does individual therapy. The parole officer cannot be expected to act as a shadow for such an individual, but should insist on frequent reporting. The officer should precipitate unexpected encounters. Care should be taken that the offender does not take a job, either in a paid position or as a volunteer, which increases his exposure to children, such as school custodian, carnival worker, scout leader, maintenance worker, Little League coach, and the like. The parole officer should insist on strict abstinence from alcohol and drugs, particularly drugs of the stimulant group (see Chapter 21). There is one possibility to which the officer must always be alert. Cases have been reported in which children have been killed by this type of chronic offender, not in the commission of an assaultive rape or as part of a sadistic offense, but out of fear of apprehension and return to the penitentiary.

INCEST

The *American Heritage Dictionary* defines incest as, "Sexual union between two persons whose blood relationship is so close that their marriage is illegal or forbidden by law," While incestuous relationships undoubtedly occur between adults, the type of relationship which is of concern to the courts and to the corrections worker is that between an adult and a child. The adult involved may be father, uncle, grandfather, or sibling.

Stepfathers, adopted fathers, or foster fathers are involved with greater frequency than are natural parents. Such a relationship may not be incestuous but the same psychological connotations are present. Both homosexual and heterosexual relations may take place. An incestuous relationship between a mother and son is an extremely rare occurrence unless one or both are psychotic.

Incest represents a special form of pedophilia. There are important differences, however. In may instances there are strong bonds of mutual affection involved. While accurate statistics are unavailable, it would appear that, in at least 50 percent of the cases, the adult is under the influence of alcohol, at least during the early stages of the relationship. Sexual relations may go on for years, until the child leaves the home. At times successive girls in the family are involved as they become pubescent. At times the father uses the excuse that he is teaching his daughters the facts of life or that he is gentle and considerate in initiating them into sexual activity, whereas another male would be rough and uncaring.

One of the surprising things about such a relationship is that it can exist for so long with the mother seemingly oblivious. Investigation will frequently reveal the mother has been told by her daughter (or daughters) but has refused to believe it. Probably more frequently she has known for some time, but for her own purposes either has done nothing about it or has passively gone out of her way to foster it. The motives for this behavior are almost as varied as the women involved. The frigid mother may be glad to have her daughter relieve her of a sexual burden. It may be a way of holding onto her husband who is threatening to leave. It may be a weapon by which to blackmail her husband. The motivation may be completely unconscious, but the frequency with which the pattern emerges is amazing.

As for the girls, it is surprising how many do not protest, beyond the original statements to the mother. Here, too, the motivations are diverse. At times the girl enjoys the relationship, while simultaneously feeling guilty about both her enjoyment and her feelings of having displaced her mother. At times she may be unconsciously aware of the motives underlying the mother's seeming indifference and, out of loyalty to the mother, is reluctant to tell anyone else. At times, she may be afraid to say anything because of the father's threats, or, like the mother, she may hesitate to deprive the home of the breadwinner. At times her only possible recourse is through behavior designed to reveal the situation indirectly.

Certain patterns of behavior should alert the juvenile court worker to a silent plea for help. Such a pattern invariably denotes an impossible home situation, and at times the basic problem in this situation is an incestuous relationship which the juvenile is unable to report openly. The cue to such a situation is an offense committed with little attempt at concealment, at a time when a previous offense is still awaiting disposition or adjudication. This is particularly meaningful if the second offense occurs in the interval between the release from detention for the first offense and final disposition.

A.J. was a thirteen-year-old girl brought to the juvenile detention home by the police on a charge of purse snatching. She had seized the purse of a woman waiting in line at a check-out stand in a large supermarket. Because of the physical arrangement of the store, it was impossible for her to avoid apprehension. A.J. had been released from detention just two days prior to her current offense. She was awaiting adjudication for a similar offense, which occurred the day before her original detention. Naturally, she was detained at the time of the second detention hearing. She would give no plausible explanation for her behavior, she did not insist on being sent home, nor did she appear to be upset by being detained.

As this particular court applies the doctrine inherent in the Gault decision, no social investigation can be performed until after an adjudication hearing. There was a delay of several days before A.J. was found delinquent for the first offense. A probation counselor was assigned at that time. A.J. assured her counselor she was just trying to get money to buy new jeans. At a home visit, her parents volunteered no information which might explain A.J.'s strange behavior. The youngest child, she was described as having been a well-behaved girl who had given her parents no trouble. They denied any difficulties in their relationship with each other.

Everything was fine.

The counselor was not convinced. Something did not add up. She obtained the address of A.J.'s oldest sister, B., age nineteen, now living away from home. At first the sister corroborated the parents' story, but in response to the counselor's obvious sincerity and desire to be of help, she suddenly broke down and started to cry. The true story then emerged. Things had been going well at home until B. was about twelve years of age and A.J. six. The father became involved with another woman and wanted a divorce. The mother refused, ostensibly on religious grounds. The father finally gave up the other woman and remained at home, but the mother began to drink. B. did not know if the mother and father were still having relations with each other, but when she was seventeen, the father started making advances to her. She rebuked these overtures and reported them to the mother, who did nothing except to increase her drinking. It was at this time that B. left home.

A.J. had always been close to her father. Two weeks before her first detention she came to B. and told her that, from the time B. moved out, the father had been making advances to her. She, too, had informed her mother, but nothing had happened. Some two months before that conversation with B., A.J. had started having relations with her father. Although she implored B. for help, she swore her to secrecy because she did not want her father to go to prison. When B. had not found a solution, A.J. then tried to get herself arrested. Released from detention, she immediately repeated her offense. This was her attempt to solve her problem and be removed from the home without implicating her father.

Incestuous homosexual relationships between a father figure and a male child are generally not tolerated by the mother, once she is aware of the situation. Male children who are involved in homosexual relationships with father figures are much more apt to be psychologically damaged than are females.

A.K., twelve years old, is a case in point. His father, who was truly polymorphous perverse, had forced A.K., as well as his younger brother, to commit fellatio on him, and he had also practiced cunnilingus on the five-year-old daughter. The mother's reaction to this was to divorce the father without filing a child molestation charge or mentioning his behavior in her complaint. She continued to allow him to have visitation rights with the children, until he started dating an eighteen-year-old girl. This was apparently the last straw. She filed a complaint with the police. (As an aside, which throws some light on his personality structure, it might be mentioned that during his psychiatric examination, A.K.'s father bragged about his youthful fiancee. He finished his encomium with the remark, "She sends me. I'm a butt and breast man myself.")

A.K. had an acute schizophreniform psychosis and had to be hospitalized. Each time he seemed to be on the verge of recovery, his father would visit or phone, implying that once he was remarried he would take A.K. out of there. At that time the father was still awaiting disposition on the charge of child molestation. Even after the father's removal from the community, A.K.'s symptoms persisted.

It has generally been held that the psychological damage is less when the girl involved is still very young, or even prepubertal, as long as the mother is obviously condoning. In the latter instance, it would seem as though the mother's assent lessened the girl's feeling of guilt and made it easier for her to maintain her psychological equilibrium. As for those younger girls in whom actual intercourse has not taken place, the same factors mentioned in discussing the victim of pedophilia would seem to determine their future mental health. However, even when the family situation is stable and the child herself seems well-adjusted, there may be lesser degrees of further damage.

Mrs. A.L., a twenty-seven-year-old, married woman, the mother of three children, sought help with feelings of diffuse anxiety. For two years she had been suffering recurrent feelings that something terrible was bound to happen, some nameless doom hung over her. Although previously sexually responsive and receptive to all sorts of foreplay, she had, for this same two year period, become progressively disinterested in sex and was actually disgusted when her husband attempted to stimulate her genitals orally in foreplay. On discussing her life situation at the time of the onset of her symptoms, it was learned they had started about the time her uncle was released from a state hospital for the criminally insane. As she was urged to talk about this, the vague feeling emerged that she was somehow involved in his having been there. Repeated exploration brought forth the sudden memory that he had involved her in sex play when she was four years old, and this had been the reason for his commitment. When she become aware of the connection between her anxiety and his discharge, she commented that he had not attempted to contact her in these two years. At that point the anxiety attacks disappeared.

However, the frigidity and associated sexual symptoms persisted. Headaches began to replace the anxiety attacks. In the midst of a therapy session, while relating how close she had been to her aunt, this uncle's wife, she suddenly burst into tears. When she finally regained control, she related a vivid memory of a session with her aunt immediately after the trial. The aunt had turned on her, almost viciously, and accused her of being responsible for the uncle's behavior. This outburst had culminated in, "How in the world could you let him do that filthy thing to you?" The frigidity had commenced with the husband's first usage of oral-genital foreplay following the uncle's release. Conjoint therapy with the husband and wife rapidly alleviated her remaining symptoms.

One other form of incest occurs, probably with greater frequency than has been reported. This is incest between siblings. Except where there is a marked disparity in age of the two participants, this is dealt with by psychiatrists and social agencies with greater frequency than by the law.

Role of the Corrections Worker in Incest

As in pedophilia, making recommendations for disposition for incestuous offenders is an extremely difficult area for the probation officer. The problem is frequently compounded by the ambivalent, at times paradoxical, attitude of the wife. Where the incestuous experience has been homosexual, she frequently demands her husband be given the utmost penalty of the law. She is unable to understand "what got into the man," and how she "could ever have married such an animal." Further discussion will sometimes reveal it is the homosexuality, rather than the pedophilia or the incestuous nature of the pedophilia, which is so upsetting to her. On the contrary, if the relationship has been heterosexual, even if more than one daughter has been involved, the mother may fight to have her husband return to the home. If anyone should be removed from the home, she prefers it to be the daughters. (It is the author's impression that this is more frequent when the man is not the natural father of the girls, but a second or third husband.) In part this may be an attempt to assuage some of her own guilt. The mother's wishes to have her husband home must be balanced against the possibility of the children feeling that they are being punished when they are the ones removed.

In those cases in which the offender has served his sentence, is about to be released on parole, and is planning to return home with wife's blessing, it is incumbent on the parole officer to involve the Children's Services Board or Child Welfare Agency in an evaluation of the home before allowing him to return. The attitudes of the children to the return are of equal importance as those of the wife.

Juvenile court workers encounter a situation where incestuous feelings, rather than incestuous behavior, are present and influence the behavior of the girl. This is most apt to involve girls in their early adolescence. Two aspects of this situation are seen. In the one, the girl who has previously been a relatively obedient child, making a good adjustment at home, in school, and the community, suddenly seems to be in utter rebellion. She is particularly negativistic in relationship to her father, disregards his wishes, disobeys his commands, and almost seems to hate him. At the same time she becomes "boy crazy," sometimes to to the point of promiscuity. The dynamics here involve the sudden reactivation in early adolescence of the normal five or six-year-old's attraction to the father. This is now eroticized by the push of adolescent sexuality. The girl is frightened by this desire toward the father and must put as great a distance as possible between them. The situation is even more intense when the male involved is a stepfather, because the erotic wish is apt to be more conscious. Then, the rationalization is frequently brought into play, "You're not even my father, you have no right to tell me what to do." The parent, bewildered by the behavior, is apt to react in ways which increase the girl's rebelliousness, and eventually her behavior leads to court involvement.

The reverse of this situation occurs when it is the father who has to struggle against his own desires towards this budding sexual object, who used to be his little girl and sit on his lap. It is now apt to be more than just her lips that brush against him in the goodnight kiss. He has a great need to protect himself against the desires which arise within him. Projection is an easy defense to fall into. "All those guys out there are just waiting to get her, and it's my duty as a father to protect her." He, therefore, clamps down hard. He objects to every boy she brings to the house. He imposes unreasonable curfews. He finds innumerable, petty reasons to ground her. Under these conditions, many adolescent girls are driven to rebel, to become defiant, to sneak out, run away, or get involved in drugs. Eventually such a girl also finds herself in juvenile court.

Either of these situations are easily misinterpreted and can be compounded by improper handling. The alert worker can recognize them and be a tremendous help, either directly or by moving the family towards therapy.

RAPE

Rape is defined as sexual relations with another by force. Statutes vary from state to state. In some states, only vaginal intercourse with a female is recognized as rape. In some states, penetration is not necessary. In some states homosexual rape is called sodomy. (Except in pedophilia, homosexual rape is rare outside of penal and other institutions.) In all states, the general statutory intent is the same: to make it an offense to take sexual liberties with another without that person's consent. Rape is not listed as a sexual deviation in *DSM II*. Absence of such a listing implies there is no specific condition which can be labeled "rapism," unlike those conditions labeled exhibitionism, voyeurism, fetishism, etc.

This does not mean that psychiatrists have not been interested in rape as a form of deviant human behavior. Many articles have been written in psychiatric journals about the nature of the act, the personality and motivations of the rapist, and the nature and personality of the victim. At one time a perusal of the psychiatirc literature would almost have conveyed the impression the victim had as much unconscious motivation to be raped as the rapist had motivation to perpetrate the act. Fortunately, that viewpoint has largely been abandoned. There are a small proportion of victims who do appear to "be asking for it," by frequenting potentially dangerous places at inappropriate times, by accepting rides from strangers met in a bar, or on the street. The great majority of the victims, however, have little to say in their choice as objects, The current thrust of psychiatric preoccupation with the victim has to do with minimizing the psychological trauma inflicted on her. It is hoped that support systems will be set up in each community, commencing with the moment of examination at the hospital, going through the report to the police and their investigation, to the trial and its aftermath.

It was stated in the introduction to Chapter 11 that rape is more an act of aggression than it is a sexual act. This is certainly true in those rapes which occur as byproducts of a felony; breaking and entering and armed robbery are the two most common of these. It is also true when the victim is terrorized and badly beaten. In many instances, rape is an assertion of male domination; the prevailing motive is to make the woman submit. This is particularly true if the question of *machismo* is involved. In many of these instances, the woman will be forced to perform acts whch may be repugnant to her, such as fellatio, or to submit to anal intercourse. Cohen and Seghorn,[2] in their discussion of those offenders in whom the act of rape is viewed as another aspect of aggression report the very surprising and otherwise unreported finding that these individuals show the fewest ego defects and the most adequate social and occupational histories. They also state that the recidivism rate for rape is very low in such males. This is surprising in view

---

[2]As abstracted in the Sandoz, "Psychiatric Spectator".

of the fact that previous convictions for aggressive offenses increase the possibility of recidivism of offenders involved in other sexual deviations. Such aggressive behavior is also thought by most writers to increase the possibility of the rather unusual progression from less to more serious sexual offenses.

Increasing evidence is being presented of a relationship between rape and alcohol. In the past, the emphasis was frequently on the intoxication of the victim. Today, assertions are being made that as high as 50 percent of males are under the influence of alcohol at the time of the act and that as high as 35 percent of rapists are chronic alcoholics.

In some instances, the use of force in the sexual act is necessary to insure the male's potency. Certain men may have marked feelings of inadequacy and inferiority. They persuade themselves women enjoy being taken forcibly, and the struggle is a pretense. Many of these men, if the woman struggles hard enough or screams, will run. At times, however, submission through fear will lead to the reinforcement of the belief the woman herself wished for the act. Rapists have trapped themselves through this self-delusion.

> A.M. was a seventeen-year-old black male, the son of a dominating mother and an indifferent, at times alcoholic, father. He had grown up with marked feelings of resentment against women bossing him around. This resentment against women was increased when as an adolescent and experimenting with sex, he found that he was unable to maintain an erection long enough to have satisfactory intercourse. The girl involved in one such unsuccessful attempt had spread the story among her girlfriends of what had happened. This rapidly spread to his masculine peers. He was ribbed unmercifully about this. He decided the only way he could regain any prestige at all was by having sexual relations with a white woman against her wishes. Accordingly, armed with a knife, he lurked in the parking lot of a supermarket, found a solitary young woman laden with groceries coming out of the store, put the knife to her back, and directed her to get into her car. He had her drive to a secluded alley where, under threat of the knife, he raped her. Once the act was committed he continued in conversation with her, and in utter fear of

him, she consented to anything he was saying. What he did
ask was, "Well, didn't you like that? Come on, you'd better
tell me you liked it, now didn't you like it?" She said, "Yes,
she did like it." Where-upon, he asked for her name and
telephone number, and she gave it to him. Naturally, she
reported this to the police, but there were no clues as to the
identity of her assailant.

However, one week later the phone rang and it was A.M.
He identified himself and said, "How would you like some
more of that stuff?" Sensing an opportunity, she said she
thought she would and asked where could they meet. He set
up a date outside the same supermarket. She notified the
police, who were in hiding when she arrived. A.M. did not
appear and, after waiting for thirty minutes, she went home.
Following her return home, he called and said, "Well this
time I just wanted to see if you'd do it. Now I know you will,
how about meeting me tomorrow night? Same time, same
place." The victim again agreed and again notified the police. This time, when she arrived there, A.M. appeared within
a brief time and was immediately apprehended by the police.

No inferences should be drawn from the case of A.M. as to
the incidence of interracial rape. Statistics on this aspect of the
problem are inconclusive. It also should not be inferred that
definite evidence of either sexual deviation or psychopathology
is to be found in the case of all rapists. Psychopathology can be
demonstrated in almost all cases where an offender commits a
series of rapes over a period of time. Such an individual may
rarely be found to be actually psychotic. Psychodynamic factors
will also be found to be operative in cases of particularly sadistic and brutal rapes. Almost invariably the dynamics will
involve intense hostility to all females, sometimes serving as a
displacement of hostility to the mother or wife. (Being married
is no assurance against committing rape.)

Gang rape serves as an excellent illustration of the wide
range of personality types who may be involved in this behavior. (Gang rapes must be carefully distinguished from *gang
shags* in which a cooperative woman, most commonly a teenager, has sexual relations with a series of males in each other's
presence.) At the present time, the highest percentage of gang
rapes appear to be perpetrated by members of the more clan-

nish and aggressive motorcycle clubs, but they are certainly not confined to this group. In those circumstances, one or two highly antisocial, aggressive individuals will generally be found to be the ringleaders. Some of the participants are involved more out of fear of being considered weak or unmanly than out of any more complex motives. Alcoholism usually plays a large role in these cases.

Role of the Corrections Worker in Rape

Even in those jurisdictions where forcible rape is a probatable offense, it is rare that an individual found guilty of rape is placed on probation. Hence, the role of the probation officer will usually be limited to writing a presentence report. Psychological and psychiatric examination is mandatory prior to sentencing in those states which have sexual psychopath laws. More than just the usual presentence report is required, if it is to be of value to the examining clinician. A detailed statement from the victim is important, not only as to what was done by the rapist, but also as to what was said. Record of past offenses, both sexual and nonsexual, are of great value. Particularly significant is the history of family relationships during the offender's childhood. The extent of alcoholic involvement is also important. If the offender is married an effort should be made to obtain the wife's view of the nature of the marriage, their respective roles, and any problems which may have arisen.

Since such very differing psychodynamic patterns are found in the rapist, there are few concrete suggestions which can be made to the parole officer. As is the case with other aggressive offenses, rape is statistically an act of younger men. As a general rule, if an offender paroled for this offense is under the age of thirty-five, he will require more careful observation and is entitled to more careful consideration for possible therapy. Whatever, the age, the parole officer should be alert to signs of build up of hostility and resentment and attempt to defuse them. This can be done by exploration and/or allowing the parolee to talk about his feelings freely. A combination of these emotional responses and evidences of resumed or increased drinking are real prognosticators of possible recidivism. If the parolee is married, an attempt should be made to work conjointly with the wife and the offender, particularly in an attempt to obtain the cooperation of the wife in avoiding any semblance of belittling her husband during arguments.

SADISM (302.6)

Sadism (302.6) derives its name from the notorious Marquis de Sade who flourished at the time of the French Revolution. His name was inextricably linked to cruelty during sexual satisfaction by his thinly disguised autobiographical novels which describe such behavior. Sadism refers to the specific sexual deviation in which sexual gratification is obtained by inflicting pain on another. The term is widely used (or misused) to include those who seem to enjoy making others suffer whether through cutting remarks, depriving them of harmless pleasures, or forcing them to perform uncomfortable tasks. Such behavior frequently does not have its roots in sexual deviation and does not apply to the subject under discussion here. Some acts of rape may be truly sadistic in that the major gratification is in the fusion of inflicting punishment and sexual gratification.

The offenses committed by those who have the sexual deviation, sadism, range from physical abuse and bodily mutilation to especially brutal and violent murders in which the sexual component may be only symbolic or may be blatantly obvious. Offenders in this group are notoriously apt to have committed multiple examples of the same offense prior to apprehension. Some have become almost legendary: Blue Beard, Jack the Ripper, the Boston Strangler. A remembered event of my hometown was terrorized by an offender labeled Jack the Whipper, because he used a bullwhip on any young woman he found on the streets after 10:00 PM. In Toledo, the Collingwood Slasher preyed on young student nurses in a limited area of the city, slashing them across the breasts with a knife. At times the offense consists of throwing acid at a woman's face in order to disfigure her. In sadistic or so-called lust murders, the victims may be found with breasts cut off, genitalia excised, or foreign objects placed in the vagina or rectum. These acts of degradation or mutilation may sometimes be demonstrated to have taken place before the victim's death, sometimes after. In those cases in which there had been coitus, the sexual act was usually performed while the victim was alive, but not necessarily so. There is one sort of sexual deviation in which the abnormal desire is for sexual relations with a dead woman. This has been immortalized in a bawdy limerick. This deviation is called *necrophilia* — love for the dead. This is not necessarily accompanied by sadism and some such individuals occasionally find employment as undertakers' assistants, and in this way find methods of satisfying their craving without having to resort to murder.

Sadism does not always have to reach the described degree of intensity to figure in legal proceedings.

> Mr. A.N. was referred for examination after he had been arrested on a charge of assault and battery filed by his wife. The actual offense occurred on the Fourth of July. During the course of the family celebration, Mr. A.N. had written his initials in the driveway in gun powder obtained from several Cherry Bombs. He had then handed a match to his wife with instructions to light the gun powder, with full knowledge of what would happen. (There was no fuse.) She was severely burned about the face and hands in the resultant explosion.

> Mrs. A.N. told a story of being repeatedly bound and beaten by her husband prior to sexual intercourse. Since she "loved him," she had taken no action against him until this final painful experience. During his examination, he revealed he took great pleasure in putting kittens in the washing machine and observing them through the glass window as they struggled unsuccessfully to stay alive. (This story received partial confirmation from the local animal shelter which had finally refused to allow him to have any more kittens when they were unable to ascertain what he had done with all those he had previously taken from them.)

> Of interest to those who believe sadism is closely allied to the struggle over toilet training, Mr. A.N. reported that after each such washing machine episode he had a sudden urge to defecate, and that following the Fourth of July incident he developed an intractable diarrhea which was still present at

the time of the examination six weeks later.

In all these instances, it is obvious severe psychopathology must exist. On those occasions in which the sexual behavior is more symbolic than obvious, (ripping, whipping, slashing, acid throwing), the offender may rationalize his behavior by saying he is attacking seductive, immodest, or careless women in order to remind them and others like them of the error of their ways. This is, of course, an example of the same sort of mechanism discussed in the section on incest in which the father projects his desire on the daughter. There is a great deal of controversy as to the psychodynamics of sadism, most of which is irrelevant here. What is relevant is that it is bound up to an ambivalent love/hate feeling about women, a feeling with its roots in the first three years of life. Mr. V. described in Chapter 8 had an undoubtedly sadistic element operative in the development of his obsessive-compulsive neurosis and his ultimate offenses.

Compared to other sexual offenders, there is a relatively high proportion of psychotic individuals in this group. Even where frank psychosis does not exist, there is generally very severe psychopathology. It is in this particular area that some of the most heated battles are fought in the courtroom over the question of the insanity of the defendant.

Role of the Corrections Worker in Sadism

These battles do not usually involve the corrections worker. Where he does get involved is once again by way of the presentence report in the time period between a finding of guilt and imposition of sentence. Again, the final recommendation is generally made by the clinician, just as the final disposition is always made by the judge. Of particular interest to the clinician are the history and details of prior arrests and mental hospitalizations, when these are present. As with married rapists, the description of the husband's behavior vis-à-vis his wife can be extremely significant. Rigid ascetism as far as all *pleasures of the flesh* is concerned (particularly sexual prudishness), fire setting, and cruelty to animals are said to be of particular significance in the childhood history of these people.

It is frequently stated that sexual offenders have the lowest recidivism rate of all antisocial offenses. If the two most common offenses, exhibitionism and child molestation, which have the highest recidivism rate of all sexual offenses, are omitted, the recidivism rate for other offenses is obviously quite low. One very plausible explanation for this is that most of these remaining sexual offenses carry severe penalties, and the offenders are much older when released from confinement. Certainly, this is true of sadistic offenses. Like the murderer, the sadist if released at all is usually well over forty-five years of age before getting out of the penitentiary and the potential for recidivism is reduced.

ROLE OF THE CORRECTIONS WORKER IN SEXUAL OFFENSES

The importance of refraining from value judgments when dealing with the sexual offender should be stressed. In almost no other area of human behavior is there so great a range of attitudes. These may vary from tolerance to disgust, if not downright revulsion. People in corrections, as in all other fields of human endeavor, come in all sizes and shapes, with all sorts of experiences, feelings, and attitudes. For the most part they would not have become engaged in this work without a strong desire to help others. Yet, it seems to be commonplace to expend untold energy working with a habitual burglar or confidence man, but unusual to find the tolerance necessary to put as much effort into the attempt to rehabilitate a child molester. The latter may be much more desperately eager to change his ways, to conform to society's expectations, but it becomes harder to do so if he is met with a poorly concealed attitude of contempt or disgust on the part of those who are theoretically there to help him. It is much easier to empathize with someone like Mr. V. (see Chapter 8) who is obviously ill, no matter how revolting the offense, than with Mr. A.C. (see Chapter 11). "Why doesn't he just drop into a bar and pick up a girl like anyone else might do?" or even, "Why couldn't he just masturbate until the brothels are opened again?''. It is sometimes very difficult to feel that such an act as exhibitionism is not completely an exercise in free will.

There is another important factor which enters in at this point. It is doubtful that many of us, even in the deepest corners of our minds, have ever been tempted by the thought of killing, dismembering, or eating a woman. Yet the urge to show ourselves (exhibitionism), to peep at others (voyeurism), and to touch an attractive bottom in an elevator (frottage) is certainly not an alien one, and we have learned many substitute behaviors to help confine these urges. It is a difficult task for the father of a nubile, adolescent daughter to suppress any feelings of desire as she snuggles enticingly against him to say goodnight. When another gives expression to these urges which are familiar, we do not say, "I might have done that myself." Instead, by a mental mechanism called *reaction formation* we deny and repress further the urge within ourselves, over-react, and want to "throw the book at him." Fortunately, a slow change in the direction of understanding seems to be occurring in the attitude of society as sexuality begins to be treated as just another facet of life.

Just as homosexuals are increasingly "coming out of the closets," so too is the knowledge growing that no one is free from sexual urges, licit or illicit. In 1976, a considerable controversy developed as to the propriety of a candidate for the highest office in this country making a public statement to the effect that he, too, has sinned by lusting after strange women in his heart. The corrections worker, to deal effectively with this area of professional duty, must have the candidate's honesty in order to prevent personal problems from interfering with effective professionalism.

Chapter 13

BEHAVIOR DISORDERS
OF ADOLESCENCE (308)

GENERAL CONSIDERATIONS

IT is, of course, possible that any of the conditions discussed to this point may occur in adolescents. However, it is unusual for the younger adolescent to develop any of the major mental disorders. As far as schizophrenia is concerned, onset is sometimes seen in early childhood. Occasionally, hebephrenic schizophrenia will develop in the early teens, but this is much more usual in the late teens. Catatonic schizophrenia rarely occurs before the age of nineteen or twenty, and paranoid schizophrenia is almost never seen in teenagers. Manic depressive disorders, as such, rarely manifest themselves before the early twenties. Even though *DSM II* does not include a specific heading for adolescent depression, this condition does occur. The form it takes is different from that seen in adults, and will be discussed later in this chapter.

Adolescents can be mentally retarded or brain damaged, and this will have to be taken into account whenever an adolescent is seen. Conversion hysteria and dissociative hysteria are not rare in teenage females. When present, they take the same form as the illness does in adults. **Behavior Disorders of Adolescence (308)**, the classification now under discussion, are, in a sense, incipient personality disorders which occur in the adolescent. As a general rule, we do not like to label adolescents as antisocial personalities or passive-aggressive personalities, etc., although they may show all the traits that are manifested in those conditions.

There are six behavior disorders of childhood or adolescence listed. Two of these need only brief mention because they are rarely seen by the corrections worker. One is **Withdrawing Reaction in Adolescence (308.1)**. The characteristics of this per-

239

sonality disorder are about the same as those of the schizoid personality. On rare occasions, one of these individuals comes in contact with the juvenile court for impulsive sexual acting out, a form of behavior which has been described in Chapter 10 under the heading of Pedophilia. **Overanxious Reaction of Adolescence (308.2)** is almost never seen in court settings. The symptomatology of this condition is characterized by chronic anxiety with overblown fears, tendency to sleeplessness, various psychophysiological responses, such as blushing, sweating, rapid heart rate, etc.. These people are immature, are extremely conforming, are always looking for praise or approval, and therefore almost never come in conflict with the law. The remainder of the behavior disorders of adolescence will be discussed in detail, as well as the manifestations of depression as it is shown in adolescence. The Borderline Syndrome, which was described in Chapter 10, is being seen with increasing frequency in adolescence. Its manifestations in this age group do not differ from those encountered at a later time.

HYPERKINETIC REACTION OF ADOLESCENCE (308.0)

Those young adolescents who, as children, have been classified in the group of hyperactive, hyperkinetic, or minimally brain damaged children, are labeled as **Hyperkinetic Reaction of Adolescence (308.0)**. As a usual role, the syndrome of the hyperkinetic child, also called the minimally brain damaged child (MBD), has pretty well run its course by early adolescence. However, a fair number of these youngsters between twelve and fifteen still find their way into juvenile court settings. As the name implies, the hyperkinetic adolescent is characterized by a marked increase in activity. These children have been overactive from birth. They are the sort of children who, as soon as they are able to move around, are the bane of their parents' existence. They are into everything. They have a short attention span. They are extremely restless and easily distracted. For this reason they have difficulty in learning, even though their basic intelligence may be normal or even superior. As they grow older, they get into constant fights with their peers, who cannot understand their inability to play at any one game for a period of time. Since their parents are not quite sure how to handle them, they tend to be punished severely for behavior they cannot help. As a result they become more and more rebellious and less and less tractable. When they get into school, they run into constant difficulty with their classmates.

When the condition is recognized and a multidisciplinary treatment is available and utilized, good results can be expected. If the condition is neglected or improperly treated, these children, when they reach adolescence become well known to the police and the courts. The offenses which bring the hyperkinetic adolescent to the court are numerous. They may range all the way from school truancy to arson. Such adolescents are frequently assaultive to persons and destructive of property. Although they would like to be friends with other youngsters, they find themselves isolated and react rather furiously to this. Shoplifting, automobile thefts, and unprovoked assaults, both physical and sexual, are also numbered among the offenses which these youngsters may commit.

The diagnosis is made on the basis of a longitudinal history as well as cross-sectional observation of behavior. A carefully taken history will reveal this behavior disorder actually starts in the crib and has never abated. In many instances, a half-hearted attempt at treatment by way of medication will have been made. Although some improvement may have been seen as a result of this medication, the behavior has rarely changed significantly. The difficulty with such children starts almost at the moment of getting out of the crib. Once in school, they are almost constantly in the office of the counselor or principal. The diagnosis can almost be made from the history, although the history of any particular child will have to differ from the history of siblings in order to rule out familial-cultural patterns. Boys with this condition outnumber girls by a ratio of almost three to one. The EEG does not show consistent change. Neurological examination reveals only so-called soft neurological signs.[1] For these reasons, many object to the term Minimal

---

[1]Soft neurological signs consist, among others, of minimal disorders of coordination, sensation, and automatic associated movements.

Brain Damage.

As far as the situation in adolescents with this diagnosis is concerned, they usually do not show the extreme hyperactivity seen in younger children with this condition, although the author has seen one fourteen-year-old boy who absolutely could not sit still in his chair. They show diminished attention span, difficulty in concentration, and marked distractibility. As a result, carrying on a meaningful conversation may be extremely difficult.

As far as the management of such conditions is concerned, there must have been a multidisciplinary approach. This is the condition about which so much furor has been raised in the press concerning the use of stimulant medication. Actually, amphetamines (Benzedrine®, Dexedrine®) and other stimulants (such as Ritalin®) do have an extremely beneficial effect on this condition. Paradoxically, these medications do not decrease the overactivity by sedation or tranquilization. Since they are really stimulants, they exert their effects by increasing attention span and ability to concentrate, so the child is really able to sit and pay attention to one thing for a longer time. There may be improvement if medication is relied on as the only treatment modality, but overall such treatment is doomed to failure. In addition to the medication, which helps only in the way mentioned, there should be help from learning specialists, behavior analysts, remedial teachers, pediatricians, and psychologists. All must join forces, not only to help the child, but also to work with the parents, to teach them to manage the child in such a way that the child's personality will not have been permanently affected as the condition recedes with time. As noted, the actual hyperkinetic effects disappear about the end of early adolescence and what remains in many youngsters is the scarring which is left on the personality because of the lack of proper management in childhood.

A.O. is quite illustrative of the Hyperkinetic Reaction of Adolescence. This thirteen-year-old boy was brought to the juvenile court from the Children's Home in which he had been placed by his family. He had been at the Children's Home for approximately six months. They now felt they could no longer handle him. Not only was he fighting with the other youngsters, breaking windows, and running away, but he had also started sexually attacking some of the girls in the home. The history revealed that he was the third child in a family of five. As is quite typical for youngsters with this condition, his mother's labor had been quite prolonged for a third child. Her membranes had ruptured early, so that it was a so-called "dry birth." She had been in labor for over ten hours. When the baby was born, he had difficulty in breathing and was "blue" for approximately four minutes. He responded to brief oxygen inhalation and before too long his respiratory rhythms were normal.

The mother described him as having never been a cuddly child. When held in her arms he tried to kick and get away. He was climbing over the sides of his crib before he could walk. He would fall to the floor and start screaming. If no one paid any attention to his screams, he would then start crawling around, getting into anything that intrigued him. Once he started walking, everything in the house which was breakable had to be placed out of his reach. This soon became difficult to do. Before long he learned to move foot stools, and then chairs, to climb to greater heights in order to get whatever he wanted. School was almost a total disaster. He was finally excluded and received home tutoring.

Placement in the Children's Home was an act of parental desperation. When locked in his room in an effort to control him, he would immediately open the window, grab on to the telephone wire which ran on the side of the house next to his window, pull himself hand over hand to the telephone pole and then down to the ground. After three or four such efforts his family was convinced that he was going to kill himself, and stopped attempting to cope with him by themselves. They asked the cooperation of the Children's Service Board who admitted him to the Children's Home, from which he was transferred to juvenile court.

In the office, A.O. was charming, attractive, but kept up an incessant line of chatter. From time to time he got up from his chair and explored various objects in the room including the cassette recorder, stacks of charts, etc. Interestingly, he went to a table which held a stack of papers containing statistics on childrens' offenses. He read the list with quite some gusto, pausing from time to time to say, "Oh, auto theft, I've done that." "Oh, shoplifting, I've done that." "Oh, assault, that's me." This was done with a great deal of pride.

By the time adolescence is reached and the characterology has been fixed, the corrections worker has an extremely difficult task in dealing with such a youngster. An attempt should be made to have him placed in a special class in school. If still under age fifteen, attempts should be made through the physician to attempt a trial with one of the above-named medications as a part of an overall treatment plan. Discussion with the family is imperative. By this time, most families have thrown up their hands and are practically screaming, "Take this kid out of our hair." It takes much tact, patience, and diplomacy to persuade such a family to try again, and mobilize all the services needed to understand and help the youngster. It may be necessary to remove the adolescent to a setting where behavioral modification techniques may be employed. These should focus on positive, rather than aversive, reinforcement, i.e. reward rather than punishment. Sometimes, training the family in disregarding the target symptoms which are so annoying and concentrating on the youngster's strengths, praising and reinforcing them, may be enough assistance to allow the family to foster a more normal adolescence for this disturbed youngster. Placement in the usual juvenile training institution is completely counter-productive.

RUNAWAY REACTION OF ADOLESCENCE (308.3)

There is a general tendency to remove so-called *status offenders*[2] from juvenile court jurisdiction and to assign their management to other, more socially oriented, community agencies. Those with **Runaway Reaction of Adolescence (308.3)** are usually considered status offenders. Nevertheless, they continue to be seen frequently by corrections workers. Typically, these children come from chaotically disturbed and rejecting homes. More subtle, but equally as devastating, rejection can be seen in

---

[2]A status offender is one who commits acts which would not be considered illegal if committed by an adult.

rigidly organized homes as well. The original flight from home is a reaction to this unpleasant situation, or even the threat of one. Thus, a test in school, for which the teenager is unprepared, may become a stimulus to run. A misstep at school may precipitate a runaway to avoid punishment at home. At times this becomes an excuse rather than a reason. "I stayed out until two o'clock in the morning and knew my father would beat me up if I went home." The reason for staying out is never made clear.

Such a reaction poses serious problems. The adolescent may be exposed to dangerous, even life-threatening situations while on the run. Equally important is the risk of being involved in criminal behavior, thereby transforming a status offender into a delinquent. Antisocial behavior, such as stealing, prostitution, or drug pushing, may be the adolescent's maladaptive way of coping with the reality of the need for food and shelter. The stealing may be part of the psychological pattern of stealing to replace lost love; the objects may be stolen from a parent or teacher preparatory to running away.

Such adolescents must be carefully differentiated from those who are running, not from something, but to something. This latter group are seeking excitement, have learned the streets are more fun than home and, instead of staying away for only one or two days at a time, will be on the run for weeks or months. Not uncommonly, such adolescents also become involved in more serious crimes. Investigation will sometimes reveal the fact that while the home conditions are quite harsh and traumatic, they have, in many instances, been exaggerated by the adolescent to justify the act of running away. The major motivations are the joys of "running to" and the adolescent's own rebellious stance. This latter group of adolescents is not composed solely of those who are subsumed under runaway reaction of adolescence. Many of those in this group are much too aggressive and have too much ego-strength to be so classified. Many of them fit better in the next group to be described.

Incestuous advances by an adult in the home may sometimes be a strong motivating force in adolescent runaways. Incestuous feelings coming to the surface, as described in Chapter

12, may be involved even more frequently. There is an entire group of adolescents in whom the runaway reaction is, in reality, an attempt at flight from conflict which is occurring within the adolescent, a conflict which may never have reached consciousness. This should be suspected whenever a runaway reaction has developed in which the counselor cannot demonstrate a pattern either of running from or of running to. In those instances, professional help of a higher level of psychological expertise may have to be sought.

An isolated episode of running away which lasts from a few hours to one or two days is present in the developmental history of almost everyone. Certainly, in these circumstances, a crisis intervention model which combines a shelter house with workers to mediate the underlying problems is preferrable to juvenile court intervention. This is particularly true if the system has effective liaison with members of other disciplines who have the competence to aid the adolescent running from inner-conflicts. The system breaks down when the problem lies in a chaotic home, which no model of social intervention will change, and the social agency lacks authority to remove the child permanently. A juvenile probation officer may be involved in this situation, as well as in those situations where the status runaway offender commits truly delinquent acts.

In many of those situations in which the juvenile court becomes involved, a truly paradoxical condition may develop. The adolescent, who has run from the home, the school, the community, strenuously resists all mandated removal from the home. The parents, who have caused the reaction by their rejection, fight tooth and nail to oppose removal by the court. This struggle reaches its utmost severity when the proposed removal is to a foster home rather than to a state operated institution. The reason for this strange event is that for the adolescent, the home, however bad, represents the familiar. At the same time, verbalization of the wish to leave is impossible in the presence of the parents. "It will hurt my parents too much." To the parents, foster home placement labels them as "bad parents," incapable of raising their child. Placement at the juvenile rehabilitation center proves that, "No one can be expected to handle that brat." A group home is sometimes an acceptable compromise.

When the adolescent is returned to a home which has not changed, and cannot be changed, the probation officer is left with very few tools with which to work. Every effort must be made to bolster the adolescent's strengths to help cope with the pressure of the push away from home and the pull to the streets. Close coordination with school personnel, a counselor when available, faculty when no counselor exists, is important in attempting to modify the curriculum to give the youngster a chance at success, not to mention the need to help the adolescent to learn some of the things needed for survival in the world. A job within the capabilities of the adolescent, at times a part of a combined school/work program, may be a way of both gaining a feeling of success and for furnishing an accessible alternative in which to spend more time away from the chaotic home. Involvement in organized sports may be an excellent ego-strengthening medium for well-coordinated adolescents. Federal grants for local education currently depend on equal participation of both sexes in all activities, so sports are becoming as important an outlet for the female adolescent as they are for the male. As in the management of those who attempt to cope with their problems by the use of alcohol or drugs, it is essential that the probation counselor not be dismayed by an infrequent repetition of the runaway pattern. Patience and tolerance are extremely necessary qualities in dealing with this kind of adolescent.

UNSOCIALIZED AGGRESSIVE REACTION OF ADOLESCENCE (308.4)

Unsocialized Aggressive Reaction of Adolescence (308.4) is a diagnosis which includes the largest share of adolescents with psychiatric diagnoses seen in juvenile court. The unsocialized aggressive reaction of adolescence is usually seen as a predecessor of the antisocial personality. At times, the differentiation from the antisocial personality is extremely difficult to make. It may be the label of unsocialized aggressive reaction has been placed in order to avoid giving the child the more formidable diagnosis of antisocial personality. There is a danger that once the latter label has been applied it will never be dislodged.

The characteristic behavior of the unsocialized aggressive reaction may be gathered from the name itself. Disobedience, rebelliousness, and aggressiveness are cardinal behavior traits of this condition. These do not occur on the basis of poor attention span as in the case of the hyperkinetic child. Unsocialized aggressive youngsters, when they are motivated, can concentrate very well and can maintain the same activity over long periods of time. They are physically and verbally aggressive. In this characteristic they closely resemble the aggressiveness of the explosive personality. They carry a grudge over a long period of time, and can be quite harmful to the person, or quite destructive to the property, of those whom they dislike. They usually have a history of temper tantrums starting in early childhood; they tend to steal without any feeling of violating other people's property rights. As mentioned in discussing the background of the antisocial personality, these people have never had any consistent discipline from their parents, they feel rejected and basically inferior, and at adolescence have not developed even the rudiments of a conscience. The great majority of them are quite muscular. It is difficult to continue to be aggressive when the physique to do so successfully is lacking.

A.P. was seen at juvenile court for psychiatric examination on a request for transfer to adult court. A.P. was a sixteen-year-old male, currently before the court on a charge of armed robbery and kidnapping. The youngest of five children, his father was alcoholic and employed only sporadically. His mother was sexually promiscuous. There was quite some doubt as to his paternity. This was frequently a subject of heated arguments (in his presence) between the father and mother. He had been suspended from school for truancy, absenteeism, and fighting. Finally, he was expelled from school at the age of fifteen. He had had several previous juvenile court contacts for assault and battery, malicious destruction of property, car theft, criminal trespassing, and breaking and entering. In almost all of these offenses he had been alone, although on rare occasions there had been one codelinquent.

His current offense occurred at two in the morning. With his girlfriend he had thumbed a ride from a passing motorist. The motorist pulled over, and as he opened the car door, A.P. pulled out a gun and demanded the man's wallet. He then motioned the man to slide over in the seat, put his girlfriend in the back seat, took the wheel of the car, and started to drive off. As they were driving down the street, a police car was seen approaching. The victim leaned over and blew the horn constantly to attract the cruiser's attention. A wild chase followed in which the car was finally forced over to the curb and A.P. was arrested.

He had obtained the gun in quite a characteristic fashion. He had been approached by a young man who offered to sell him a gun for thirty-five dollars. A.P. demanded to see it and have the action demonstrated to him. The man broke open the cylinder to show that the gun was loaded, put it back in place, and showed A.P. how to take the safety catch off. A.P. took the gun in his hand, examined it, broke it open, placed a bullet in the firing chamber, then calmly turned it on the vendor and said, "I've got the gun. Get your ass out of here."

Such youngsters on the probation officer's caseload pose an extremely difficult problem in management. They are incapable of being loyal. They are incapable of forming any deep relationships. Any attempts to change their behavior through the formation of a relationship are futile. In this connection, a further discussion of A.P. might be quite illuminating.

While A.P. was in detention in the juvenile detention home, awaiting a decision on the request for transfer to adult court, an indigenous youth worker from his area came in contact with him, worked with him steadily, and felt he was making tremendous progress with the youngster. He, indeed, felt this boy should not be transferred to adult court, that he had too great a potential, and he was just a downtrodden youngster, who, if given the chance, would show he had reformed. His request was refused by the court and A.P. was transferred to adult court. The worker immediately arranged for bond and had him released to his custody. Within three weeks, A.P. was rearrested, this time on a much more serious charge, that of attempted murder in connection with a drug theft.

These are the youngsters who fill the so-called training or reform schools, sometimes called industrial schools, the juvenile rehabilitation centers run by the state and federal government. The recidivism rate among them is extremely high. Whether this is a function of the behavioral disorder itself or whether it is a function of the deficiencies of various institutions is a widely discussed question. Some good results have been claimed for the use of the G.G.I. technique or its successor, Positive Peer Culture. One of the outstanding defects in the system is the lack of attempts to modify the home while the adolescent is away or, if this cannot be done, to find a new home. This is almost always coupled with a defect in the postrelease follow up. Parole officers have had no previous contact with the adolescent and have an overburdened caseload. It has been my experience that youngsters apt to benefit from these group techniques are not in this group of behavior disorders, but in the next one to be discussed.

GROUP DELINQUENT REACTION OF ADOLESCENCE (308.5)

It has always been my opinion that there is a question as to whether this so-called behavior disorder properly belongs in the classification of psychiatric disorders. This diagnosis is applied to a majority of those adolescents seen in juvenile court who come from the high crime, inner-city areas of big cities. These are youngsters whose widespread delinquent activities are carried out in groups. Sometimes these are large, formally organized gangs; sometimes they are just a collection of neighborhood boys, less frequently girls, who know each other and run around together. They have highly developed group loyalty. They tend to steal as a group, skip school as a group, run away as a group, fight others as a group, etc. Sometimes this behavior can become extrememly antisocial. This has been particularly the case in the last few years when lethal weapons seem to be so readily available. In their own way, these youths are reacting not in an antisocial but in a dyssocial fashion. In many instances their behavior is adaptive rather than maladaptive. In rare instances it is a form of self-preservation.

This is the youngster generally thought of by the public when the term juvenile delinquent is used. For this reason, it is often impossible to carry on a reasonable discourse as to the causes and prevention of juvenile delinquency, since the characteristics of these youngsters are so different from the characteristics of other youngsters who become involved with the courts. Yet, it is these youngsters about whom most of the statistical, sociological, and criminological studies have been done. The outcomes of these studies have been in many ways fascinating. They demonstrate, for example, that such youngsters are not only not amenable to psychological or psychotherapeutic treatment, but their behavior may actually worsen if so treated. These studies also demonstrate that these youngsters are much more apt to settle down and become stable citizens later in life, if not caught up in the juvenile justice network. On the other hand, those who go through what are called rehabilitative centers, accumulate a long record, and are officially labeled juvenile delinquents have a greater chance of becoming adult felons.

In the management of these youngsters, the more innovative techniques are certainly necessary. These include outreach workers, indigenous workers, group therapy (particularly using the Guided Group Interaction or the Positive Peer Culture techniques), unstructured education, using youngsters themselves as counselors, vocational training, drop-in centers, and similar rehabilitative modalities. Most important is to find ways for them to be financially productive without the need for recourse to the rip-off.

ADOLESCENT DEPRESSION

It has been said that this is the age of depression, just as the period between the two World Wars was called the age of anxiety. Nowhere is this more evidence than in adolescents. The fact has not been widely advertised, but suicide is the third highest cause of death in adolescents, being exceeded only by cancer and accidental death. As a matter of fact, among college students, suicide is the second largest cause of death. The reason that we do not normally think of depression as being an adolescent syndrome is that it is manifested in quite a different way in the adolescent than it is in the adult.

For a long time it has been known that hostility is an outstanding characteristic of depression. Indeed, the analytic schools of psychiatry claim depression is a result of hostility and agression which is turned inward against the self rather than outward on the environment. There would seem to be an inverse relationship between expression of hostility and depression. Those countries which have high rates of homicide have low rates of suicide, and vice versa. Japan, which has possibly the lowest homicide rate in the world, has the highest suicide rate. In England, where the homicide rate is also low, the suicide rate is relatively high. Interestingly, in England, homicides appear to occur in about 50 percent of cases as part of either a suicide pact, or the killer commits suicide immediately after having murdered his victim. The United States, which has an appallingly high rate of homicide, has a relatively low rate of suicide, although this is beginning to climb. (Most recent figures reported show 2.5 suicides per 100,000 population.) Nowhere is this relationship between hostility and depression seen more clearly than in the adolescent. Adolescents, in reaction to situations which might normally be expected to produce depression, react by hostility, resentment, and acting-out behavior. This acting-out behavior may take many forms, but it is usually in the form of retaliation against the environment, generally in the form of crimes against person or property.

No one has ever collected any statistics as to the percentage of adolescents before the juvenile courts who are depressed. As far as I am able to learn, no one has been able to do a psychiatric study of every youngster coming before a juvenile court. I see a large number of depressed adolescents in the course of my work as consultant to the Juvenile Court of Lucas County. It must be realized, however, that this is a slanted sample, because I see only a very small percentage of those children who appear before the court. The children seen are selected because the referees or probation counselors feel that they are unable to discover sufficient reason in the child's environment for the child's behavior. In the adolescent it would appear that a complete ventilation of hostility must precede the ability to show or manifest depression in its usual form of depressed mood, tears, retardation, or agitation. In the adolescent what we see is anger, which almost seems to be blind, striking out in all directions. It is is only with some difficulty that the adolescent can be brought to look through this anger to its underlying cause. In a large number of cases depression will be found to underlie it.

A.Q., a seventeen-year-old male was examined because of child abuse. While babysitting for a two-year-old boy, he had beaten him so badly that the child had to be hospitalized for thorough examination which revealed a greenstick fracture of a collarbone. This was the second time in two months that A.Q. had harmed the child while babysitting. The child's parents, who were distant relatives, had been aware of the first episode, but since the child had not been seriously hurt and since they were fond of A.Q., they had merely talked to him. He was obviously repentant at that time, could give no excuse for his behavior, promised that it would never happen again, and begged for another chance. He had been so obviously sincere and had always seemed to be so fond of the two-year-old, that the chance was given to him.

A.Q. was the second of five siblings. His father was alcoholic, brutal, punitive, and seemed to single A.Q. out for special abuse. The father was a long distance truck driver who was rarely home other than on weekends. Occasionally and without warning, he would leave the family for weeks. His behavior was unpredictable. At times he would take the children on picnics, fishing, or swimming. At those times he was good to them. A.Q.'s mother was kind but ineffective. She was totally unable to protect herself or the children from the father but for years was unable to leave her husband.

When A.Q. was seven-years-old his younger brother, six, was killed when run over by an automobile. He had been with A.Q. a couple of blocks from home, had disobeyed, and run out into the street. A.Q. protests that it was really not his fault, but at the time he was petrified at the thought of what his father might do on his return home from the road. To A.Q.'s amazement, the father did not punish him. Possibly, it would have relieved him of an inner sense of guilt if he had been punished.

Through the years the mother had made several abortive attempts to divorce the father. Finally, much to everyone's surprise, she did. A.Q. was then fifteen. The father, after a series of scenes, went back to his hometown, a short distance away, and moved in with his mother. During the following year, he would take the two younger sisters to visit with him for week-ends and over long holidays. He never took A.Q. or his older brother, who worked and felt quite independent. A.Q. felt isolated. When he did see his father, he was grilled about his mother's relations with other men. She did not date at all, but the father told A.Q. frequently, "If I ever see her dating a man I'll kill them both."

About one year before the child abuse episodes, the mother did start going with another man, someone whom A.Q. liked and who was kind to him. One Saturday night after they had been going together about two months, this man came over to take the family to a drive-in. His station wagon would not start, and they decided to stay home and watch television. The father came in unexpectedly to pick up the girls, saw the man, turned on his heels, and walked out. An hour and a half later he came back and pushed through the door with a gun in his hand. He shot at and wounded the mother, who then ran out the door. He then turned and with one shot killed the other man. He started out of the door to follow the mother, but A.Q. and his brother barred the way. He put the gun to his older son's chest and forced him away from the door. By then the mother was out of sight.

A.Q. followed his father out of the house while his brother phoned the police. The father returned from searching through the neighborhood and sat on a bench in the yard. The two girls started from the house toward the father. He shouted to A.Q., "Don't let them look." As A.Q. held the girls against his chest, he looked over his shoulder and saw his 'father put the gun to his own head and kill himself.

A.Q. could not seem to cry. His mother recovered after a

prolonged and financially crippling hospitalization. A.Q. showed no obvious signs of depression. He turned to religion. At bible class he met a girl, one year younger than he. As their relationship developed, the intensity of A.Q.'s dependence on her frightened her parents. They insisted they break up. It was shortly after the girl informed A.Q. that she intended to listen to her parents that the first episode of child abuse happened. The girl (ignorant of this occurrence) vacillated between obeying her parents and talking to A.Q. in bible class and over the phone. She finally told him she was seeing another boy. He confirmed this by seeing them together and argued with her desperately but unavailingly. The following day the serious episode of child abuse occurred. The underlying depression was directly responsible.

One alternative to violent acting out as a reaction to depression in adolescents is suicide. In many instances, adolescent suicide follows a pattern first described by Teicher. Many of its features are similar to the patterns seen in A.Q., but there are also marked differences. According to Teicher, there are three phases to this pattern. The first, or developmental phase, occupies the early life of the adolescent. This is marked by frequent separations and losses. Four or five father figures may succeed each other in ten to twelve years. The father may be in the penitentiary. The mother may die, and a series of stepmothers or foster mothers follow. The family is extremely mobile, and the adolescent may have attended six to twelve schools before reaching high school.

In such an unstable setting, the push of adolescence arrives and the second stage, the stage of escalation, sets in. The youth begins to rebel and family friction increases. The more demands placed upon the youngster, the greater the rebellion and the more intense the friction. Finally, both sides give up. The parents, as it were, wash their hands of their child and the child in effect says, "I don't care."

The stage is now set for the third phase. At this point an affair starts with a peer of the opposite sex. All of the adolescent's time and energy is involved in this love affair. As a result, the few friends previously acquired are neglected, parents are scorned, and for the adolescent the world consists only of the two of them. The partner is unable to tolerate the intensity of these needs and demands, and terminates the relationship. At this point there is literally nowhere for the adolescent to turn. All bridges have been burned. Suicide is then the only logical way out.

Those who work with delinquent adolescents should be thoroughly conversant with this pattern and always on the alert to spot it. At times good judgment than calls for enlisting professional help. At all times, when dealing with the acting-out adolescent in whom an underlying depression is suspected as the cause of the behavior, it will be necessary to make the adolescent aware of the anger just beneath the surface in order to get at the deeper depression.

There is classic triad of mourning. When a dearly loved person is lost the first stage is shock. "It can't happen. I won't believe it. It's impossible." The second stage is anger. Usually this runs a three phase pattern of its own: anger at the departed for leaving; anger at the environment for allowing it (the doctor did not do all he could, the nurse did not give the right medicine, etc.); anger at oneself (I should have done more, I should have been better during the dear one's life). This leads to the third stage of grief and mourning, with resolution.

The adolescent has trouble getting past the second part of the second stage, anger at the environment. This is why the acting out. Help in verbalizing this anger, instead of acting it out, permits progression to the next stages, a recognition and expression of the underlying grief, and then restitution.

OTHER REACTIONS OF ADOLOESCENCE (308.9)

The single **Other Reaction of Adolescence (308.97)** which is most important for corrections is the manipulative adolescent. Generally, such manipulation is part of a budding hysterical personality disorder. Such an adolescent will have played her (such youngsters are generally female) father off against her mother, her school teacher against her school counselor, and now she is eager and willing to play the same game with her probation officer. The only way to stay even with such an adolescent is to refuse to take any statement for granted. "My school counselor said I can drop out of school if it's okay with the court." "My mother says I can spend the weekend with my girlfriend if I have your permission." "Don't you think my mother's being unreasonable not to let me go to the junior prom?" (The mother may just have grounded her for shoplifting the prom gown after having made her take the gown back.) "I can't make my appointment tomorrow, can you possibly come out here?" "I like you so much better than that old referee. She is unfair." "Will you take my girlfriend on? She just can't stand her counselor, and I told her how wonderful you are." There is only one way to stay ahead in this game. Take nothing for granted. Check every statement, no matter how reasonable. Do not be flattered or seduced. Finally, let the adolescent know you know, not sneeringly or laughingly or punitively but calmly and matter-of-factly, and always with the implied attitude that you expect it to stop. Only when it stops can any real progress toward behavioral change be made.

There is one more mechanism which is operative in delinquent adolescents of which the probation officer must be aware. It cannot be classified as a behavior disorder, since it can be seen in almost any sort of youngster. This was first described in 1952 by Zurek and Johnson and has been elaborated by them since. They refer to this mechanism as a *superego lacuna,* which can be roughly translated to "a hole in the conscience." Superego lacunae have also been discussed in Chapter 9. Collect phone calls to a nonexistent family member, to let the other members know of a safe arrival from a journey without the need to pay a penny for a long distance call, rob the phone company of millions of dollars in revenue evey year. The rationalization is, "They are a big company; it won't hurt them." This indicates a real superego lacuna.

The delinquent sort of lacuna is put in the child's conscience by the parent with whom the child identifies most closely. Not uncommonly, the parent is completely unaware of what is going on. The child is responding to a parent's unspoken wish.

The mother who married at fifteen, raised nine children, and feels robbed of a chance to have had her fling says to her teenage daughter, "That man is ten years older than you. There's only one thing he wants when he asks you out." When she then lets the daughter go out with him, she is obviously permitting the daughter to give him what he wants and is creating a superego lacuna. The father who did not get his driver's license until he was thirty because the poverty in his family was so great that no car could be afforded, says to his fifteen-year-old son, "You know you can't drive the car without a license." When he then asks the son to back the car out of the garage, to put it away, or lets him take the wheel on back country roads, he is creating a superego lacuna.

When delinquent behavior persists in cases where by all logic it should not, then it is necessary to look for the superego lacuna and see what parental wish the youngster is filling. Until it is out in the open, and the parent's behavior stops, the child's will not. At times such unconscious parental behavior may result in more serious problems.

> A.R. is a twelve-year-old girl sent from juvenile court to an inpatient adolescent unit for thirty days observation. A.R. had been arrested for possession of marijuana after the neighbors had complained to the police about wild parties going on in the home. Investigation at juvenile court revealed her to look as though she should be fourteen or fifteen and to think of herself as though she were eighteen. Her parents had been divorced when she was eight, and A.R. had been placed in her mother's custody. She had so successfully manipulated the parents, one against the other, that at age eleven she had succeeded in being allowed to go to live with her father.
>
> The reason she thought of herself as eighteen was readily apparent. The father was a traveling salesman who was away for days at a time. During those times A.R. was left alone with no supervision. It was during these times the noisy parties occurred. It was learned in the hospital that A.R. had been extremely sexually promiscuous. While many explanations for this behavior were possible, the real motivation became apparent one day when she was found with a quantity of the raunchier magazines. According to her, they had been

brought to her by her father. When accosted with this, his answer was, "Well, the attendant asked me to bring her something to read." The almost openly seductive nature of this act pointed directly at the superego lacuna which led to A.R.'s promiscuity.

PART TWO
INTERVIEWING AND CORRECTIONS

Chapter 14

PRINCIPLES OF INTERVIEWING

GENERAL CONSIDERATIONS

THE question may properly be raised about the validity of attempting to apply the interviewing techniques of psychiatry to corrections. The probability of the corrections worker coming into contact with increasing numbers of grossly abnormal people has already been discussed. More pertinent is the fact that the relationship of the psychiatrist to large numbers of patients is identical to that of the corrections worker to the greatest proportion of clients. These patients and clients do not want to be in a relationship. In the case of the patients, they are frequently seen either in the psychiatrist's office or at the hospital, not because they want to be there, but because a spouse, a relative, a friend, or a court has persuaded them they must be there. In the case of the client, it is a choice of the lesser of two evils: either going to or remaining in a penal institution or being on probation or parole. The same resentments, hostilities, fears, misapprehensions, and desires to mislead are present in each of the groups coerced into the relationship. At the same time the assumption is made that identical motives are present in psychiatrists and corrections workers. These motives include a genuine desire to be of help, to make the relationship a more meaningful one than that of cursory reporting of facts, and to effect, where possible, a change of attitudes.

There are, of course, also very definite differences. The corrections worker is always an officer of the court and is always viewed that way by his client. (Being an officer of the court does not imply that the corrections worker is a police officer or a detective.) Probation officers do not have unlimited quantities of time at their disposal in which to obtain the necessary information on which to base a presentence report. The psychiatrist seeing a patient in treatment may utilize an almost unlimited number of sessions before arriving at a final evaluation. The probation officer in a presentence investigation starts from scratch, with little but the police report from which information can be obtained. A psychiatrist before seeing the patient sees the report of the referring physician, frequently has the investigation of a trained social worker, and usually is able to talk to interested relatives. If the examination is mandated by the court, the probation worker's presentence investigation report may even be available. However, in those cases in which the first visit is under duress, the psychiatrist is generally under even more time pressure than the corrections worker. In those cases in which treatment is to be involved, the psychiatrist, without any salesmanship, must persuade the reluctant patient that there is interest, understanding, ability to help, and no desire to take over and run the patient's life. Generally, in court mandated investigations, there is opportunity for only one interview, and that is limited by the exigencies of scheduling to an hour or an hour and a half. The obvious differences in the two situations, that of the psychiatrist when first seeing the patient and of the probation officer when first interviewing a client, pale before the striking similarities.

This and the following chapter will derive in a great measure from a series of articles which were written for *Federal Probation* and reprinted widely by HEW, the State Departments of Corrections of Indiana, New Jersey, and Illinois, by the United States Navy Training Class for M.P.s, and by several social work courses. However, thirteen years have passed since that original publication. My previous views have been modified in certain areas, variations of techniques have proved helpful in special situations, and I have had the benefit of a myriad of new examples which attest to the utility of the basic techniques. This will not be just a rehashing of old material.

The statement was made in the introduction to this book that an attempt would be made to avoid taking a doctrinaire position which asserted the primacy of any one psychiatric theory over another. The statement was also made that no attempt would be made to make psychiatrists of correction workers. Both of these promises will be kept. There is, however, a body of assumptions which pervades almost every school of psychiatry, no matter what terminology is used in the description of these assumptions. Some understanding of these three basic postulates is necessary to fully comprehend the suggestions about interviewing which may be applied to corrections.

The first of these is that individuals tend to act, and react, in ways which are consistent for them. No one person's behavior is completely consistent, but the odds are good that future behavior can be predicted from past behavior. The second assumption is that unless something is done to change this behavior it will persist, even ·though it may be illogical, maladaptive, and unwanted. It makes no difference whether this maladaptive behavior is conceived as being unconsciously motivated, reflexly conditioned, positively reinforced, or the act of the child within. It makes no sense from a common sense point of view. The attempt must be made to see it through the eyes of the offender, as difficult as this may be.

The third postulate is that not only is the behavior itself a repetition of past behavior, but the attitudes of the client are also a repetition of past attitudes. In the area of corrections, this is particularly important as far as attitudes towards authority are concerned. No matter how workers tend to structure their own attitudes, clients see them through the glasses of the past. The workers are viewed in the same light as past authority figures were. More importantly, the reactions to the officer are a carry-over from these past attitudes. This means that, no matter how unpleasant, seductive, insulting, provocative, submissive, or ingratiating the attitude is, the officer must be able to recognize it as still directed against that past authority figure, real or conceptualized, and not against the officer in person.

There is an important corollary to this. Corrections workers are humans also and sometimes are just as blind in seeing in themselves a carry-over of their own past attitudes and behaviors. Any officer who feels an unusual degree of dislike for, or attraction to, a particular offender, or feels sudden anger or emotion, must stop and ask, "Why?" Is there something in the officer's own past which is causing these reactions? For example, a worker who had been involved in a struggle for freedom from extremely dominating parents might have consistent reactions to clients caught up in this same struggle. These reactions might be empathic, "I know what's going on," or might be contemptuous, "I could settle my problems without outside help from somebody; the offender who can't must be a weakling." The male officer who is struggling against feelings of having been dominated by his mother and henpecked by his wife may find himself unaccountably made angry by the loud, aggressive offender who has his wife under his thumb. Every effort should be made to recognize these illogical reactions and to bare their roots. If it is impossible for their origin to be traced, every effort should be made to see they do not enter into the officer's decision-making process.

Finally, the officer must have a genuine respect for the basic humanity of all people, no matter how distorted their behavior. (As noted, that behavior may be as handicapping to the client as it is to society.) If this situation is recognized and the necessary leadership is applied in the proper way, it may be possible to change old attitudes and behavior. This leadership must not be arbitrary, intolerant, or punitive, or the result will be merely to reinforce the probationer's feelings about past traumatizing, authority figures. The worker must avoid arguing, belittling, or ridiculing the client. There are times when the officer must be firm, but this must be done without sarcastic, demeaning, or seductive remarks.

FORMING A RELATIONSHIP

The most significant aspect of any interview is the formation of a relationship. This holds true if only a single interview is contemplated, as in a presentence investigation for a nonprobatable offense, or when a series of interviews is to be expected. In some respects, the nature of the relationship is dictated by the fact that the worker is an agent of the court. That fact is never far from the client's mind. If being an agent of the court is seen by the worker as the central core of the relationship, the initial interview will develop along the lines of laying down probation conditions and letting the client know in no uncertain terms that the worker is boss and no nonsense will be tolerated. The relationship will then be strictly authoritarian.

The worker may see the relationship as one in which emphasis is solely on the reality-oriented concepts of funnelling the client into community resources in order to attain successful rehabilitation, i.e. Vocational Rehabilitation, Welfare (for temporary aid), educational work toward a GED, or even to improve functional illiteracy, etc. Under those circumstances the relationship will evolve along the lines of the worker as helper and the client as beneficiary. This too will become obvious in the interview. If, however, the worker is still idealistic enough (and that term is not being used in a derogatory sense) to want to go beyond these forms of relationship into one in which attitudinal changes on the part of the client can take place, then a different sort of relationship must be formed.

This is not to judge these various types of relationships. Certainly, it is obvious to all who have spent any time in corrections, and it will quickly become obvious to those who are just beginning, that the nature of the relationship depends not only on the desire of the corrections worker but also on the wishes, capabilities, and intentions of the offender. The attempt to form a relationship, and the nature of that relationship, between a parole officer and a three time loser (who merely wants to get his parole time over and done with) is going to be completely different from that formed between a parole officer and an individual just released from his first stay in a penal institution, sincere in his resolve it is going to be the last. Little time will be spent in describing techniques for the former situation. Nothing can be more discouraging than trying to lead a series of horses to water, none of whom will drink. This implies that the corrections worker has the experience and the knowledge to spot the individual who means what his words seem to be saying, and who is not hiding a wish to change behind a fear that "I can't," expressed as, "I won't." It is equally important that the officer also have the ability to spot the con that only too often lies behind the "you gotta help me to go straight." Hopefully, aids in this recognition will appear as these chapters unfold. Their main thrust is going to be toward forming a relationship with those who really desire to change. From all that follows individual workers will have to choose that which seems to be most comfortable for their personalities. The best techniques in the world are only techniques, unless they fit the worker.

There are five important aspects in building a relationship quickly. They must be treated sequentially for purposes of discussion, but they are all going on simultaneously. These aspects are: conveying a feeling of respect for the other as an individual; showing interest; maintaining a nonjudgmental attitude; being empathic and understanding; letting the other person talk. These must not become obtrusive techniques. Unfortunately, there is no such thing as a cookbook method of building a relationship, i.e. take five minutes of this, three minutes of that, and mix thoroughly with a dash of the other, simmer, and serve with a grain of salt. Much of what follows may seem quite elementary. It is amazing how much of what is done on an empirical basis can be done even more effectively once the rationale for its use is clarified.

CONVEYING RESPECT

The Use of Names

Regarding the simple matter of the use of names, how should a client be addressed, first name, last name, Mr., Mrs., Ms.? This sounds trivial, but it may set the tone of the entire interview, indeed of the entire relationship. Where there is a wide barrier in age (unless one is dealing with a child, or a very young adolescent), first names should rarely be used in the first interview. A twenty-two-year-old probation officer calling a fifty-year-old probationer, "Jack," robs him of his self-respect and dignity. A fifty-year old probation officer calling a twenty-two-year-old probationer, "Jack," sounds like, "All right, you young punk." More importantly, this use of first names may stimulate undesirable thoughts of the child/parent relationship, and all the probationer's resentment, hostility, and rebellion may be displaced from the parent onto the officer. This is especially true when the two participants in the dialogue are of opposite sex. Then, whatever sexual feelings which may have been involved may also be stimulated at no matter what level of consciousness.

Race also plays a part in the significance of the usage of names. This varies from region to region, from city to city, and even from time to time. At one period the use of an unadorned last name, Smith instead of Mr. Smith or Brown instead of Mr. Brown, may be an insult. At another it may be a token of friendly intentions. The worker should stay abreast of what is current in that particular community. The same thing is true in the use of racial designations when talking about other members of the same race. Is the preferred terminology Black, Negro, Afro-American, Colored, or Bilalian? Should it be Chicano, Spanish-American, Mexican? There is apt to be a good deal of sensitivity about this and the worker should respect it.

Where the worker and the client are approximately the same age, it is good practice to ask the simple question, "What would you like me to call you?" Among other things, this gives the client some say in setting the tone of the relationship. If the client chooses the use of the first name, it carries the implication that the officer's first name may be used as well.

This may sound like a good deal of bother about a very minor issue. Actually, it is an important one. It sets the tone of the relationship from the start, whether it is going to be authoritarian, patronizing, or egalitarian. More than anything else, it bespeaks the corrections worker's acknowledgement of the dignity of the other person as a human being; that person is not a number, not a body in a caseload, but an individual, a person with a name and a unique personality that goes with that name. It is also good technique to call the person by name at least two or three times in that first interview. This is also helpful in fixing the name in the worker's mind. It is a serious break of technique to fail to remember a name or to use the wrong name during the first interview. It is especially serious to say Tom repeatedly if the client has stated he prefers Mr.

Smith. It is quite possible that if a series of interviews are held, the use of the name will change as the nature of the relationship develops.

Choice of Language

As the interview transpires it is sometimes very difficult to continue to project the original attitude of respect for the other as a person. The very words that the worker uses can either foster or destroy this effort. To talk to an illiterate person in the verbiage of a college professor is an obvious put-down. To talk to that person in the same illiterate, even vulgar, way shows an equal amount of disrespect. The correct speech is in simple words, correctly pronounced, and used with proper grammar. If the individual uses street jive, the proper response is to use a phrase from that speech occasionally, to demonstrate familiarity with it, but not to use it constantly, which sounds like mockery, again a lack of respect. For many people, one of the most difficult things to respond to is a foreign accent. They either find themselves imitating the accent, which surely sounds like a takeoff, or responding to it in pidgin English, which makes their speech no more comprehensible, but makes the recipient feel foolish. Another common bad habit is to reply in a very loud, carefully enunciated tone, as though the listener were a hard of hearing child. None of these generate the feeling of being respected.

Discussing the Purpose of the Interview

A further way of showing respect for the client as an individual (and equally as a way of conveying interest) is to make sure the client knows what the purposes of the interview are. Workers are so certain of what the goal is they forget the client may not know anything about it. A perfunctory statment can fall awfully flat. Often the tone of the interview is quite different if the client is seeing the officer for the first time for a presentence investigation, for the first time as a probationer, as a parolee, or whatever the interview is for.

One very good method of discussing the purpose of the interview is to ask, "Do you know why you're here?" The answer is often surprising. "The judge said I had to come." "To keep from going to jail." "To see if I'm smart enough to be on the streets." "To find out if I really did it!" (This from someone who has just been found guilty, or has pled guilty or no contest.) If the answer is the correct one, then the next statement should be either, "That's right. Let me tell you exactly what that means," or it might be, "That's right. Could you tell me what you understand by those words?". Which of these two answers to use depends on a quick estimate of whether the particular individual needs to seem in control or seems to prefer to be somewhat dependent at the beginning of the interview.·

That this is in no way an academic question can be seen by the case of A.S. Under the Ohio Revised Code, in an attempt to conform to the United States Supreme Court ruling about the use of capital punishment, the death penalty is mandatory in certain types of murder unless mitigating circumstances can be demonstrated. These mitigating circumstances are spelled out precisely by the code. One of these is that the defendant at the time of the crime was suffering from mental illness or defect not sufficient to justify a verdict of not guilty by reason of insanity, but sufficient to have some bearing on the murderer's behavior.

Mr. A.S. was ordered to be so examined after having been found guilty of murder in the commission of a kidnapping. He insisted, in spite of the verdict, that he was innocent, but an examination for mitigating circumstances was ordered by the court. A.S. was originally seen at the county jail by a social worker. He refused to talk at all on the grounds that his attorney was preparing an appeal and had ordered him not to talk. After some conversation back and forth with his attorney, A.S. agreed to see the social worker but would answer only in terms of, "yes," "no," "I don't know," or other terse, nonrevealing answers. He halfheartedly performed the first few tests for a psychologist administering the Weschler in the jail. He then gave random answers, put forth no effort, and refused to do any more. Brought from the jail to the Diagnostic Center for a Rorschach and other projective testing, he listened to the statement about lack of confidentiality and said, "You can't make me answer any questions," turned on his heals, walked out the door, and instructed the deputies to return him to the jail.

It was arranged for him to see me the next day, but a call from the jail stated he said he would have to be knocked out and restrained before he would agree to the visit. Again, the cooperation of his attorney was enlisted, again A.S. stated he would cooperate; again the social worker traveled to the jail, and again the same monosyllabic answers. He did agree to keep the newly arranged appointment and at the proper time appeared at the interview accompanied by the deputies.

He was obviously sullen and hostile when brought into the office. Addressed as Mr. S., he was asked if he knew why he was being seen. In a sullen fashion he replied his attorneys told him he had to do so. He was here, but that did not mean he was going to say anything. The reply to this was that he had a right to know what was going on. The aspect of the law pertaining to psychiatric examination was then explained in detail. I made it clear that I did not have to pass on his guilt or innocence. All that was necessary was to try to find out what sort of person he was. Also, because of the lack of confidentiality, I felt at perfect liberty, indeed under an obligation, to report to the court as much of the conversation as he felt necessary, and Mr. S. should govern himself accordingly. As this verbal interchange proceeded, a dramatic change was transpiring in Mr. S. His hard, hostile look softened; his rigid shoulders relaxed; his hands, held tightly clasped, fell apart; he made himself as comfortable as his handcuffs would permit. Finally, he was told that absolutely no promises could be made regarding whether his talking would be of the slightest benefit to him. The next hour was spent in a completely cooperative discussion of Mr. S's life, although he continued to insist he was innocent of the charges. At the end of the interview I offered my thanks, and again reiterated there could be no promise that this would be of any benefit to him.

At that point he asked me to please apologize to the others who had seen him. He stated he had been bitter over what he felt to be a raw deal. No one had taken the trouble to sit down and explain what was going on to him. All anyone had said was what he said could not be confidential, and he had no real idea of what use was to be made of the material. He then agreed to retake the tests.

It should be stated at this point that the next day a call was received from Mr. S's attorney saying A.S. was not so sure he wanted to go ahead with the testing, but that was still probably his, the attorney's fault. He was still not sure about his future course and did not want his client incriminating himself in case of an appeal. He said his client would call if he again changed his mind. The significance does not lie in the outcome of the case. The example is being used to demonstrate that the initial honest explanation to the client of what the examination is about conveys a feeling of respect, of being seen as an individual. It gives the client a feeling of being a human being in his own right.

CONVEYING INTEREST

There are many different ways in which interest in a client is demonstrated. All of these will remain just technical maneuvers unless they are supported by a genuine interest. Just as the worker generally attempts to be alert to the probationer or parolee who is trying to con, so too the client very quickly becomes aware of the worker who is just utilizing a series of techniques. No amount of technical knowledge can mask a disinterested tone of voice, bodily set, or facial expression.

The Physical Setting

Some techniques used in conveying interest are quite obvious; others are more subtle. The setting in which the interview takes place can be utilized as a symbolic way of showing interest. The average probation worker has little say over the physical surroundings. In many places two or more workers share an office; in others all personnel are in one large space, sometimes without partitions or dividers. Even where only the semblance of privacy is possible, it is important that the focus of the interview is obviously directed to the client alone. The desk top may have some personal touches, photographs, appointment book, desk set, plants, but the only official material there should pertain to the client being interviewed at that time. This may entail sweeping fifteen folders into a desk drawer just the moment before the client walks in, but if it is an interview by appointment it should be apparent that the worker's time and interest are at the moment devoted only to the client. If the meeting is unscheduled, material on the desk should be pointedly pushed to one side as the client walks in. This simple procedure says quite loudly, "You are the only one who matters to me at this moment."

The same general principle holds true for phone calls. Time spent with the client belongs to that client and should not be interrupted for anything except an emergency. If there is no possibility of having incoming calls intercepted at a central point, the first comment on answering the phone should be, "I'm busy now, if you'll leave me a number I'll be glad to call back." If it should be an emergency, this should be indicated to the client who is sitting there. The most damaging phone calls are those which are personal. "Yes, I do love you." "Sure, I can meet you for lunch this noon." "Yes, I certainly would like to play tennis tomorrow night." All these may show interest in the caller, but display a lack of interest in the person sitting in the chair. The same thing holds true for the coworker or supervisor who disregards the client and says, "May I see you for a moment about something?" This must be discouraged, even if it becomes a matter which has to be taken up at staff meetings. There are occasions when a matter is urgent enough so that such an interruption is mandatory. If so, its urgency should not be minimized by a parting witticism, so that what the client hears is the worker and another official laughing. Then, not only is there a feeling the interruption was frivolous and unnecessary, but there may even be a question as to whether there was a personal reference in the laughter.

The Importance of Undivided Attention

Interest is also shown by undivided attention to what is being said. Any physical activity not related to the interview is taboo. This seems so obvious it should not need mentioning, but there have been complaints of activities as out of place while conducting an interview as cleaning fingernails, eating fruit or nuts, repairing a desk lamp, or reading mail. At one point, it was necessary for personal health reasons that I stop smoking. Since I was accustomed to smoking better than two packs a day, this was extremely difficult. The first several weeks it was bearable only if I were doing something with my hands. I started the habit of rubbing two small stones together in the same way people use worry beads. Within two to three days, a difficult choice had to be made: I could either simply say nothing about it, in which case there was a real problem in the relationship with patients who viewed this activity as a loss of interest in them, or at the beginning of the interview tell them what was going on and run the risk of having them think, "I have a crackpot for a psychiatrist." The second course was chosen as the preferable one.

Note Taking

This matter of distracting physical activity brings up the question of taking notes. Record keeping is an essential part of any interview. This is particularly true in corrections where the reasons for any recommendation to the court, or for any change in the status of an offender, must be well documented. Information is transmitted in many ways during an interview, all of which will be described. The author finds it impossible to assimilate this flow of information and still take notes. To do so would entail many things. First, there is the danger that the process of notetaking may become the dominant issue in the interview. This poses the very real risk that the client may feel, "Taking notes is more important than I am." Secondly, it is almost impossible to get everything down and still observe all there is to observe. Third, it becomes necessary to either constantly interrupt the client's flow of thought in order to keep up with what is being said or else to let the flow of thought proceed and lose what *is* being said while recording what was said two minutes ago.

Usually this dilemma is resolved by one of two equally unsatisfactory methods. Either the interviewer stops writing in order to devote full attention to something extremely interesting or important which is being said or else these are the only occasions when notes are taken. Either method tends to be quite disconcerting to the client. Another potential drawback is that an individual already worried about the outcome of the interview, e.g. someone undergoing a presentence evaluation, may clam up almost completely at the thought that every word uttered is being written down. There is, of course, a certain body of factual data which no one can be expected to remember without immediate notation. This includes such things as names of parents and siblings, significant dates, schools attended, jobs held with length of time and reasons for leaving. In most instances this material should be deferred until after some attempts have been made to attain a modicum of rapport and most of it should be obtained in one stretch.

There is one essential precaution to be taken if notes are not used. Time must be spent as soon as possible after the interview in noting all the significant material which was covered. For a busy corrections worker it is commonplace for one client to follow another into the office in a seemingly endless stream. Depending on the memory of the worker, it is imperative this stream be interspersed with periods of recording. Few people can remember more than three consecutive interviews without forgetting significant material, or, even worse, confusing one interview with another. Tape recording entire interviews has been suggested but is extremely impractical. It takes as long to listen to the taped interview as to conduct one. If secretarial help is available, the recorder may be used for notes immediately after an interview. It takes less than half the time to dictate than it does to write. A distinct advantage of waiting until after the interview to record, whether orally or in writing, is that it forces the worker to organize impressions of the interview into a coherent and meaningful whole. This must be weighed against the chances of omitting significant material. Should the worker feel notetaking is essential to avoid this danger, the notetaking should be as inconspicuous as possible.

The Manner of the Interviewer

The physical setting of the interview, the individual attention of the listener, taking or not taking notes are all overshadowed in importance by the general manner of the interviewer. Many factors enter into this. The facial expression should be pleasant, without seeming to be frivolous or unconcerned. Eye contact is important from time to time but should not be constant. There are many cultural differences about this matter of eye contact. Middle class individuals feel eye contact expresses honesty. Many lower class people, particularly inner city residents and especially blacks, feel constant eye contact is an affront, challenging, and hostile. Relatively primitive people, some from Caribbean areas, some from rural backward areas of this country, and many immigrants from eastern and southern Europe, equate eye contact with some form of the evil eye. There even may be a fear that an attempt if being made in this way to suck the individual's spirit. The bodily set should be relaxed. Leaning forward in the chair from time to time indicates an intensification of interest.

The quality, intensity, and intonation of the voice play an extremely important role in conveying interest. Even the most routine questions should not be asked in a perfunctory tone of voice. The overall impression should be firm and forthright, while still warm. This excludes both a prosecutorial insistence or a buddy-buddy attitude. Above all, there must be no periods of inattention which are brought to a crashing halt by intense silence while the client awaits a response to a remark to which the worker has not really listened. At times when attempting to evaluate the emotional status of a client, it is helpful to close the eyes and just listen to the tone of voice. If this technique is used, it is imperative that within a very short period of time some verbalization must be made to demonstrate that the closed eyes do not imply the worker is falling asleep. None of these methods of conveying attention by paying interest means anything unless there is genuine interest.

Interest is also conveyed by the appearance of being unhurried. No one likes to be rushed through an interview. (A client with something to hide may try to do the rushing.) This unhurried manner does not mean that an interview is needlessly prolonged or allowed to drag on endlessly, nor that fifteen or twenty minutes is wasted on sports, the weather, or a meaningless topic before getting down to the meat of the interview. It does mean that regardless of pressure of time, the worker remains calm, unhurried, and relaxed. Little happens when the officer is curt, brusque, and impatient. If interviews are conducted on a timed basis, i.e. a fifteen, twenty, or thirty minute slot set aside for that particular client, some warning should be given three to five minutes beforehand that time is running out. If the interview is on a time-as-needed basis, this should be terminated by a remark such as, "Well, that pretty much seems to be it. Is there anything else you think I ought to know today?" Or, "Do you see anything coming up that seems like trouble?" If there is a decision to be made, the concluding remark might be, "Why don't you think it over and let me know in . . . (time sequence)." Each person will find closing remarks which best suit that individual's personality.

Remembering Details

Memory for material which has been related is probably the single most important factor in conveying interest. A reference at a later point in the interview to something mentioned earlier is the most convenient way of demonstrating this memory. The converse of this proposition is equally true. Nothing is more damaging to the client's appraisal of the degree of interest than to be forced to repeat the same piece of information or to correct the same misconception two or three times during an interview. "He really didn't give a damn or he'd remember." "She can't be very interested or she wouldn't ask me the same question she did ten minutes ago." "He couldn't have been listening while I told him that before." These are the common thoughts which a client has when such an episode occurs. The accompanying feeling may seriously interfere with any attempts to form a relationship.

It is equally important to carry this knowledge from one interview to the next. There are only two basic reasons to put an interview on paper. One is to aid in writing a report, the other to jog the memory. Hence, a client seen previously should *never* (and never must be stressed) be seen a second, third, fourth, or *n*th time without a careful review of the record. With a probationer or parolee it is helpful to refer in one interview to material discussed in a previous one. If this is about an important topic, a new job, taking an exam, being evaluated at Vocational Rehabilitation, it should be introduced at the beginning of the interview. "How's the new job going?" "Did your grades come back on that test?" "What are they planning for you at Vocational Rehabilitation? Do you think you'll like that deal?"

This reference to something important in the individual's life always implies a real interest on the part of the officer. It is sometimes equally impressive to use material which is not particularly essential but which is relevant to the topic under discussion. "Is that the rappy you talked about last time who was the only guy in the pen you could trust?" This must be used sparingly because otherwise the individual feels, "I can't tell him anything because he remembers everything and it might be held against me."

The same precaution which applies to failing to remember a detail within an interview also applies to forgetting something of significance from a previous interview. Should this occur, any expression of surprise should be avoided. A statement might be made such as, "I'm sorry, I'm a little bit mixed up on that. Would you fill me in on it." Above all, arguments as to whether the information had or had not been given previously should be avoided. This does not apply, of course, to material under discussion which has to do with a misstep on the part of the client, which has now been uncovered, when it is plain that it was not reported previously.

Minimal Responses

There is one final technique for conveying interest. Regardless of whether the client is answering a question or is talking about a self-initiated topic, no one likes to have words drop into a vacuum. There must be some sort of response from the interviewer. Even if words are flowing like a stream, they should be replied to with a nod, a smile, a grunt, an "mmh hnn," or "Is that so?", anything which conveys a response. This should not divert the flow of thought (unless intentionally), but should make the person aware the words are being heard and understood.

The Nonjudgmental Attitude

A third tool in building the relationship is the consistent maintenance of a nonjudgmental attitude. This is a concept that is frequently misunderstood. A nonjudgmental attitude does not imply an approving or condoning attitude any more than it implies a condemnatory attitude. It means exactly what it says; it speaks of attitude not behavior. The corrections worker's position as an officer of the court mandates continuous reaction to all observed and reported behavior. That reaction may include the decision that the behavior is serious enough to warrant application for revocation of probation. What a nonjudgmental attitude involves is that this decision is taken without any implication to suggest the probationer is bad, incorrigible, or untrustworthy. This matter of being nonjudgmental also does not preclude an atempt to make such an episode a learning experience for the probationer, by pointing out that certain behavior entails certain consequences and that the same behavior has led to the same consequences in the past and will do so in the future. Such confrontation can be done without moralizing, preaching, or condemning.

Particular attention should be paid during the initial interview to the maintenance of this nonjudgmental attitude.

"What were you like as a kid?"

"I was a hell-raiser. I got sent away because I couldn't stand my stepmother, so I kept breaking up her things and running away."

This does not call for, "Serves you right," or "It doesn't seem to have taught you much to have been sent away." A non-judgmental answer would be, "What made you dislike you stepmother so much?". This is a direct response that says, "I heard you." It also says, "I'm willing to believe there are two sides to the question."

This attitude should also carry throughout all contacts with the client. "I got fired because I was late for work again," should not evoke an, "I told you so," or "That's a stupid thing to do," or "Won't you ever learn." A response should be made that responds to the statement and conveys interest without passing judgment. "I wonder why you can't seem to get up on time?" not only would fill the above criteria but might also be a first step in moving the probationer off dead center.

It is equally important not to pass judgment on others. If the response to the last question is, "She used to cheat on my old man and I couldn't stand it," the response should not be along the lines of "She must have been a real slut." This might appear to be a good way of communicating interest, and in effect saying, "I'm on your side, I don't blame you." In a sense it does. At the same time it does some things that could be quite destructive to a relationship. First, the probationer may think it is an easy step from passing judgment on the stepmother whom the officer does not know to passing judgment on the probationer himself. Second, he may think, "I can tell that poor fish anything I want and it will be believed without any confirmation.." A better answer would be, "How did that make you feel inside when you thought she was cheating?". This does not pass judgment on her. While not in any way intimating that the client is lying, the use of "thought" instead of "learn" implies that both parties have the benefit of the doubt. Finally, it helps to begin a process which is of utmost significance in dealing with offenders, that is, the attempt to get them to recognize and identify feelings and to connect specific feelings to specific behavior.

Understanding and Empathy

Communicating empathy and understanding are two other

means of building a relationship. Empathy involves the capacity to put oneself in another person's shoes, to see a situation from that point of view, and particularly to be aware of the other's feelings. Until recently it was believed that empathy was an inborn ability like artistic talent or mathematical genius. It has been shown recently that, while some people may have a natural ability to empathize with others, it can be taught and learned. Only if this empathy is conveyed to the client can it be of help in building a relationship and facilitating the flow of an interview. If empathy is present, it is usually conveyed without awareness that special techniques are being used. There are many ways in which this is done. Offering a tissue to a tearful client conveys the message, "It's all right to cry, we all have to relieve our feelings sometimes." This is particularly helpful in the case of a hard-boiled individual whose eyes begin to fill. If the tissue is brushed away, it should not be reproffered, but the box should be placed in close approximation to the individual. Almost invariably, it will be used a little later, even if somewhat surreptitiously. If the offer induces a flood of tears, silence is frequently the best response. If the silence seems to induce tension then a simple, "Go ahead and cry and get rid of it," may be used.

Another method of communicating empathy is a remark such as, "That must be hard for you to talk about," when a particularly sensitive area is being discussed. "You obviously don't want to talk about that now, maybe we can get back to it later," may also be utilized. (Obviously, this is not to be used when this is a definite effort to duck talking about something which must be talked about. "Is it true you were drunk last night?" "How is it I haven't seen you in six weeks?" The reference is to an event in the past which threatens to evoke feelings the individual cannot cope with now.)

The next most important technique for communicating empathy is to rephrase the client's feelings and reflect them back.

"I was so mad I could have killed him."

"You were *really* angry."

"When she left me I just didn't feel anything was worth anything."

"You felt kind of empty inside."

A great deal of care must be taken that it is the actual feeling that is being reflected and not a statement of how the officer thought the client should feel. It is certainly possible, and sometimes desirable, for the corrections worker to indicate what *action* should be taken by an individual; it is never permissible in a good relationship to tell another person how that person should *feel*.

Inextricably linked with empathy is understanding. Only too often in corrections, the client enters the interview situation with the feeling, "Nobody understands me; nobody ever has understood me; nobody really wants to understand me." At the same time the client completely overlooks the fact that, "I don't understand myself; I never have understood myself; I'm really a little bit afraid to try to understand myself." In spite of this, there is almost invariably the wish for "somebody to understand me." The worker must be able to convey both the desire to understand and the ability to do so.

The desire to understand is conveyed by the questions asked and the manner of asking them. A relentless interrogatory may convey a desire to understand, but it certainly does not convey a desire to use that understanding in a way helpful to the person being interrogated. Those questions directed at feelings and motives convey the greatest wish to be understanding. In the example used in the last section, the question, "What made you dislike your stepmother so much?" was directed toward motive; "How did you feel inside when you thought she was cheating on your father?" is devoted toward feelings. Both indicate a desire to understand.

In that situation, the ability to understand would have been conveyed by, "That must have made you feel all upset and uptight inside," rather than, "How did you feel?" Such remarks should be reserved for those occasions when there is no question about the correctness of the feeling expressed. There may have been a deeper, unconscious feeling involved here, that of being frightened by, "If my stepmother were so loose with her favors, maybe she'd give it to me." Such a feeling might be at the root of the runaway behavior, but this depth of understanding should be utilized with the greatest of caution and only if a relationship has been well established and the worker is prepared to deal with the probationer's reaction to the interpretation.

It is better to proceed slowly with exploratory rather than empathic remarks until the real personality of the probationer is better known. At that time the officer will be more aware of how this particular probationer feels in these particular circumstances. At times an empathic association may be too right, too early in the relationship. It may spotlight a feeling the probationer is unwilling to acknowledge. The statement of the officer is then contradicted and defenses go up. The probationer becomes afraid of the officer's ability to spot true feelings and becomes wary and on guard. This is particularly apt to be true in the adolescent, especially the adolescent boy. The officer may recognize that the interview situation has the youngster a little frightened. If the officer starts empathizing with the boy's concern with a remark such as, "It must be a little frightening talking to me for the first time," the specter of being *chicken* may be raised, and the adolescent has to deny this. His guard is likely to go up right away, and there is the danger of losing contact with him, at least for that interview. Under these circumstances, it is sometimes of help to aid him to project his feelings with a remark like, "It's perfectly natural for lots of people to be uptight in a situation like this, but you don't seem to be very upset." This helps to put him at ease and may even allow him to verbalize, "I was a little bit when I first came in, but I'm not now." He is able to feel the probation officer is understanding and is not going to put him down because he was a little afraid.

Frequently, the probation officer is presented with the sort of person who is basically insecure but who tries to keep up a front of self-sufficiency and assurance. In dealing with this sort of person, it is a help in conveying understanding to ask, "Maybe you could help me to understand what was going through your mind when . . . ," or even, "To help me to understand what you are feeling when . . . ," rather than the usual, "How did you feel?" or "That must have made you feel . . .".

This implies the desire to understand and feel with the individual without any possible challenge to the worth of these feelings. It does not threaten the facade of self-assurance while still conveying the desire to understand another's feelings.

In addition to these methods just described, or even at times instead of them, a nod, a smile, an assenting murmur all help to convey understanding and empathy as well as interest. The facial expression of warmth or the interest conveyed in the tone of voice may be all that is necessary. Certainly, these nonspecific measures are preferable until enough understanding of the probationer has accumulated to allow the officer to be sure of the correctness of the verbalized observations.

Resisting the Temptation to Interrupt

There is one other indispensable step in this process of creating the sort of atmosphere in which a relationship which fosters communication can develop. That step is letting the client talk and not cutting the flow of communication short by interruption. This does not contradict the principle of conveying interest by making the appropriate comments or assent rather than letting words fall into a vacuum. The two principles are actually quite different. These assenting phrases are made to facilitate the flow of thought. Interruptions are designed to stop it, correct it, or change its direction. Certainly there are many times when they are not only useful but essential. At this point attention is being focused on those interruptions which may be harmful. Two general situations which tempt interruptions occur with the greatest frequency. The first arises out of impatience, annoyance, irritation; the second springs from interest and the desire to pursue a topic which the probationer seems to have left up in the air.

An example of the first type occurs when the probationer starts talking about relatively meaningless topics and the worker is eager to get to material of significance. The probationer refers to something which might seem to be of importance, only to drop it immediately and resume the apparent chit-chat. This could be extremely annoying, and it is a great temptation to interrupt at this point in order to get back to the topic which seemed to be so meaningful. With most clients this temptation should be resisted in the evaluative interview. It is always possible to introduce the interesting topic at a later time. It is rarely possible to anticipate the direction the seemingly trivial talk may have taken if allowed to go unchecked. It may be the client would have arrived at far more meaningful material if allowed to proceed at will. It may be the probationer is working up to a topic which is extremely sensitive and difficult to approach, and this seemingly meaningless material is a way of temporizing while gauging the extent of the worker's interest and ability to understand. An interruption may increase the difficulty to the extent that the really significant material never emerges. The client may even seize on the worker's interest in the topic which was offered and withdrawn. Talking about this question pleases the officer, but gives the probationer a chance to duck the really significant material which was painfully being approached. With relatively little experience, it does not need much additional expenditure of time to differentiate between the individual who is trying to build up to something significant and the individual who is talking to kill time and evade the real issues. Ways of dealing with that type of person will be explored in a later chapter.

The following is an example of the second type of situation in which interruptions are most likely to be harmful. The probation officer has been asking questions designed to elicit factual material and asked, "What jobs have you held?"

The probationer answers, "Well, let's see. Right after I quit school I went to work at McDonald's. I didn't like that so I quit after three months. Then I got a job at the glass company. That was good pay, but after about six months I couldn't stand changing shifts every two weeks. Then I went to work at the hospital. I met my wife there. She's a real hard woman to figure out. Sometimes I don't know what she wants out of me ... "

This digression to the character of the wife is obviously not going to give the officer the listing of jobs needed for a presentence report. But it should not be stopped. It may furnish all the significant material necessary to determine a client's attitude toward male/female relationships, the feelings which led to his behavior on the day of the offense, and even some estimate as to his stability and how that may effect a recommendation for probation. Talking in this spontaneous manner, a client is much less on guard than in answering direct questions about all these subjects. Interruptions then must be used with caution.

At first glance it may seem that the techniques which have been described are extremely time-consuming and must lead to a completely unstructured interview situation. Neither of these assumptions is valid. The apparently time-consuming side excursions, as was just noted, frequently turn out to be shortcuts to the main highway and are actually time-savers in themselves. Certainly, these techniques are timesaving when attempting to establish a relationship meant to exist over a period of time. Nor does their use necessarily lead to an unstructured interview. Directions will be given in Chapter 16 for the use of nondirective techniques in a structured interview.

Chapter 15

THE ART OF LISTENING

GENERAL CONSIDERATIONS

THE corrections worker must make use of all available help in attempting to understand the client. This implies a consistent and thorough use of all sensory modalities and correlating the information received through them with all the knowledge about human behavior which has been gained through study and experience. This chapter will be concerned with the various observations which should be made and the information which can be obtained from them. Much of this material may seem to be belaboring the obvious, but unless the habit of making systematic observations is formed much meaningful knowledge may be overlooked. It goes without saying that these observations should be made unobtrusively. No one enjoys the feeling of being a laboratory insect pinned under a microscope and wiggling for the edification of the viewer. Once that sort of atmosphere seeps into an interview, no amount of perfection in the use of other interviewing techniques will allow a positive relationship to be formed. As a general rule, the corrections worker comes to the interview with some information about the client. This may consist only of some statistical data, the details of the offense, and the past arrest record. The type of observations to be discussed should enable the worker to modify and expand the impressions gained from that original material.

VISUAL OBSERVATIONS

The observations fall into several categories, the first of which is visual. It takes practice and effort to acquire the ability to look at someone and see everything meaningful which can be observed. This ability is facilitated by the use of a mental list

288

of questions. The implications of the answers are filed away and checked against the flow of information coming from other senses and from a consideration of what is said. These questions start with a general impression which the individual makes on the probation officer. Does this person appear attractive or unattractive? As a general rule, to which there may be exceptions, there are marked differences in self-concept between attractive and unattractive people. As a result, the former do not have to avail themselves of the same sort of defenses and compensatory reactions as do the latter. Is there anything bizarre about this individual's appearance? Is there any evidence of physical defects which might have had some bearing on personality development? These include such things as extremes in height or weight, buck teeth, harelip, squint, defective extremities, premature baldness, facial acne with resultant scars, overly large or overly small breasts in a woman, or other defects of this sort.

A.T. was a sixteen-year-old male referred from juvenile court after his second arrest for exposing himself. He was as bald as the proverbial billiard ball and had apparently been so since birth. He was an only child. Large sums of money, which his parents could ill-afford to spend, had been expended in efforts to grow hair on his head. Other youngsters teased him unmercifully. When he was thirteen his parents had bought an expensive wig for him, but this action came too late. His baldness was so well known that the wig served only as an object for others to snatch and pass around in an endless game of keep-away. A.T. had withdrawn more and more into a fantasy world populated by invincible characters, such as the Six Million Dollar Man. He was constantly engaged in drawing engines of destruction, capable of destroying the world. His father had been aware of A.T.'s habit of exposing himself (although only arrested twice, neighbors had frequently complained to the father about this behavior). He attempted to cure this habit by taking the boy to a prostitute. She had aggravated the situation by bursting into uncontrollable laughter upon seeing him.

A.T.'s exhibitionism was one expression of his hostility and contempt for a world which had rejected him because of his physical deformity.

CLOTHING

While these speculations are going on about the implications of the general physical appearance, attention should be paid to the clothing. Many individuals seen by the corrections worker will be seen in settings where uniform attire is mandatory. Approximately 80 percent of the people whom I observe are brought from jails and juvenile detention. In each instance they are wearing clothing furnished by the institution. Yet the differences in appearance are striking. These are some of the questions which should be asked about clothing, and some of the implications which the answers carry. Is it neat, or slovenly? If it is neat, is it fussily meticulous? This may be the first clue to a rigidly compulsive type of character organization of a sort which may make the worker's attempt to modify behavior patterns much more difficult. If it is slovenly, does this mean carelessness, indifference, depression, or deterioration? Is there a lack of personal cleanliness? This may represent a personal or cultural factor. Is there anything bizarre about the person's attire? Even in an institution, attire may be embellished by the inmate in such a fashion that it screams schizophrenia to anyone who looks carefully. How is the clothing worn? It certainly says something pretty obvious about the *machismo* attitude of the male who comes to an interview with his prison coveralls unbuttoned to the fifth button and carefully rolled back to disclose a hairy or tatooed chest. Certain inferences can be drawn about the female who on a cold day has her blouse well unbuttoned and is wearing no bra.

In those instances where the individual comes to the interview from home rather than jail even more information can be gained from the choice of clothing and the manner in which it is worn. Is it representative of a certain group about whom some inferences might be drawn? Examples of this might be the insignia-laden leather jacket consistent with certain types of motorcycle clubs; the hip-hugging, genital-accentuating, tight jeans of certain gay males; the stereotyped garb of the street prostitute, which varies from time to time and city to city. Is the clothing loud and flamboyant, or unobtrusive and mousy?

In either case does it represent the personality of the wearer, or the personality which the wearer wishes to portray? As Buttercup remarked in Gilbert and Sullivan's *Pinafore,* "Things aren't always what they seem, skim milk masquerades as cream; highlows pass as patent leathers; jackdaws strut in peacock's feathers."[1]

If the individual is a woman, is her dress appropriate to the occasion, or is she overdressed in a manner suggestive of a consciously or unconsciously seductive attitude to the male probation officer, and possibly to all men? It must be stressed that all these observations must be checked against other obtainable facts. A woman who is wearing her only outfit can scarcely be accused of being overdressed or seductive; a fourteen-year-old boy wearing his brother's hand-me-downs hardly reveals his own personality.

Other things about the attire which should be noted is the presence or absence of jewelry, its quantity and character. In some areas, a large gold earring on a male denotes homosexuality if it is worn on a certain ear; the particular ear varies from location to location. Some people wear religious insignias either in pendants around the neck or in the form of pins. Others wear cult identifying marks such as the Star of Isis and Osiris which identifies a witch or a wizard. Again, not only is the individual piece of jewelry significant, but it's appropriateness to the occasion should be noted.

Hair, Nails, and Skin

Personal preferences in those aspects of bodily appearance over which an individual has control should also be assessed for meaning. The significance attached to hair style, beard, moustache, and other hirsute adornments in males is no longer as clear as it formerly was. Still, the presence of long hair or crewcut, corn-pickers, braids, or Afro, Fu-Man-Chu, VanDyke, U.S. Grant, or other beards should be noted and an attempt made to assess their significance. It is important in

---

[1]*Authentic Libretti,* Gilbert and Sullivan Operas, Crown Publishers, New York, 1939, p.80.

either a male or female whether the hair is orderly or unkempt. In a woman, the use, nonuse, or misuse of makeup is worthy of note, as is the appearance of the fingernails, long or short, painted or unpainted. If painted are they in a striking or garish tone, or a pale muted one. In either sex, badly bitten nails indicate a high degree of tension and anxiety. The cleanliness of the nails must be weighed against the occupation of the possessor. Dirty nails do not carry the same meaning in a service station attendant as they do in a banker.

Just as the significance of hair style is changing, so too is that of the tattoo. Even though the number of those who are tattooed is increasing, some estimation of personality can still be made from the number and style of the visible tattoos. LOVE and HATE tattooed across the backs of individual fingers of each hand still tend to identify the violence-prone male, or one who wishes to give that appearance. The Pachuco Cross in the webbing between the thumb and the forefinger is still seen, either as a remnant of the old Pachuco Gang or in imitation thereof. Crudely executed, monochromatic tattoos, whether initials, names, or design have almost invariably been acquired during the teens. Sexually suggestive tattoos, like the open shirt, would suggest the *macho* male. Tattooing is a growing fad with women but is still generally confined to those areas of the body seen only in the bedroom or at the pool. Visible tattoos on a woman tend to indicate an exhibitionistic trait and sometimes serve as a clue to the hysterical personality.

Mannerisms and Behavior

Mindful of the tentative conclusions of personality drawn from these observations, attention should next be directed to the general bearing, manner, and behavior of the client in the interview setting. The list of possible observations in this category is almost endless, and only a representative sample will be discussed. There is the swaggering gait and high held head of self-assurance, or even cockiness. There is the furtive look which points to slyness. There is the hang-dog guilty look; the on-guard, wary, suspicious look; the timid, hesitant look, which proclaims lack of self-confidence; the appealing look, which says, "Treat me like a little child"; the submissive look; the downcast, moist-eyed, depressed look; the heavy-eyed, seductive look; the silly look; the angry, hostile look; the vacant look of the deteriorated individual; the wild-eyed look of the psychotic; and on and on.

It is certainly important that the corrections worker be alert to the meaning of all of these varied clues and that they be used in forming tentative conclusions which will help in being empathic. It is especially important that attention be focused on the feelings which they arouse in the worker. If a cocky person makes the officer bristle, a defiant one evokes anger, or a submissive one contempt, then the question, "Why?" must be asked. The officer must be able to recognize inner reactions, must have some idea of where they originated, and must have developed effective means of dealing with them, so that they do not interfere with the process of building a relationship. At times these gut feelings may be of help in diagnosis. In most people, a schizophrenic arouses some feelings of uneasiness; a manic stimulates a desire to laugh with rather than at; a depressed person elicits feelings of either sympathy or aversion (there are some depressed people who exhibit a hostile dependent reaction); a severely paranoid person usually induces mild anxiety or even fear.

Repetitive mannerisms or *tics* should also be noted as examples of behavior. Tics may only be a sign of general tension (rarely they are seen in withdrawal symptoms of cocaine or narcotic addiction), but they also may have a symbolic significance. This symbolism may point to important areas for further exploration. For example, a repetitive screwing up of the eyes may represent an attempt to blot out something the individual had seen or the denial of some unavoidable, unpleasant, environmental situation. Repetitive, jerky, wrinkling up of the nose may be the only expression of a profound feeling of disgust. A frequent turning of the head to one side with elevation of the shoulder closest to the chin may be the warding off of a blow. A kicking out of one leg jerkily from time to time may symbolize aggression. Any such mannerism should be carefully noted, and its possible meaning evaluated. (There is a disease process, seen largely in children and adolescents, called Gilles de la Tourette's Disease, which is characterized by constantly recurring tics, and the frequent, explosive expression of curses and obscenities.)

Emotional Responses

As the interview progresses, the officer should take note of any signs signifying a particular emotional response on the part of the client. General signs of tension are quite obvious — foot tapping, nail biting, hand wringing, restlessness, fidgeting, tremor, sweating. Almost every client will display some degree of increased tension during the first interview, and probably during the early periods of subsequent interviews. If the interview is progressing satisfactorily, and the relationship is developing properly, these signs of tension should begin to disappear. If they do not, the reason for their persistence should be questioned. Is this anxiety characteristic for the client and unrelated to the interview situation, or does it mean the approach will have to be changed in order to put the client at ease? It is also quite significant if these signs of tension recur after they have once disappeared. Generally, this indicates some subject with real meaning to the probationer has been touched, either directly or by means of internal associative processes. The area under discussion when this observation is made should be noted carefully, to be explored more fully at the appropriate time.

There are signs indicative of more specific emotional reactions for which the worker should be on the alert. These include the clenched jaws and hands, paling and flushing of anger; the little moue and wrinkling of the nose of disgust; the moist eyes of sadness; the blush of embarrassment; the dilated pupils, deep rapid breathing, and frequent swallowing of fear. This list too could be expanded indefinitely. (A way of pinpointing the response of those who blush or flush derives from the fact that once such an erythematous response is produced, it lingers. The area will shrink or expand depending on the degree of emotional response. The more intense the response, the wider the area covered.) In every instance of emotional reaction, the officer should be asking, "What is bringing this on?".

Signs of Drug Use

One further aspect of visual survey must be noted. It is impossible to make a diagnosis of drug abuse solely on the basis of what is seen, but several clues may be found. The habitual narcotic user will show pin-point pupils, which remain smaller than normal for several months after drug abuse has been stopped. The presence of needle *tracks* on the back of the hands or interior surface of the forearms, particularly just beneath the bend of the elbows, is certainly another very suggestive sign. The abuser of cocaine or speed will show dilated pupils, even if the room is relatively bright. These people will also tend to be quite thin, even to the point of emaciation. Motor movements may be jerky, and there is generally an observable increase in psychomotor activity, with a degree of restlessness. Tracks may also be seen with the person who *shoots* rather than *pops* or *snorts* the drugs. The chronic gasoline sniffer shows reddened eyes and a runny nose. Red eyes are also prominent during marijuana smoking but disappear shortly after any episode.

AURAL OBSERVATIONS

Vocal Quality

Concurrently with the visual observations, there should be equally thorough aural observation. What is under investigation here is form rather than content. What does the voice reveal about the probationer's personality? Is it slow and hesitant, that of a timid and insecure person? Is it forthright and confident? Is it angry and hostile — constantly or only when certain topics are under discussion? Is there an edge of resentment, of surliness? Is every statement made tentatively, as if with a question mark at the end, while the client awaits the worker's reaction as a clue as to whether the statement should be modified or not?

CHOICE OF ROLE

What roles are taken in the dialogue? Does the individual initiate and carry more than a fair share of the conversation? Is this because of the basic need to dominate any situation, or is it because of fear and an attempt to conceal this fear behind a facade of self-assurance? Is there silence until the probation officer takes the lead? Does this imply the probationer's concept of their respective roles of officer and probationer in the interview, or does it mean dependence and nonaggressiveness? Could this represent a fear of initiating a conversation lest it reveal too much? Is there deliberate evasiveness? The following is a verbatim excerpt from an interview with an evasive individual.

Mr. A.U. was being examined for competency to stand trial. He was twenty-years-old, had spent at least seven years in correctional institutions, and had about a tenth grade education. He is accused of breaking and entering, robbery, and murder. The question at issue at the moment is his understanding of the charge against him. This segment is well into the interview and is typical of the entire time spent with him.

Q. What is murder?
A. Somebody gets dead.
Q. How?
A. Could be any way.
Q. If he's killed in an automobile accident, is that murder?
A. Could be.
Q. What if it were a one car accident, the dead person was the only one driving, and he skidded and hit a bridge abutment?
A. I don't know.
Q. What does murder usually mean?
A. As far as I know, somebody's dead.
Q. How did he get dead?
A. How did he get dead?
Q. Yes.

A. He just dies.
Q. And that means murder?
A. You said he got killed in a car, didn't you?
Q. What does murder usually mean?
A. To tell the truth, I don't know.
Q. Does it bother you that you don't know?
A. No.
Q. What does breaking and entering mean?
A. *I* broke into something. (Note the I in response to the general question.)
Q. What does that mean?
A. Anything I guess.
Q. Anything special?
A. I don't know.
Q. What does robbery mean?
A. You take some money.
Q. From where?
A. Anywhere.

This is scarcely an example of building a relationship during an interview. It is, however, a classic example of the individual who is trying to be evasive and succeeding.

Speech Defects

While the form and quality of the speech is being observed, attention should also be paid to defective speech. Speech defects may have as much bearing on personality development as physical defects do. Some details to be observed are stammering, lisping, transposition of syllables, baby talk, inability to pronounce certain letters. Do these result in teasing and social isolation? Does the baby talk represent mental retardation or the persistence of childish emotional patterns? Can it possibly be regression, either as a result of mental illness or as a result of the stress of the interview? Does the individual use *neologisms* (that is, are new words coined)? This does not have to be as consistent as Lewis Carroll's famous, "'Twas brillig and the slithy toves did gyre and gimble in the wabe,"[2] but many

---

[2]Carroll, Lewis, "Through the Looking Glass," in *The Complete Works of Lewis Carroll*, Modern Library Edition, p. 153.

schizophrenics and some deteriorated, senile individuals will coin new words, the former because of autism, the latter in an attempt to replace the forgotten words.

Quality of Language

In this systematic appraisal of the picture which the individual presents to the world, the worker should next listen to the general quality of the language used. This furnishes valuable clues to the general intelligence and cultural level of the client. This language should then serve as a key to the language used by the officer. It should be tuned to a level which the probationer can comprehend and at which he can feel comfortable. Naturally, this should never be done in such a way as to become condescending or derogatory. The comment was made earlier about being careful not to imitate the speech of another unconsciously and thus appear to be derisive. An attempt should be made to phrase questions, explanations, and comments in understandable terms.

The particular group to which a client belongs may be suggested by the language used with about the same accuracy attained from observation of attire. This may be a universal although ever-changing jargon, such as the *gay* speech of the homosexual or the *cool* speech of the hep-cat, or it may be a specialized form of a group in a particular neighborhood. The example of this latter group which comes most easily to mind at this moment is the variation from community to community of names applied to particular drugs or methods of using them. It is important that the worker be familiar with all these terms and understand them. It is of help in communication if such terms are used by the officer from time to time to indicate understanding. This usage should not be at the same frequency as that of the probationer. This would either imply condescension and mockery or place the relationship on a footing in which the worker is in danger of losing the leadership role.

The officer should be on guard against the use of technical terms. These will have become second nature and a part of the natural speech of members of the profession. However, they will carry an entirely different connotation to those outside that group and may even have fear-inspiring overtones.

There are important implications to other aspects of the probationer's language. As was noted earlier, most people exhibit some degree of tension during the early stages of an interview. The relaxation of this tension is an indication that the interview is going well. In the same way many probationers use a somewhat stilted and formal speech in the early stages of the interview. It is as though they were on their best behavior in order to impress the probation officer. Lapsing back to a more customary speech pattern may be interpreted as a sign of relaxation and the beginning of a relationship. An occasional individual will consistently use highfalutin language which is totally out of of character and may be misused almost to the point of being ludicrous. This is most likely to appear in people who are of borderline or mildly mentally retarded intelligence and is generally interpreted as a means of bolstering a poorly developed ego-concept. Where a formal and more stilted language, replete with big words and phrases, is used consistently and appropriately, it connotes either an individual who has pretty well effected a partial retreat from the real world into a world of classic books or connotes an individual who is a real phony and believes that this is the way that educated upper class people talk.

USING OTHER SENSES

Man's sense of smell has atrophied since his primitive days as a hunter. This may be a severe handicap in many areas but the nose plays only a minor role in interviewing. It used to be stated that a schizophrenic odor existed, but it is now generally concluded this is the net result of the reluctance of the deteriorated schizophrenic to wash and the clinging odor of the back ward. The use of the sense of smell is limited to a few specific areas. The detection of the odor of alcohol is obvious. (Incidentally, this may linger on the breath for twenty-four hours after the last ingestion of alcohol.) At times the acrid sweet smell of marijuana may linger in the hair or clothing of an individual. More commonly, marijuana usage is suggested by the persistence of the scent of incense, which is frequently used in conjunction with marijuana smoking. The intensity, as well as the quality, of a woman's perfume or body cologne may tell something about her. The odor of personal or oral uncleanliness needs no mention. Some people claim to be able to smell fear. Where such a smell exists, it would seem to be the result of the perspiration which so frequently accompanies fear. In certain individuals the so-called apocrine glands, which are sweat glands emanating a peculiar odor, would appear to be stimulated.

The touch and kinesthetic senses are brought into play largely in the evaluation of the handshake. This ritual should be a part of the beginning and termination of every initial interview and may frequently be employed in later ones. Not only is the form and quality of the original handshake noted, but it may then be compared to the terminal one to see if any changes have occurred. A dry, brisk handshake at the beginning of the interview, followed by a terminal, moist, limp one suggests the individual has become emotionally involved and drained. This may be from fear or from relief and will have to be interpreted in the context of the interview. Certain adolescents and young adults, if they have approved of an interview, will change the conventional handshake on greeting to the thumb shake on parting.

Listening to Silence

Another aspect of the art of listening must be recognized. This is the matter of listening to silence. There are several types of silence which may occur in the course of an interview. The most common type in the original interview is the silence of rumination before answering a question. This silence almost talks. The worker can almost hear the client saying silently, "Should I talk about it or shouldn't I?" or "Would *this* be the better answer, or *that?*" Every correction worker has this experience while awaiting an answer, of watching the wheels turn in the client's brain. This, of course, means the worker must take every answer with a grain of salt. The disappearance of such silence generally indicates a growing ability to trust the worker. At times it is a sort of resignation, an "Oh, hell, he's going to find out anyway. I might as well tell him."

A second type of silence, also apt to occur in the first interview but by no means confined to it, is the long silence denoting anxiety and tension. Sometimes this occurs following a terse answer to a question, when the interviewer is expecting more. Sometimes it occurs after a nonspecific question; sometimes when the interviewer remains silent awaiting an observation from the client. These silences are almost always accompanied by signs of increased tension and indicate the interview is not progressing well. Early in the interview, it is difficult to tell whether this is due to the failure to create an atmosphere which will facilitate communication, or whether it is due to the client's usual difficulty in talking. In either circumstance it should not be allowed to persist. The tone of the entire relationship tends to be established in the first interview. It can be changed in later sessions, but it is more difficult to do. The silence should be broken with a remark indicating that, "It is hard to talk to a stranger," or "Maybe we can come back to that later. What about . . ."

A long silence which occurs in an established relationship should be allowed to continue. If there is tension present, it is an indication the client is attempting to talk about something which for one reason or another is quite difficult. Any direct question may furnish a means of avoiding that topic completely. At times the growing tension may cause the client to just blurt the topic out. Occasionally, at that point in a therapeutic relationship it is not unusual for the individual to suddenly get up and leave. The topic will be covered then on return, whether the return is immediate, or not until the next session. In an established relationship, a silence can occur without any tension. These silences may say, "All right, that topic is wrapped up, I wonder where I'll go from here." At times the client may act as though in a reverie. This should be probed by, "Would you like to share your thoughts with me?".

Another type of silence which occurs frequently is the *block*. Blocking is the term used to describe the phenomenon of sudden silence happening when an individual stops talking in the middle of a sentence and seems unable to continue. The manifestations of blocking have been described in Chapter 5. As a usual thing, the block indicates the individual has touched on material, either directly or through association, which is so threatening there is a complete inability to continue the thought, let alone utter it.

At times the material under discussion immediately preceding the block serves as a direct clue to its significance. At other times the mental associations of the worker may lead to the origin of the block. At other times no significance may be immediately obvious. It is generally not good technique to explore this immediately with the probationer; it will only increase the repression. A moment or two should be allowed for the recovery of composure, and the interview continued by repetition of the last word or two which had been said. If there is a response to this then the interview should continue to the next natural break in the conversation. At that time an inquiry might be made as to the reason for the block. "I wonder if you could tell me why you seemed to go blank like that?" An inability to respond to this question indicates a need to introduce another topic. The subject under discussion at the time of the block should be filed away in the worker's mind for reintroduction at a later time. Frequent blocking is sometimes the first clue to possible schizophrenia.

The worker must be on watch for another type of silence. This is the silence of omission, the thing which is not said. There is a dialogue between Sherlock Holmes and Inspector Gregory, which goes as follows:

" 'Is there any point to which you would wish to draw my attention?'

'To the curious incident of the dog in the night time.'

'The dog did nothing in the night time.'

'That was the curious incident,' remarked Sherlock Holmes.'"[3]

---

[3]*Silver Blaze, The Complete Sherlock Holmes,* Sir Arthur Conan Doyle, Doubleday & Company, Inc. New York (s.d.), p. 347.

The dog didn't bark because the intruder was someone well known. The same sort of silence occurs in interviewing. A very common example in corrections occurs when a life history is taken in chronological fashion. Very frequently the number of years spent in various occupations do not add up to the number of years since the individual started to work. Translating this into dates will quickly bring out a specific period of unemployed time. Usually this has been spent in a penal institution. Or, the statement will be made, "I entered the Army in 1961 and got out in 1963." When pushed for specifics, it becomes, "I entered in December 1961 and was discharged in January, 1963," which does not add up to even a minimum tour of duty. The explanation is usually a dishonorable discharge, about which there was a silence which screamed for exploration. Or consider the male client who is being followed on probation for a drug bust, and who comes in every two weeks and always starts with, "Well, I'm still clean, and I sure feel good." If he then comes in and starts with, "My wife hasn't been feeling well," or "What'd you think of the World Series?" his silence about drug usage screams, "I'd better ask what is going on."

A dramatic instance seen in practice is that of Mrs. A.V. She was talking about her husband and how she felt she had let him down. She had described him in every detail. He was the best man in the world, kind, generous and understanding. He was handsome and a man among men. She told of his hobbies, his business, his virtues. He was such a perfect husband and a perfect father. She could not possibly live up to him. On first meeting him, the most noticeable thing about him was his artificial leg. She had not said a word about that.

LISTENING TO MEANING

It has become a classic legend about psychiatrists, the tale of the two psychiatrists who meet on the street. As the story goes, the first one says, "Good morning, how are you today?", and the second one thinks, "I wonder what he meant by that." The aim of this section is to make the counselor also "wonder what he meant by that." The discussion up to this point has been concerned with nonverbal communication which is extremely important. Throughout this observation with the eyes, ears, and nose, however, a different type of listening should have been taking place, the sort of listening to which all these other observations serve as litmus paper to test the accuracy of what is heard. Someone who says, "Oh no, that doesn't make me angry," while both hands are clenched into fists so tightly that the knuckles are white, is either not in touch with inner feelings or is lying. So this sort of observation is extremely important while listening to meaning.

Equally important is something which has been described as *listening with the third ear.* At any one moment, an individual's verbalizations are progressing at three levels. The first level is concerned with the face value of what the probationer says. It is the way reality is viewed, past, present, and future. It is full of, "what I said and did to him, and what he said and did to me." If this is accepted at its face value, probationers and their behavior will never be fully understood.

Communication at the second level is determined by characteristic attitudes and defenses. It is at this level that the worker strikes pay dirt. The meanings implicit here are revealed by the choice of topic for discussion, by the manner of description, by the emotions concealed as well as those displayed, by habitual distortion of the environment, by the use of all the nonverbal methods of communication which have been discussed under Observation, and particularly by the method of relating to the probation officer as compared to the description of the methods used in relating to other important figures in the individual's life. It is by attention to this level that the worker discovers the defenses which are characteristic for this individual, e.g. projections, rationalization, displacement, compensation, fantasy, identification, denial, etc. It is at this level also that the individual's attitudes are most clearly seen, attitudes towards society, authority figures, parental figures, the opposite sex, peer group, religion, education, and work. Frequently, these can be inferred directly from the way the individual relates to the worker. The attitude to the worker is a reflection of attitudes towards others in the environment. Here, too, is where the individual's more obvious motives can be seen, such as need for status, recognition, personal aggrandizement, affection, sympathy, sexual gratification, material gain, even punishment, and the strength of these drives can be assayed. This does not mean the corrections worker should be playing the role of psychiatrist, psychoanalyst, or psychologist. It does mean utilizing all the education and competence at the officer's disposal to recognize, identify, and weigh these factors.

Those other disciplines are concerned with the third level. This is the unconscious level which is made up of forgotten, traumata, repressed wishes, unacceptable drives, and disabling conflicts. This material is revealed through dreams, slips of the tongue, free association, and the psychologist's projective tests. In some people the roots of behavior are so deeply imbedded at this level that alteration in behavior can be brought about only by referral for more specialized treatment designed to deal with this third level. For the purposes of the corrections worker, this level may be ignored, although there are times when the unconscious meanings become so clear they shriek out loud for attention. The case of Mrs. L. in Chapter 6 who stole only baby clothes and then only under certain circumstances is a good example of this.

Two other examples will help to clarify the concept of listening at various levels.

Mr. A.W. is a twenty-four-year-old white male. He had been arrested for sale of marijuana. He had been placed on probation and referred for treatment. Preliminary contacts led to a suspicion of character disorder. On this particular session he came in wearing a loud plaid jacket, a scarlet shirt unbuttoned to just about his belt, matching scarlet slacks, and bright blue suede shoes. He spent a large part of the interview describing in explicit, almost clinical detail a recent sexual encounter with a young woman. At the last moment, after much foreplay (described almost as though by a blow-by-blow fight announcer), he had refrained from actual penetration because she was a virgin. The girl had professed herself as being quite thankful and grateful for this act.

What is he revealing? On the first level he is relating a presumably reality based encounter, which he appears to view as extremely ego-satisfying. He is a great guy. He has a way with women. He is compassionate. He will not let this woman lose her virginity to please him, and she is grateful. What can be inferred at the second level? He obviously wants approval from a father figure (the therapist). Is that something he did not get as a boy? (It is learned at another session that this is a true conjecture.) Why did he bring this subject up in the first place? The shirt unbuttoned to the waist and the need to relate this conquest strongly suggest he has marked feelings of masculine inadequacy and has to be seen by others as an extremely competent male. Why the pride in refraining from intercourse? That makes him look like a man of principle, but is there anything more? Possibly, this is an over-compensation for feelings of guilt over sexual activity. It might also be that stopping at this point might be tied in with his weak masculine image. Maybe he was afraid he might fail if he attempted to complete the act, and he used the defense of rationalization. (It is learned later that he is still a virgin.)

The third level is approached by asking why does he have to tell this story in such clinical detail. The clothing suggests an exhibitionistic streak. The excessive use of detail sounds as though he were attempting to have the therapist act out the role of voyeur. Indeed, later sessions confirm a feeling of a polymorphously perverse individual.

> The second example is that of Mr. A.X. He is a twenty-two-year-old male accused of forceful homosexual assault on a minor. According to the social history, he is an adopted child, and neither he nor his foster parents know anything about his natural parents. Yet when he is asked what he knows about his natural parents, he replies, "Well, I understand that my father was a rich businessman, and my mother was a society woman. They had an affair, and I popped out of it." This last phrase, "and I popped out of it" is accompanied by a moue and a wrinkling of the nose.

What does this seem to mean in terms of the three levels? On the first level he is making what seems to be a simple statement about his parentage. What meanings might the corrections worker be able to infer from this at the second level? The need to invent the story as to his natural parents is partially an expression of the universal need for identity, "Who am I?" "Where did I come from?" It is also evidence of the use of fantasy as a defense and of his need for status. The contemptuous tone of the second sentence reflects a feeling of being rejected by the natural parents and a certain degree of hostility to this. At the third level, the use of the phrase, "and I popped out of it" and the accompanying emotional tone of disgust, demonstrated by his facial expression, suggests deep feelings of disgust engendered by the female genitalia, possibly disgust over the whole business of procreation, and may point to some of the roots of his homosexuality.

Listening in this fashion is a demanding task but it is not only worth the effort in terms of better understanding and ability to work with the individual, but adds a quality of intellectual excitement necessary to maintain enthusiasm in what is frequently a discouraging task. As the worker listens in this same way throughout an interview, or in a series of interviews, with the same client, certain themes, attitudes, and defenses begin to be recognized, running through the probationer's conversation over and over again with minor variations like the main themes of a symphony. This serves to transform a series of minor and seemingly unrelated or isolated instances into a meaningful interrelated whole. This does not mean that the worker must probe for the deep unconscious meanings of what is revealed. It is quite possible to understand and work with most probationers without ever getting into that level.

SUMMARY

It is hoped that this systematic way of evaluating all that goes on in the interview, both verbal and nonverbal, will have done two things. First, it will offer the worker an explanation for why it is so often possible after one interview to make very definite statements about an individual's personality and character, without any clear idea of where these strong impressions came from. The second is that it will prompt the worker to begin to make observations in an organized and purposeful fashion, so that the source of those positive impressions is clear and capable of being documented; and the impressions themselves will be more reliable.

Chapter 16

THE CONDUCT OF THE INTERVIEW

GENERAL CONSIDERATIONS

THE description of interviewing techniques in the last two chapters has laid the ground work for the discussion of the evaluative interview. The purposes of this interview may vary widely, from the need to write a presentence report, to the first visit with a newly assigned probationer or parolee, through the first session by a jail or prison counselor with a new arrival. Naturally, there will be variations in the way the interview progresses depending on the ultimate goal. For purposes of convenience they will be described as one interview whose purpose is twofold: (1) to develop a relationship and (2) to obtain a picture of defendants and their backgrounds from which a report can be written, while at the same time inferences can be drawn concerning the dynamics of the antisocial behavior. These should be going on simultaneously. To quote Keve, "Of course, the most important step in the investigation process is that first interview with the defendant, and if you handle it skillfully, you not only have the basis for a truly competent report, but you also have gone a long way toward launching the treatment job that must develop later."[1]

This initial interview may be done in one session, commonly taking two or three hours, or may be split into several sessions of one hour or less. Which route is followed will be a function both of the officer's preference and the exigencies of the schedule. My own bias is for the split interview approach, where possible. It allows for clarification of confused material, without prosecutorial or third degree tactics. It also allows for waiting to ask about emotionally charged material until after some feeling of mutual trust has developed.

---

[1]Keve, Paul W., "The Probation Officer Investigates, 1960," quoted in *Federal Probation*, September 1963.

309

This area of trust is one that sets corrections aside from most other helping fields. The corrections worker has the dual task of representing the system while helping the client with material issues and assisting the client to change those attitudes leading to conflict with the system. This bifurcated role leads to a series of ethical dilemmas which have to be discussed with each new defendant before the relationship can get off the ground. Perhaps the first dilemma has to do with the matter of helping. Does the worker have a right to try to change the attitudes of someone who does not want those attitudes changed, or does responsibility stop when the potentially harmful effects of the attitudes have been delineated? A second problem lies in differentiation for the client of the worker's attitudes toward feeling and behavior. The defendant must know he can confide his feelings about anyone or anything to the worker and they will be respected and kept in confidence. On the other hand, the client cannot expect the worker to listen to planned or executed illegal behavior without taking some official action. The worker may get to like and respect the defendant as a person, but it must always be clearly understood that liking and respect cannot be used to get the worker to blink at antisocial behavior. The worker must point out to the client that probation or parole conditions have to be observed by the client and upheld by the worker. This may be in spite of the fact neither of them had a hand in setting those conditions, and neither may agree with them. In the presentence evaluation, the worker must make it clear that even while asking for answers to some extremely personal questions, there can be no guarantee that these answers can be kept confidential.

How is it possible to lay all this on a defendant and still expect cooperation and trust? As I see this situation, the question should be phrased in the reverse. How is it possible to expect anyone to cooperate, not only during the initial interview, but also in the future, unless all this has been laid on the table from the beginning? The solution lies in complete honesty and frankness from the start. The remark of a worker to the effect that, "You may tell me as often as you want, you think I'm a son of a bitch, but I don't ever want to hear you call me a son of a bitch" has already been quoted. That epitomizes an honest relationship which can grow into a truly therapeutic one.

BEGINNING THE INTERVIEW

The original introduction must include several areas. Identification comes first. "I'm John Jones or Mary Smith." The overall purpose is next. "I've been asked to do a presentence examination," or "I'll be your probation officer or parole officer." Then the purpose of the particular interview, "I'd like to find out as much about you as I can today." Before proceeding, there should be a discussion of the issues just described. During this discussion, the idea of wishing to be of help as well as merely serving as a watchdog should be introduced. This must be done rather off-handedly so as not to inspire jeers of derision, expressed or concealed. There should never be the slightest hint of a patronizing or condescending attitude. Nothing arouses more scorn in an individual in this situation than the thought of a "do-gooder" entering the picture. The techniques which have been described in the last two chapters should have been in use while these preliminaries are going on. These techniques should be those which both facilitate the formation of a relationship and aid the observations of the worker.

It might seem desirable at this point in the interview to pause and try to find some common ground of interest, sports, hobbies, news events, anything which might help the client feel at ease. This common ground might serve that purpose, but it is rather hard to empathize with answers about the weather, the World Series, or the job market. Some officers find that *they* are more at ease with this approach, in which case its use may be justified.

If it is necessary, the talk should be focused on the client. "How do *you* feel in this kind of weather?" "Who do *you* like in the Series?" "What do *you* think your chances are of getting a job?" The focus from the beginning should be on the *client* and the reactions displayed, regardless of the topic. Where feasible, the small talk should be omitted. At this point the interview proper should get underway. This should be as broad and nonspecific as possible. "All I know about you is what they sent over from the court. Would you like to tell me about it?" Not, "about what you did," or "about the robbery," or "why you got busted," but about "it." "Would you like to talk about what brought you here?" not "How did you ever get in a mess like this," or not, "I see you got five to ten, suspended and are on probation. You must have pulled a big one to get five to ten." The reason for this indefinite approach is that it gives the individual a chance to talk about what is deemed really important right from the start. That talk might not be what the officer expects, but it might provide valuable leads to some of the real factors in the situation.

A.Y. will illustrate some of the advantages of this broad opening. A.Y. was twelve years old when seen following an arrest for shoplifting. It was known this was the latest in a series of offenses dating back several years, starting with taking coins from his mother's purse, fighting at the drop of a hat, stealing from other youngsters in school, stealing from teachers, and culminating in the shoplifting which was a pretty clumsy attempt. When asked to, "Tell me about it," he replied, "Well, the way I see it is that somebody's got to say no to me and make it stick." As he talked, it became apparent he saw himself as the prize in the struggle between his parents, who were contesting with each other over and through him. It became a question of which one could do the most for him, cover up the most for him, both from each other and from the authorities. If one said he could not do something, he had only to go to the other to get permission. If both said no, he would do it anyway, secure in the knowledge no punishment would follow. If a punishment were imposed, it would not be carried out, or if one threatened punishment, the other would protect him from it. He was literally afraid of what he might be tempted to do if controls were not applied. Each offense was a renewed way of asking for controls. All of this, except the statement about controls, which was implied rather than overt, came out spontaneously in response to the question, "Would you like to tell me about it?"

Another example of the sort of answer which may be received to this sort of open-ended question is shown by Mr. T. cited in Chapter 8 in the section about hysterical dissociation. Mr. T. is the man who had killed his wife with a shotgun when he fully believed he intended to kill himself. When he was asked to, "Tell me about it," he did not respond with, "I killed my wife but I didn't mean to." Instead, he started with the change in his life when he first met his wife in high school and proceeded to talk uninterruptedly (except for nods, "um-hms," "Yes, go on," etc.) unfolding the entire story until he was arrested in his father's home.

Pitfalls and Tests

It is obvious that not everyone will respond in this way to such a nondirective opening, and the problem posed by those who do not will be discussed at a later point. With those people who originally seem to respond well to this approach, the handling of this stage of the interview, this first outpouring in response to the opening question, is frequently crucial in determining the success or failure of the entire evaluation. It is here that the need to be interested, understanding, and above all nonjudgmental is so important. At this moment, the worker knows nothing of the needs, attitudes, motives, and defenses of the probationer except what has been learned in the primary discussion, and the probationer is equally as uninformed about the officer. Frequently, the first statements the individual makes may be a test to see how the worker will respond. The following is a good example of how this testing may be carried on.

Mr. A.Z. was interviewed with absolutely no prior knowledge of his situation. He was seen in private practice. His appointment had been made through a call to my secretary by his attorney, who would not even divulge the nature of the charges against his client. He was a forty-five-year-old white male. After the preliminary introductions he was asked if he would like to "tell me about it." His response was, "Well, Doc, you see, I have quite a problem. I'm one of those guys, if he's been without a woman for some time and he gets a few drinks, then he always wants to go looking for guys who like other guys."

The tone of voice with which this was delivered and the searching facial expressions accompanying the words indicated an expectation, and a fear, that the response would be couched in some judgmental fashion. This was obviously a test of whether he could find acceptance and understanding. At this point it would be too risky to attempt to convey understanding. As yet there was nothing known about him which provided any leads to understanding. The response, then, had to be one which would indicate acceptance, and a desire to understand. This was an answer where the tone of voice was just as important as the words. There could be no indication of shock, and yet at the same time it could not be matter-of-fact because that would minimize the tremendous importance this problem posed for him.

The response was, "How does that make you feel?" His reply was, on the surface, a matter-of-fact statement, "It makes me feel like hell," but the tone of voice and quizzical facial expression turned this statement into a question. He was really saying, "You must think I'm pretty terrible, awful, way out, can't be helped, don't you?" Any attempt to empathize with the surface statement with some such remark as, "An urge like that sure must shake you," or "I imagine you do feel like hell," would only serve to confirm the suspicions implicit in the tone of voice and facial expression. Again, this was a way of testing. The answer given was, "That must be an uncomfortable way to feel. Suppose you tell me a little bit more about it." This contained no judgment that he was good, bad, abnormal, or depraved, but it did indicate interest to know more about him. He was able to relax, let down his guard, and at least for then stop testing.

At this stage of the interview, responses must be phrased very carefully with a full awareness that testing may be going on.

CONTINUING THE INTERVIEW

The client who accepts the interviewer's response to these first tests should be allowed to continue talking until that subject is temporarily exhausted. It is generally wiser not to push for elaboration of specific details about this topic, either when the probationer is talking or when the flow has ceased, but simply to make appropriate remarks which indicate understanding and interest in what is being said. The reason for not pressing for amplification at this point is that not enough is known about the individual to evaluate the willingness or ability to expand on what has been said. When the topic has been exhausted some sort of summarizing remark should be made which will serve as a transition to obtaining other material for the social history or presentence investigation. A typical remark might be, "Well that seems to give us a good picture of the way you feel about it, suppose we explore your background a little. Possibly that will help us understand why you feel that way," or "Well, I would like to understand better why you might have these feelings. Suppose we try to learn a little bit more about it." It is then easy to proceed to, "Tell me a little about your family" or "your job," or any other topics which should be explored. Notice again that a nonspecific question is used even when exploring specific topics, thus, "Tell me a little bit about your family," not, "Who is in your family?" "Tell me about your job," not, "Where do you work?", etc.

One immediate advantage of this nondirective type of approach can be seen from what has already been discussed. The initial question or questions may lead directly to the root of the problem with which the officer will have to deal. There is another more subtle and more far reaching implication of this approach, the benefits of which are not so immediately obvious. However, it may be of even greater significance as the relationship between the probationer and the officer continues. Right at the beginning of the relationship this approach makes it clear that this is not a situation in which the officer is going to do something to or for the probationer. Rather this is to be a situation in which they do something together. The role of the probationer is equally as important as the role of the officer for the successful conclusion of their mutual task.

While this nonspecific question and answer routine has been going on, the worker should be attuned to the first voluntary introduction of a new topic at the initiative of the person being interviewed. What does the introduction of this new topic mean to this person? Is there an association between it and the topic which has just been under discussion? Is this association obvious, or obscure? Is it clear or must the officer guess at the significance of the introduction of this new topic? Is it a sign the probationer is now more at ease and secure and hence can talk of things which have more meaning and urgency? Is the subject so pressing it must be introduced, even though it seems inappropriate? On the contrary, is it possible the subject previously under discussion was so threatening it became essential to get away from it, and this new topic is just a red herring designed to divert the officer from something about which the probationer cannot yet talk? If, while the officer is answering these questions mentally, interest and understanding in the probationer is shown and no judgments passed, the probationer will continue to relax, and the interview will proceed more and more easily.

What the officer learns during these early stages about the individual is determined by the pace at which the interview has proceeded, the material covered, and the depths to which it is explored. By utilizing those various aspects of listening previously discussed and evaluating the information obtained from them, the officer should have formed a rough, but hopefully reasonably accurate, picture of the individual and the individual's needs, particularly as those needs relate to the interview situation. The supposition is that the officer will then utilize the knowledge of those needs to facilitate the interview.

While this sort of scrutiny must be most intense during the early phases of the interview, the officer has to continue to be alert to modify first impressions as the interview progresses. Thus, the officer notes how noncommittal or how descriptive are the answers to questions, whether the probationer is only following the officer's lead or branches off on inner associative patterns. The officer observes whether the probationer is watching intently to see what effect the responses have on the officer, and whether these responses are then modified in terms of what the probationer believes the officer's reaction to them to be. Does this flow spontaneously or is it always necessary to do some prodding?

It is from observations of this nature in these early stages of the interview that the officer begins to determine how the needs of the probationer may be most satisfactorily met. Is this a passive, rather dependent sort of person who is going to require a great deal of help in the interview situation or an aggressive independent one who, once reasonably at ease, will relate much better if left largely unguided? Is the individual continually wary and on guard, so that the questions will have to be carefully phrased so as not to evoke suspicion? Is there a great deal of hostility which will have to be overcome before the client gets really involved? Is there a great deal of loquacious, rambling, verbal production for which focusing will have to be utilized? It is with the answers to this type of question in mind that the officer proceeds to elicit the background information.

THOSE WHO RESPOND DIFFERENTLY

It would be extremely gratifying if all people responded in a revealing way to, "Would you like to tell me about it?". Unfortunately, this does not always happen. Sometimes the probationer has some difficulty in responding to this sort of nondirective question. A fairly frequent answer in presentence interviews is, "I didn't do it. My lawyer said it would go easier for me if I didn't try to fight it." Or, "I just copped a rap for somebody else." Or, "I didn't do it, it was one witness' word against mine, and they believed him." There are innumerable variations to this theme. It is very unwise in the initial phase of the first interview to express either belief or disbelief in such statements. This opening gambit should be met with, "I'm sure you have good reason for thinking the way you do. Why don't we try to learn a little bit more about you, and then come back to it later." Or, "I'd like to know a lot more about you than just whether or not you're guilty. Let's talk a little about you."

Another common response to, "Would you like to tell me about it," is silence. The client obviously has difficulty in responding to this sort of open-ended question. This is particularly true of certain adolescents, of borderline or mildly mentally retarded individuals, and of street-wise defendants who are leery of volunteering anything which is not specifically asked. As has been noted earlier, such a silence should not be allowed to persist in an initial interview. As soon as this sort of resistance is noted, it should be met with a remark like, "Well maybe you'll want to tell me about it when you get to know me better," and then other more neutral questions are asked. This neutral question should not be small talk but should be one that presumably has no emotional overtones. If the client is confined, "How are you getting along in jail?" This then might be followed by, "Is this your first time in jail?" If the answer is "No," then some inquiries about what happened in the intervening time are appropriate. As the silence disappears, it is then possible to say, "I'd like to know something more about you, would you like to tell me about yourself?"

This brings up the next type of response apt to be obtained from those who do not respond at length to, "Would you like to tell me about it?" This response has the general theme, "about what?". If it is simply that, an answer might be, "Would you like to tell me a little bit about yourself?". If the answer to this is, "What about myself?", it might be answered with, "Anything you want to tell me." If this does not bring an answer, then it is wise to shift gears and get into more specific questions. The nature of these questions will be discussed in a moment.

A variation of this may be tried with adolescents still in school. If there is no answer to, "Anything you want to tell me," it is sometimes helpful to ask, "What would you write if you were asked by your English teacher to write an essay on the topic, 'All About Me'?" If this draws a blank, more concrete questions should be asked. Obviously, a battle is going on and no contest of wills should be allowed to enter the interview situations.

In any of these instances, when more concrete questions are to be used, this might be a good place to get the specific factual matter out of the way. For awhile very definite questions may have to be asked, "How old are you?", "Are you married?" etc. As soon as possible the technique previously advocated for continuing the interview should be utilized. Thus, not, "How many brothers and sisters do you have?" but, "Tell me about your family." Not, "Are your parents living?" but, "Tell me about your parents." Not, "What school do you go to?" or "Are you working?", but "Tell me about school," and "Tell me about your job." These are examples of specific questions raised in a nonspecific way. This leaves an opening for the client to develop any amount of significant material in that area or even to move from there into another area spontaneously. The goal, insofar as is possible, is not to ask questions that can be answered by "yes" or "no" or by one or two words.

Commonly, just this small amount of stimulus will serve to initiate an exploration of meaningful and possibly problem laden areas. There will always be a small number of individuals who are unable to respond to these approaches and will give specific answers to specific questions. This may be so for any number of reasons. These may be introverted or severely inhibited individuals who have a great deal of trouble expressing themselves. Calvin Coolidge, our thirtieth President, has become notorious for his laconic use of words. Anything more than a "yup," or "nope," or "might be" from him was considered unusual. Some people are extremely literal, accustomed to thinking only in the most specific and concrete terms. Some are extremely defensive, afraid of revealing too much if they say anything beyond the most economical answer to the question. Whatever the reason, it is necessary to deal with people on their own terms. A complete question-and-answer routine may have to be followed for some time before any loosening process sets in. These are frequently the most exhausting interviews to conduct.

DEALING WITH THE CONCRETE INDIVIDUAL

Many individuals respond only to specific questions, and then only in a specific and concrete fashion with no verbal expression of feelings and attitudes. It becomes a real task to convert this sort of response into one which will be more meaningful and through which a relationship can be established. In dealing with this kind of person, it is crucial that the officer remain watchful for the first answer which contains material over and above the question asked. If, when this happens, the alert officer responds with the proper degree of interest, and particularly with no judgmental implications, a significant milestone will be passed.

Once this first tentative ball has been tossed to the officer and expertly fielded and thrown back, the defenses come down faster and faster. For example, a question and answer interview may have been going on. Only simple answers have been given to the questions asked. Then the question is asked, "What does your wife think about your drinking?" The answer is, "She doesn't like it. She bawls the hell out of me. *Then I go out and take another drink.*"

Here, for the first time, there has been an answer which goes beyond the question asked. The individual has volunteered a reaction which has not been requested. It might be quite tempting to use this opening to point out that this is exactly the wrong thing to do: "That doesn't get you anywhere," or, "That just makes the situation worse." These remarks do point out the inadequacy of the reaction, but they also pass judgment at the same time. This is exactly the sort of response clients are expecting, anticipating that here, too, is another individual who will weigh them on the balance of rational behavior and find them wanting. This temptation must be resisted. Some way should be found to convey understanding, if not acceptance. "It kind of gripes you when she jumps you?", or "You wish she'd keep her mouth shut," might be appropriate remarks. Just as with the person who responds immediately to the first question, who tests with the loaded response, so too with the individual who waits for some time before testing. In this instance, too, once this first test has been passed, the individual will almost always open up more and more.

At times this first test, or even a subsequent one, may be even more direct and more pointed. For instance, in the example just used, the individual may add to, "Then I go out and get another drink," the direct question, "What would you do?" This type of loaded question puts the officer directly on the spot. Any direct answer will be wrong. The reply, "I guess I'd do the same thing," condones the behavior. This may spoil any future chance to change this particular pattern. At this time, before a relationship has been established, a reply embodying a more effective way of dealing with the situation might be interpreted as critical and judgmental. A reply which intimates such a situation could not happen to the officer injects a "holier than thou" flavor into the situation, and no relationship can flourish in such an atmosphere. A psychiatrist might well reply at this point, "I wonder what makes you ask?" This is not good technique for a counselor.

The way out of this dilemma is to evade the question, and attempt to focus on the underlying feelings. The answer might be phrased in such terms as, "I'm not quite sure what I'd do. I suppose it would depend on how I felt. Does it kind of gripe you when she chews you out?" Again, this response conveys empathy and understanding, without compromising the officer's position.

Earlier in this section one specific question was suggested to be put to adolescents still in school. It should be noted that for many adolescents, particularly the unsocialized aggressive type, the whole style of interviewing may have to be changed. This type of adolescent responds very poorly to nondirective questions, even to those which are open-ended. It may be necessary to involve them in an argument in order to capture their attention at all. Early confrontation (always without moralizing) about the effects of their behavior on themselves, as well as others, may frequently be helpful. The inclusion of the effects of the behavior on themselves displays interest, whereas if it is confined only to the effects on others it shows a lack of concern for them as people. Care must always be taken to steer a neutral path between the adolescent and the parents until there has been time to evaluate the situation fully. Any disapproving remarks about either the adolescent or his parents should only be made when all are present. If argumentation is used as a device the officer should always be ready to admit it when an argument has been lost. One final caution in dealing with adolescents, they should always be told the absolute truth. Any time the interviewer is not willing to do this, the subject should not be discussed.

FOCUSING THE INTERVIEW

With the type of individual who has just been discussed, there is no problem in focusing. Each specific question serves as the focus. The problem with these people is not focusing, but generating enough spontaneity to allow the identification of important factors in the genesis of their problems. Focusing also presents no problem in those persons who respond to the nonspecific questions asked, exhaust the area, and then just wait for another stimulus to explore a different field as thoroughly. With these people it is a question of which fields to explore, to what depths, and in what order.

Focusing in the initial interview only becomes a problem with those prople who respond to the original invitation to "tell me about it," with a seemingly endless stream of somewhat disconnected material. In such instances, the determination to be made is whether or not the stream of talk will cover most of the significant topics which need investigation. If the answer is yes, it is equally probable that this stream of talk will also open many areas that the interviewer might not have thought to broach, areas which might be quite important. Under those circumstances, there is no great need to attempt to focus in the initial interview. Instead, there should be an attempt to sort out and classify the meaningful material. Its significance to the probationer should be assessed. Feelings and areas of concern which have been isolated in this interview should be noted for elaboration and clarification in later interviews. Instead of attempting to focus, there should be continued usage of the previously described techniques to express interest and facilitate the flow of thought. The worker nods, smiles, says "hm hm," repeats the words immediately preceding the pause, empathizes with feelings, or rephrases a statement to intensify its meaning.

If such an individual is being seen in a continuing relationship (for example on probation), it is wise to attempt to focus subsequent interviews on just one or two meaningful topics which have been introduced in the first interview. For example, during the first interview, a male probationer may have referred to, or touched on, such diverse subjects as his feelings of being a failure, his reaction to his antisocial behavior, his dissatisfaction with his wife, his feelings about what he considers to be unreasonable attitudes of his parents during his childhood, the undisciplined attitudes of his son, the seemingly inordinate demands of employers, his fantasies of being a white-hat, big Cadillac dude, the high cost of living, his feelings about an older brother who made it through college while he did not even graduate from high school, the different feelings he has for his daughter than for his son, etc.

At the next interview, an attempt should be made to focus on just one or two of these topics which seem to be of real significance. Thus, if the probationer refers to his parents' attitudes again, the officer might make some such statements as, "You mentioned something about that last time. Would you like to talk a little bit about what you thought they really expected of you?" At appropriate moments in the response, the question will then be interpolated, "And, how did that make you feel?" If the probationer tends to drift from this area of the parents' expectations before it is fully explored, the new topic should be acknowledged. The discussion then should be brought back to the parents and their attitudes. This may be done by means of pointed questions, such as, "What was your parents' reaction when you brought home your grade card?" This may elicit a feeling of having failed, and an underlying feeling of resentment that it was not really failure, but that the parents' demands were too great. It is then not too difficult to phrase questions in such a way that the connection between the childhood feelings and the present feelings of being a failure become quite clear. This area can then be further explored.

If in an initial, or subsequent, interview the client seems to be really eager to talk about a topic, this should be allowed, no matter how great the worker's impatience to get to something else. This was touched on in Chapter 14 and is reiterated here because of its importance. Such an attempt to cut off the client says in a symbolic fashion, "What you want doesn't mean anything." This can only lead to resentment, a lessened feeling of self-worth, and increased resistance. Most importantly, what seems trivial to the worker, because of eagerness to get on with what seem to be more significant topics, may be preliminary to something extremely significant to the client. This material may never emerge if the client is not allowed to talk about it at will.

The number of individuals in presentence status who want to talk about their offenses is always a source of amazement. It is almost as though, once found guilty, there is a need to unburden, which they were not allowed to satisfy in the courtroom, possibly out of the attorney's well-justified fear that it might influence the verdict. Such people may have to be allowed to purge themselves in this way before even the simplest factual material can be obtained.

In the initial interview, when there seems to be no hope of getting necessary and significant material from the individual's flow of words, the question will have to be asked, "What is going on?" There are several answers to this question, and the method of focusing to be used depends on the answer given. The first possibility is that this is a part of the individual's personality, that this is a garrulous person who will ramble on as long as allowed to do so. Obviously, a good deal of time will be wasted by letting this continue. There are two ways to deal with this. The first is quite direct and is preferred by most corrections workers, possibly rightfully. It consists of interrupting at a pause for breath and asking a direct question (hopefully, in a nonspecific way). As soon as there is any evidence that the answer is veering from that topic, another direct question is asked to expand on that first question. Once the first question is answered completely, the process is repeated with each subsequent topic. As this technique is continued, the chances are good, sometimes even within one interview, that the rambling will partially stop, and it will be easier to keep the individual to the topic. Care must be taken that the interruptions and questions are not done in an authoritative fashion, or all chances of any sort of working relationship will be destroyed. There is a considerable risk that much meaningful material may never be elicited by this technique.

The second way of dealing with this rambling sort of output is definitely more time-consuming, but it would usually be my choice. This might be called nondirective focusing. This consists in essence of showing disinterest by the use of methods which are the reverse of those suggested to demonstrate interest. As the rambling proceeds, the worker instead of leaning forward in the chair leans back. Instead of "yes," or "hum, hm," there is absolute silence. The fingers may tap the desk in impatience. Yawns may be followed by closing the eyes. At first, nothing may happen, but before long this meandering current of words slows to a trickle and then comes to a dead stop. When this silence occurs, a question is asked about a topic of interest. As long as the client stays on this topic, the worker shows interest. As soon as the rambling begins, the same treatment is repeated. Before very long only topics of interest are being discussed. Obviously, this is more time-consuming than interrupting with a new question.

However, this nondirective focusing has some important advantages. It keeps the interview from developing into a question and answer session in which all the necessary facts may be gathered but the important feelings are missed. In addition, this use of disinterest serves as a counterpoint to the show of interest in significant material. It helps the probationer to learn about the areas in which the officer is interested, keeps the attention focused on these areas, and assigns the probationer the responsibility for working on them. It does this without mobilizing defenses, without any apparent domination. There is no danger of the client's developing a feeling of being shoved around. Most individuals seen in corrections are only too willing to accuse the worker of being bossy, authoritative, and inconsiderate. In this situation the client may not be completely aware of what is going on and yet may still realize that the worker is really interested in important and significant matters. The result is that the officer is able to learn about the probationer in a way which allows the latter to retain self-respect, with no feeling that the information was given involuntarily.

A second answer to, "What is going on?" is indicated when the rambling seems not only incessant, but also disconnected and disjointed. This should be quickly recognized as representing a medical problem, whether looseness of associations in the schizophrenic, flight of ideas as in the manic, or the confused deterioration of the organic patient. Under these circumstances, medical help should be requested.

There is one other possibility which must be considered in evaluating a rambling, interminable, seemingly inconsequential answer to the introductory question. That is: Is this a form of defense, a smoke screen of words, emitted, consciously or unconsciously, to avoid talking of anything of significance? The method of dealing with this sort of production depends on the worker's judgment as to whether this is conscious or unconscious. If the latter, it probably stems from uneasiness in the situation, a fear of the officer as an unknown quantity, and an attempt to gain time in order to size up the situation. In that case, no direct effort should be made to circumvent it. The worker should respect the individual's feelings of uneasiness. By means of those techniques already described, efforts should be directed toward establishing a relationship, bolstering the client's confidence, and conveying the message that the worker understands and empathizes with the feelings underlying the verbal production. With such an individual, it may take more than one interview to create an atmosphere in which meaningful interviewing can take place.

On the contrary, when it is believed that this smoke screen is conscious and deliberate and arises from an attitude of, "I'm smarter than you are; you're getting nothing from me," it must be met head on. In whatever words seem best suited to do the job, preferably in the individual's own vocabulary, the message must be conveyed, "Let's cut out the con and get on to business!" At times, it may have to be just that blunt. Dealing with such an individual in a meaningful relationship is impossible unless there is a definite understanding that the worker is not going to be fooled, will not be out-maneuvered, and has no desire to play games.

ORGANIZING THE INTERVIEW

The use of nondirective techniques does not mandate an unstructured interview. The only exception to the worker's responsibility for organizing and structuring the interview occurs when the client is effectively doing it along constructive lines. While this should occur with increasing frequency as probation continues, it is not common during an initial interview. The structuring should occur along lines which make it possible to develop a general picture of the individual. In order to do this most effectively, the worker should keep firmly in mind an outline of what areas are to be explored during the initial interview.

Each office has its own outline for an initial evaluation, presentence report, or parole summary. In general, they cover the same material, with slightly differing emphasis. The exact details are not important. What is significant is the use of the outline as a guide for areas to be explored in understanding the individual, and if possible, the reasons behind the antisocial behavior. As each topic is being discussed, three questions should be simultaneously considered: (1) "Has this topic been completely covered?" (2) "What bearing has this had on the problem that the individual is experiencing?" (3) "Does this knowledge contribute to formulation of a recommendation or a treatment program?" Used in this way, the outline is a guide to structuring the interview and does not become some sort of compartmented box meant to be filled with assorted facts, each one tucked neatly into place.

If these three questions are kept in mind as the interview progresses, the problem of whether to follow the outline, step by step, does not arise. The area covered first will be determined by the response to the opening request to "tell me about it." The outline is important in delineating the areas to be explored, and in furnishing a handy mental checklist before moving on to another area. This does not imply that if the client starts to stray from the area under discussion, brakes should be applied immediately. As soon as this side excursion has come to a logical conclusion, the probationer should be led back to that area which had been under exploration until each item in that area has been covered. Under no circumstances should zealous desire to satisfy the demands of an outline be allowed to hinder the flow of thought of a client who is bursting to talk about a specific topic or problem, no matter if nothing in the outline seems to fit that topic.

One area which is sometimes neglected in outlines and on reports has to do with the positive aspects of the individual. It is very easy to ask about rejecting, dominating, belligerent alcoholics, or otherwise imperfect parents and never include a question about a nurturant grandparent, or other relative or neighbor. It is easy to talk about school failure, and neglect athletic or other compensatory success. (Such compensatory success is not always positive without some sort of constructive channeling. One adolescent male, well known to juvenile court, compensated very well for a slight physique and an inability to handle school assignments by learning how to pick locks better than anyone in the community.) Positive personality qualities should also not be overlooked. It is usual to read reports which list *assets* and *liabilities* as, "A 1969 Ford and two hundred dollars in credit card debts." Far more significant and important are such aspects as intelligence, persistence, charm, mechanical ability, bodily dexterity, flexibility, to mention only a few possibilities.

The material necessary for a complete social investigation of the adolescent must include a school history. Before the Freedom of Information Act, a tremendous amount of valuable material could be obtained directly from the Board of Education. Not only is this now more difficult for an outsider to obtain, but it is generally less complete. With records now open to the student and family, teachers are less apt to be as free in their year-end comments as they formerly were. Many record no impressions at all. It becomes necessary then to obtain this information from the parents. In interviewing them the outline should be used in the recommended fashion. The school history should be as detailed as possible. Extra-curricular activities should be noted as well as scholastic achievements. Some parents save grade cards and these may be of help.

It is not only the quality and quantity of these achievements which are important. What the interviewer is seeking is evidence of a change in the child's habitual school patterns. This change may involve a drop in grades, an increase in absences, or a worsening in behavior. Usually, the three occur together. If such a change is noted, there should be a complete inquiry as to what was occurring in the youngster's environment during that period of time. In an impressive number of cases this knowledge may lead directly to important roots of the behavioral disturbance for which the child has come to the attention of the court.

DIRECTION AND TIMING

As various areas of the outline are being explored, it is necessary to take notice of specific topics which seem to have special emotional significance for the client. It is important not to attempt to pursue such material until any tension displayed early in the interview is no longer present. Where indicated, it is wiser, no matter how great the pressure of time, to postpone a discussion of significant material for as many sessions as seem necessary. These topics may be pursued whenever an atmosphere of trust has been established and the probationer seems at ease. This feeling may be assayed in many ways.

The client becomes obviously quieter and more composed. Foot tapping, nail biting, and unnecessary movements of the hands disappear. Bodily rigidity is replaced by relaxation. Clenched fists loosen. Lines in the forehead and between the eyebrows smooth out. Speech becomes less jerky or less bitten. Formal, precise speech is replaced by more colloquial speech. There are fewer big words, and less attention is paid to sentence structure. At times the reverse may be true. There may be less and less profanity as relaxation takes place. Hostile attitudes soften, negativistic attitudes disappear, and there is more and more spontaneous verbalization.

Just as signs of relaxation of tension are indicators of a proper time for discussion of emotionally laden material, evidence of increased tension may be indicative of what material has emotional significance. As the various areas necessary to be covered in a proper evaluation are being explored, the worker should be noting which subjects seem to call forth manifestations of increased tension, such as blocks, hesitation, bodily manifestations of emotional response, attempts to change the subject, etc. Only as an individual begins to relax, and only when the worker thinks that enough has been learned to have arrived at understanding of the basic personality mechanisms, defenses, and needs, should attempts be made to explore these emotionally laden areas. Generally, they will be found to be concerned with relationships to significant others. At times they will be seen in relationship to the offense itself. (Obviously, if a presentence report is to be written, exploration of the attitude toward the offense cannot be postponed indefinitely. Sometimes, that attitude may have to be inferred from the signs of emotional response, and from the silences, the topics which have been avoided.) Frequently these emotionally sore spots include drives and impulses (often of a sexual nature) which the individual has repressed as unacceptable. Whatever their nature, it is useless to attempt to explore them until the individual is ready to discuss them. This is demonstrated by signs of being at ease and by a developing trust.

EXPLORATION OF SENSITIVE AREAS

In initiating the exploration of sensitive areas with most people, it is better to start with an indirect approach. For example, if the area involves a relationship with another person — parent, spouse, employer, friend — the original focus should be on the behavior and feelings of that other person. (This does not contradict the statement earlier in this chapter that emphasis should always be focused on the client. That applied to the very early stages of an interview in which it was necessary to employ small talk.) If questions are phrased in a general way, it is possible to get a picture not only of how those being interviewed see others, but also of how they see themselves. This applies to their own adequacies and inadequacies in dealing with the particular attitudes and patterns under discussion. This is a place where conveying interest and empathy does a great deal to facilitate the flow of thought.

At this stage in the interview, if silence begins to occur, it should not be broken by a question or by a change of topic. Rather there should be a repetition of the last two or three words spoken before the pause, or by a restatement of the feelings expressed. A brief summary of what has been said or, "That must have made you feel..." may also be effectively employed. A lasting and effective relationship can begin to be developed only as these emotionally significant areas are being discussed. Not only is the material under discussion more open to empathy-laden responses, but the worker begins to really understand the client well enough so that these responses can be offered with reasonable assurance that they correctly interpret the underlying feelings. At this point, if the interview is progressing satisfactorily, only a cue or two about the interviewer's interests should elicit a meaningful response.

There is one exception to this general rule of not touching on sensitive areas until it is felt the individual is ready for their exploration. This exception occurs when the topic is introduced by the individual. As has been suggested, if this occurs during the opening stages of the interview no attempt should be made to push the topic beyond the point where the spontaneous development stops. If, however, an important area is introduced spontaneously at this later stage of the interview, it should be explored to the fullest, no matter how embarrassed or upset the client appears to become. The very fact this particular topic is brought up by the client means that he is eager to talk about it, no matter how difficult it may appear. This does not imply the individual should be hounded by interrogations. It does imply that encouragement should be given by all the methods discussed to this point. At times even an encouraging, "Yes, go on," may be used.

At other times it may be helpful to say something like, "I'm sure this must be hard for you to talk about. Obviously, you think things will be better if you can get it out. Won't you please try to go on." If this particular person has been noticed to have a low feeling of self-worth, it may help to remark, "I admire your wanting to talk about something as upsetting as this. It takes a lot of guts. Please go on." Whatever the technique, once people get into such an area on their own, they must be kept talking about it until there is nothing further left to say.

A somewhat different set of principles applies when the discussion on the sensitive topic is initiated by the worker because of the feeling that the client is now trusting and relaxed enough to permit exploration. Once the subject has been initiated, it should be continued as confidently, matter-of-factly, and as specifically as possible. If the topic does not seem to upset or embarrass the questioner, it will not be apt to upset the client. If the officer hesitates or generalizes, the individual is likely to interpret this as an indication that the officer is also afraid or reluctant to discuss it. This interpretation is most apt to be made in the case of a female officer interviewing a male defendant about a sexual offense. For this reason, once the decision is made that the time is right to explore a specific topic there should be no hesitation.

There are two compelling reasons for exploring significant areas thoroughly once they have been broached at the proper time. The first is that it is a great help to clients to examine these areas as completely as possible with someone in whom they have confidence, someone who is not only able to share their feelings, but also able to help to sort out those feelings and come to grips with them. Secondly, once that particular aspect of the individual's feelings and attitudes has been opened and then closed, it may be almost impossible to ever open it again. If it has been thoroughly explored, the gains obtained might be sufficient so that there is no need for the individual to reexplore it with the worker. If it has not been thoroughly discussed, the individual may think that the painful effort of talking about this significant, emotionally laden material was wasted and the worker did not consider it worth more thorough exploration. Moreover, the incomplete exploration may have caused so much embarrassment, hurt, and resentment that the topic becomes too painful to ever approach again.

THE USE OF THE RELATIONSHIP

It would be difficult to justify the amount of time devoted to the formation of a relationship if the sole purpose of that relationship were to facilitate the conduct of the interview. The relationship is probably the most important tool in the possession of the worker which can be used to effect changes in the client's behavior. It is certainly more powerful than the deterrent threat of legal sanctions. The thorough and painstaking use of this kind of relationship is truly in the domain of psychiatry, psychology, and social work, and no attempt will be made here to explore it fully. A few of the ways in which the relationship can be used by the probation officer will be discussed.

If the relationship has been progressing properly, the client will be attempting to do those things felt to be pleasing to the officer. This is first demonstrated by discussing those topics in which the officer has shown interest. This desire to please the officer then carries over into the time between visits. It has become axiomatic that the chief work in therapy goes on between therapeutic sessions and not in them. This same thing is true in counseling. Again, the first manifestations of the intersession effect are thoughts, not deeds. The client will come to the office saying, "You know that remark you made last week about how I dig in my heels and won't do anything anybody tells me to, and I said it wasn't true. I got to thinking about that and you know, you're right."

This carries with it the important corollary that the officer must be careful in every word said. It is not only the psychiatrist, in this instance the officer, who thinks, "I wonder what he meant by that?" The client, whether the relationship has been authoritarian or permissive, directive or nondirective, is constantly interpreting every word for direction as to what is or is not permitted, and what is or is not desired. (The uninvolved, manipulative client does the same thing, out of entirely different motives.) This applies with equal importance to the worker's behavior as well as speech. It is not only children who watch what their parents do in comparison or contrast to what they say.

It was stated in Chapter 14 that the client brings old attitudes and behavior patterns to the relationship. One of the most effective uses of the relationship is to point out these attitudes and patterns. "Didn't you tell me that you were fired from your last job for always being late? I notice you've been late for your last three appointments with me. What about it?" "You said you always get angry whenever your teachers tried to correct you, even when you knew they were right. Is that the same thing you were doing with me when I suggested that maybe there were better ways of getting along with your wife?".

Another way in which the relationship may be utilized is by giving the client progressively more responsibility for setting appointments, structuring the interview, and working on important areas. Again, as this is being done, the constant need to be aware of those who would con and manipulate is imperative. While the desire to please the worker may be an important factor in improving the client's behavior, the worker should always be on guard against the client who is too eager to please. While religious conversions may occur overnight, personality change takes a great deal longer to effect. It is sometimes extremely difficult to be on guard without being suspicious, to be alert without being obtrusive, and to check on questionable material offered in an interview without being disruptive of the relationship. Yet, this must be consistently done, particularly if there is the slightest feeling on the worker's part that manipulation is taking place. As was suggested in the section on focusing, any time there is a reasonable assurance of game playing occurring, it should be confronted directly, forthrightly, and without fear. There is no way of forming a relationship with a conning or manipulative individual unless this is done. Indeed, some people with tremendous experience in this field feel the only time these individuals can be benefited is if the worker not only remains constantly one jump ahead of them but consistently lets them know in no uncertain terms that the worker *is* one jump ahead and that the client is not a very good con artist.

To interview in the manner suggested in these three chapters is indeed an arduous and compelling task. At the same time, it can open entirely new areas of satisfaction for workers in a field in which satisfactions are notoriously hard to obtain. Even when the client shows no desire to change or returns to undesirable behavior, the worker can always feel, not only "I tried," but also, "I have learned something from this encounter."

Chapter 17

PROBLEMS OF DANGEROUSNESS
AND SUICIDE

DANGEROUSNESS

General Considerations

THE possibility of violence is of great interest in three areas of corrections. The first is in the presentence report, in which it is generally expected that the probation officer will make some estimate of the probability of continuing danger to the community if the defendant is allowed to remain at liberty. The second is in the institutional setting, where it is important to spot the potentially dangerous and assaultive prisoner as quickly as possible, and to be alert for any clues which may indicate that explosive behavior is imminent. The third is in the postdispositional management of the probationer, or the postrelease management of the parolee, who has been convicted of a violent offense.

It should be stated immediately that no truly valid methods or infallible signs for predicting dangerousness exist. Because of this, McClintock[1] suggests that any prediction be made from a three-dimensional frame of reference: frequency, how often has the individual been violent; location, under what particular combination of stresses and strains does violence occur; destructiveness, how dangerous to others is the violent behavior. It is universally agreed that the one best indicator of potentially assaultive behavior is a history of such behavior in the past. The more frequent the behavior, the more likely its recurrence. The accuracy of this statement changes markedly after the age of fifty. At that time the tendency to violence begins to burn out. Beyond this indicator of previous violence, the validity of any single, other sign is questionable.

---

[1]McClintock, *Crimes of Violence*, 1963.

Many studies have been done as to the incidence of violent offenses in the mentally ill. Up until recently, it was generally claimed that if alcoholism, drug ingestion or withdrawal, and the personality disorders were not considered as mental illness, the incidence of violent crime was lower for the mentally ill than for the general population. Studies done in the past ten years tend to dispute this assertion. Schizophrenics seem to be particularly implicated in violent behavior. The population studied also seems to make a great deal of difference. Those studies which focus on patients followed for a specific number of years after discharge from a mental hospital generally show a lower incidence of crime than that which exists in the general population, although the rate for violent crime may be higher. Some of these studies show that a few expatients commit a disproportionately large number of violent crimes, thus accounting for a higher overall rate in this type of offense. On the other hand, when the population of penal institutions is studied, it is almost universally found that the incidence of mental illness is significantly higher among those populations than it is for the country at large.

Dangerousness and the Presentence Report

This first area in which potential dangerousness is of significance to corrections may be approached from two angles: (1) Which of the conditions discussed in this book are most frequently associated with violent behavior? and (2) What are the more important developmental events noted in those who later commit violent acts? These acts are generally defined as murder, rape, aggravated assault, and armed robbery.

Mental Illness and Dangerousness

It should be repeated unequivocally that the mere presence of mental illness should play no role in predicting dangerous or violent behavior. Even when the mentally ill patient has already displayed violent behavior, the probability of future dangerousness has to be carefully weighed. It should always be based as much as possible on the circumstances of the particular individual and the particular offense rather than on a statistical basis. Even then, predictions are far from valid. Kozol and his coworkers, at the Massachusetts Center for the Diagnosis and Treatment of Mentally Ill, Dangerous Persons, studied mentally ill offenders intensively, spending a minimum of thirty to thirty-five hours with each patient. On follow-up for an average of almost six years, only 8 percent of those predicted to be nondangerous showed any violent behavior. On the other hand, of those released against the advice of the Center, 35 percent showed violent behavior. While the difference in these two figures, 8 percent and 35 percent, is certainly statistically significant, the presence of 65 percent false positive predictions speaks volumes as to the inability to make accurate predictions of violent behavior in the mentally ill offender.

Within the boundaries of this cautious approach, certain opinions can be offered. Of the various mental conditions described in this book, the Antisocial Personality, Alcoholism, and Schizophrenia show the highest rate of violent behavior. As might be expected, when a violent crime is perpetrated by a Schizophrenic, it is apt to be bizarre and extremely violent. Mental Retardates are comparatively rarely involved in violent crimes. Of those suffering from the Organic Brain Syndromes, those with toxic psychoses have probably the highest rate of violence. Acute Alcohol Intoxication and Pathological Intoxication are the two conditions most commonly associated with dangerousness to others. Cocaine and Amphetamine Psychoses have a relatively high rate of violence because of the combination of auditory hallucinations and paranoid ideas. In this group, the prognosis for further dangerous behavior is tied intimately to continued use of the toxin involved. The epilepsies, including the episodic dyscontrol syndrome, have an overall low potential for violence, but specific individuals will show a repetitive pattern which labels them as potentially dangerous unless the underlying epileptic condition can be brought under control. In most of the other organic syndromes, violent behavior is apt to occur as an isolated manifestation which quickly calls attention to the underlying condition and elicits reparative action.

Of the major psychoses, a small number of Schizophrenics may be extremely violent. Manics tend to be belligerent but rarely get dangerously assaultive. People with agitated depression may commit murder as an act of mercy, then attempt to take their own lives. Paranoid individuals, schizophrenic or otherwise, may of course attempt to retaliate against their supposed persecutors in what is conceived as self-defense. This is most apt to occur if the delusion is long standing, is directed against one single person or organization, and the patient feels the torment to be unbearable.

Violent behavior is rarely predicted in the neurotic individual, despite the case of Mr. V. in Chapter 8. Two Personality Disorders account for a disproportionately high percentage of violence in that group. These are the Antisocial Personality and the Explosive Personality. Those with Hysterical and Schizoid Personalities may rarely commit violent offenses. Recidivism is notoriously low for sexual offenses (2.9%) and the highest rate in this group of sexual deviants are for the nonviolent offenses. Alcoholics and certain drug abusers show the highest rate of violent crime of all those categorized as mentally ill offenders involved in antisocial behavior. One of the chief difficulties in doing any form of study which purports to make a statement about mental illness and crime is the presence of the complicating factor of alcoholism, or at least the use of alcohol at the time of the offense. It is generally concluded that alcohol does not cause violence, it releases it. As far as the Behavior Disorders of Adolescents are concerned, violent behavior is confined almost exclusively to those with Unsocialized Aggressive Reaction of Adolescence, and the Group Delinquent Reaction of Adolescence, although occasionally someone with a Hyperkinetic Reaction of Adolescence may be involved.

Developmental Factors as Predictive of Dangerousness

This is a textbook of psychiatry, so to this point the only variable mentioned in the production of violent crime has been mental illness. It is certainly apparent that the vast majority of all crimes are committed by those who are not mentally ill. It is therefore important to know whether there are factors which may have some value in predicting dangerousness in the general population. Certainly there are a host of social variables inherent in most criminal behavior, although it is impossible to weigh their significance. Crowding, poverty, hopelessness, helplessness, frustration, unemployment, and other ills are all important accompaniments of antisocial offenses. It is also certainly true that in the inner cities of many of our metropolises there exists a very real subculture of violence. In this country, if one single accompaniment of violence were to be designated, it would have to be the availability of a weapon. This is a fact to which our legislators insistently turn a blind eye.

Important and fascinating as these sociological topics are, this is a book about psychiatry. Many studies have been done in an attempt to find conditions in the developmental history, or life experiences, of an individual to try to isolate certain factors which might predict future violence. Although the majority of these studies have been done by psychiatrists, the populations studied have been found in jails, prisons, court referrals, not in mental hospitals, not even hospitals for the criminally insane. None of these studies was able to come up with one single factor, or any combination of factors, present in the history of all violent individuals. Those factors which were found may be grouped in three classes: the most frequent, considerably frequent, and those found with only a fair degree of frequency. Unfortunately, very few studies have examined the differences in rate between the incidence of these factors in violent offenders and their incidence in nonviolent offenders or in the general public.

What follows is an attempt to extract common factors from these various studies as well as from my personal experiences. The single finding which recurs most frequently is that violent offenders, as children, have been brutalized by one or both parents. Truly, violence breeds violence. In order of frequency, these are the other factors found in the class of most frequent factors: violence or murder in the family; parents assaultive to each other; head trauma with concussion (occurring before age ten); loss of consciousness; convulsions; absent mother; alcoholic parents (particularly father); temper tantrums; previous outbursts of violence; frequent fighting; a triad of fire setting, cruelty to animals, and enuresis (either of the first two are also felt to be significant if they occur alone); parental seduction; an inadequate home.

The second class, those factors found with considerable frequency, is composed almost entirely of traits within the individual rather than in the environment: social isolation; loneliness; inability to get along with others; depression; being over-controlled.

The third class, found to a lesser extent than the two previous ones contains a variety of factors: both sexual inhibition and sexual hyperactivity; self-mutilation; frequent headaches; mental disease in the family; a greater frequency of outpatient medical contacts; a preference for knives over guns; a need to carry a weapon in self-defense and panic when without it; hyperactivity; stubborness; a tendency to be accident prone; a 4-9 profile on the MMPI.

A great many people have one or several of the above-named factors in their backgrounds. Suspicion should be aroused to possible dangerousness when a large number of these factors are seen in any one individual. It will usually not be necessary to inquire specifically for many of these factors. They will emerge as a part of the life history which is obtained during the course of the evaluative interview. If they are not mentioned spontaneously, then specific inquiry should be made.

In those cases in which violence has already occurred, Kozol and his group[2] feel that in making a prediction, the individual's characteristics should be compared with the same characteristics in what they feel is the picture of the "safe" person. "Our concept of the safe person is one who appears to have developed strong conditioning against repetition of his original offensive behavior, has developed insight into his own nature,

---

[2]Diagnosing "Dangerousness" in Psychiatric Patients, special report, Roche, *Frontiers of Psychiatry*, 1972.

is relatively free of gross distortion of reality, has divested himself of hostilities and resentments, has developed a compassionate concern for the welfare and interests of others, has generally matured in attitudes of social responsibility, has an image of himself as a mature adult, specifically recognizes that freedom in the community involves responsibility as well as gratification." In contrast, the "essence of dangerousness appears to be a paucity of feeling concern for other." The presence of anger increases the patient's potential for injuring others. "Both the paucity of feeling concern for others and rage . . . may be of remote or recent origin, and may be global or selective."

It is the general experience that most probation officers, like most psychiatrists, tend to err commonly in their predictions of dangerousness and render this opinion too frequently. If no violent behavior has yet occurred, the percentage of false positive predictions tends to be extremely high. This error is the result of two factors: the desire to protect the public from the dangerous offender, and the C Y A (Cover Your Ass) syndrome. When an individual, who has been given a favorable report commits a serious offense, while on probation because of that favorable report, the officer (or psychiatrist) hears about it very quickly. On the other hand, no judgment is passed as to whether those who have been incarcerated as a result of an unfavorable report would have committed a violent act had they been free during that period of incareration.

It is extremely difficult to predict if and when violence will occur in those whom Megargee has labeled the over-controlled, those who commonly repress all aggressive tendencies. Thus, they appear basically mild and nondangerous, but it is as though with each act of repression a quantum of violence is added to the storehouse, until the individual explodes on minimal provocation. Even more difficult to predict is the sudden violent offense in an individual who may have a long record of nonviolent criminal offenses, no signs of mental disorder, and very few of the above-mentioned violence predictors in the history. I find myself currently involved in evaluating two such situations, which, since they have not been adjudicated, cannot be discussed. In each instance, alcohol features in the history.

This brings up one final statement about prediction of violence. There are many people for whom the statement can be made that the odds are excellent there will be no violent offenses committed as long as they continue to be abstinent from alcohol and certain drugs — namely cocaine and the amphetamines. The relationship of alcohol to violence is well illustrated in a paper by Mayfield.[3] He reported on 300 consecutive admissions for assaultive crimes (80% of which were homicides) to the prison system of North Carolina. Only 8 percent of the offenders were abstainers, while 36 percent were problem drinkers. The remainder were classified as drinkers. Fifty-seven percent of the offenses were committed while drinking. It was possible to ascertain blood alcohol levels of twenty-three of the victims. Eighteen of these twenty-three had also been drinking prior to the assault. Mayfield indicted the triad of alcohol, familiarity, and firearms in most homicides.

Adolescents pose special problems in the prediction of violence. At times the psychodynamics of the individual allow a fairly confident prediction as to future behavior. For example, in the case of Mr. V. in Chapter 8, it could be confidently predicted that with the repression of both hostility and sexuality, further violent behavior against women was inevitable without treatment. (This also illustrates the frustration that comes from knowing that violence will happen and not having the means to enforce the necessary treatment to prevent it.) Dr. Derek Miller, Professor of Child Psychiatry at the University of Michigan Medical School speaks[4] of, "A definable syndrome in which the attempted murder of another human being is inevitable and not due to chance alone." He first stresses the need to be alert to the indicators which have already been discussed here as a clue to further study. The specific variable which underlies the need to commit murder is a compulsion to dehumanize others. He discusses three types of this syndrome.

---

[3] Alcoholism, Alcohol, Intoxication and Assaultive Behavior, Demmie Mayfield, *Journal of Nervous Diseases,* May 1976, p. 288.

[4] Identifying and Treating the Potential Murderer, an interview with Dr. Derek Miller, Roche *Frontiers of Psychiatry,* Volume 4, Number 6, March 15, 1974, p. 1.

In the first type, the "murderous person totally dehumanizes others in his own mind." Dr. Miller refers to the use of the examiner's gut reaction as an aid to diagnosis of these youngsters. He states they arouse a "specific response of hostile anxiety on the part of the examiner." In the second type, there is only partial dehumanization of others. In this group, "Murder is inevitable because the act becomes necessary to resolve internal tensions, associated with internally mixed conflicts about sexuality and aggression. Only in murder — first in fantasy, then in fact — is he able to resolve the tensions." In the third group, "Some compulsion to dehumanize is present, but the murderer's fantasy requires the validation of peer approval to make action possible."

This section will be brought to a close by citing one more study. Guze et al.,[5] in an eight- to nine-year follow-up of felons (not necessarily violent), found, "The two factors most closely related to recidivism were the extent of prior criminal behavior and age." (Relative youth being most important.) Following these were sociopathy, alcoholism, and drug dependence. The diagnosis of *acute* alcoholism or drug usage led to a higher recidivism rate than did *past* alcoholism or drug dependence.

Dangerousness and the Penal Institution

This section will deal with those people who must be watched carefully in a penal setting because of the potentiality for impulsive and assaultive behavior. While there are certainly a large number of female prisoners who fit these criteria, the overwhelming number of studies have been done on males. For this reason, the statements made should be interpreted as being valid only for males.

The Characterologically Aggressive

These are the people who would be spotted anywhere as

---

[5]Samuel B. Guze, M.D., Donald W. Goodwin, M.D., and J. Bruce Crone, M.D., Criminal Recidivism in Psychiatric Illness, *American Journal of Psychiatry*, Volume 127.6, December 1970, p. 832.

impulsively aggressive. Diagnostically they belong to the groups labeled Unsocialized Aggressive Disorders of Adolescence or the Explosive Personality Disorders. The same careful watch would be necessary were such an individual to be encountered on the street or in a bar. Their behavior is part of their basic personality structure. The body build is generally stocky, barrel-chested, and muscular. Such individuals walk with a swagger. They are apt to be tattooed extensively and particularly to have the L O V E — H A T E combination mentioned in Chapter 15 on the back of the fingers. They will be seen to have many scars. Some of these will have been obtained in brawls, some in accidents. As high as 50 percent of these scars may have been self-inflicted. Those scars on the anterior surface of the wrists and forearms are most apt to fall in this class, but self-inflicted scars may be anywhere. Bach y Rita in one study of violent prisoners describes a man with 164 such scars. They usually speak in a loud and belligerent voice. Soft and incisive vocal tones may suggest even greater dangerousness.

From the standpoint of descriptive behavior, this is the man with the chip on his shoulder. He tries to get as much as he can by bluff and bluster. He believes firmly in a pecking order and very quickly has found his place in it, although he is constantly striving to rise. He has no scruples about sucker-punching or sandbagging someone and will brag about it afterwards. He tends to be at his worst after a few drinks of alcohol and, hence, frequently requires special attention when admitted to jail from the street. (There is some dispute as to the effect of the amphetamines on these individuals. Small doses are said to modify their behavior favorably, as in the MBD child. Large doses exacerbate dangerous behavior. This could imply that many of these people are minimally brain damaged children grown up.)

B.A. will be used to epitomize this group. B.A. was a short, stocky, sixteen-year-old, held in juvenile detention while awaiting possible certification to adult court on a third charge of armed robbery, aggravated assault, and resisting arrest. All detainees are routinely kept in their own rooms for twenty-four hours after admission to the section. Within two hours of being allowed in the open section, B.A. was found in the shower urinating on several weaker boys. This behavior continued despite the commands of the section leader to stop. He refused to return to his room when told to do so. It was only after several staff members were assembled, and it became obvious that resistance was futile, that he consented to go. The same behavior was repeated a few hours following release to the section again. Placed back in his room his remark was "Okay, you can't keep me locked up forever. When I get out I'll do what I damn please." However, this behavior was not repeated again.

The first rule in dealing with such an individual is simply to apply common sense. Neither the back nor the other cheek should be turned. There should be no attempt to out-swagger or out-tough him. It might intimidate this particular individual, as with Van Wyck Goodall's chimps, but sooner or later a guard who employs this approach is going to meet someone who will not be bluffed, and a struggle will ensue. Further, once a guard gets a reputation as a tough guy, every would-be tough guy who enters the institution is going to make him prove himself all over again. There should, of course, be no evidence of being awed by the swagger and bluster.

The second rule is to adopt an attitude of natural expectation that this individual, like everyone else, is going to obey the rules, and it is taken for granted that he will do so. This unspoken expectation that there is not going to be any trouble tends to defuse the explosive potential of these people. Any time rules *are* broken, or even skirted, the appropriate response should be made. This involves the use of enough personnel that force is not necessary. Paradoxical as it may sound, the presence of adequate security personnel is generally comforting, rather than upsetting, to an individual of this sort. It serves as a reassurance that, "We won't let you blow up, you don't have to be afraid of what you might do." At the same time it enables him to save face, which is all-important. The most significant thing is the calm expectation that the rules will be obeyed. As noted, despite B.A.'s big talk, he conformed as soon as he learned that he would not be allowed not to do so.

In some institutions it has become almost standing operating procedure to give such an individual large doses of major tranquilizers whenever trouble seems imminent, or even to administer these tranquilizers routinely every day. The use of medication in the service of the institution rather than in the service of the individual is being increasingly discouraged, and it should be. In individuals of this sort there are two medications which may be tried. Neither of these medications has any tranquilizing properties. The first instance is the use of Dilantin in the prevention of outbursts in those with an episodic dyscontrol syndrome. The second is the use of Lithium Carbonate in individuals whose acting out behavior seems to occur in clusters in response to a prolonged irritable mood. If, after sufficient observation, the medication is having no effect on behavior it should be discontinued.

The use of either individual or group psychotherapy with these people while they are still incarcerated is open to question. Either the therapist is seen as a tool of the administration or there is an attempt made to fool the therapist and, through the therapist, the parole board. Some success has been claimed for groups using either Guided Group Interaction or Transactional Analysis, particularly in instances where the therapist simply teaches the group the necessary skills and then permanently withdraws. Under these circumstances, it is claimed those offenders who genuinely wish help continue to work to improve themselves. No records are kept of whether or not they attend groups, no one connected with authority is there to report whether there is, or is not, improvement. This has yet to be employed on a wide enough scale to judge its potential usefulness.

Antisocial Personalities

The next group of individuals who are apt to have violent outbursts in jail are those with Antisocial Personality Disorders (Chapter 9). As a general rule, crimes of violence are not associated with the antisocial personality, although a small proportion of rapists and murderers fall in this group. These people usually make model prisoners. They learn the ropes very quickly (if they do not know them from past experience). They do their best to stay out of trouble with both administration and fellow prisoners, although they are not at all above inducing less knowledgeable or intelligent inmates to get into trouble, while they remain in the background. They know exactly what looks good on the record and what leads to maximum amount of "good" time for the parole board.

A compelling reason for including these people with those who are dangerous when incarcerated (in addition to their ability to foment trouble) is that they tend to crack under stress. When they do, they may blow with a bang and attack their surroundings violently, senselessly, and almost uncontrollably. These stress periods are most apt to occur at three specific times. (It will also be seen that these are the most sensitive times for potential suicide in other individuals.) These times are (1) the first thirty-six to forty-eight hours after being placed in jail, (2) the first twenty-four to forty-eight hours after having been found guilty or having been sentenced, (3) the first two to five days after transfer to the penal institution where they are to serve their time.

One other type of situation may precipitate an acute stress reaction in an antisocial personality. Because there is acute awareness of the feelings of others (note "awareness of" and not "consideration for"), the antisocial personality is quite apt to react to periods of increased tension in the institution. These may include those times when a prison break is being planned, when there is bad blood between two other prisoners who are out to get each other, when there is a general feeling of tension or imminent riot.

At any of these times, the antisocial personality may blow out of control and a short-lived, acute, psychotic episode may occur. The late Dr. Ralph Chambers, in whose hospital I received basic training about these people, used a farm metaphor to describe this behavior as, "The squealing of a pig caught under a fence." This describes not only the symptomatology, but also the fact that it is a reaction to stress. The psychosis usually clears quickly after the stress is relieved, particularly if the prisoner is removed from the stress situation. These acute reactions will also respond rapidly to antipsychotic medications.

An alert custodial staff may be able to spot such an attack developing and may be able to avoid it. Detection depends first on having made the diagnosis of antisocial disorder. The clue to an approaching attack is the development of signs of increasing anxiety in one of these people, who notoriously display a complete lack of anxiety. An alert guard will spot signs of increased restlessness during the daytime: pacing up and down; possibly tearing magazines and newspapers into strips; increased irritability. Insomnia, or restless, troubled sleep fills the night. Incidentally, this behavior, in addition to being a sign of what is going on in the individual, may also be a barometer of what is going on in the institution.

In contrast to the opinion that tranquilizers should not be used in the explosive personality, the onset of restlessness in the antisocial group is a definite indication for the use of antipsychotic medication, which may abort or lessen the intensity of an outburst. They should also be removed to the jail or prison hospital for a few days.

Psychotic Individuals

It goes without saying that people in penal settings who exhibit bizarre, psychotic behavior require careful attention. The question of violence in mentally ill offenders was gone into at length in discussing prediction in the presentence investigation. These criteria for prediction of violence apply equally in penal settings. Even the effect of the ingestion of alcohol and drugs must be taken into account in certain prisons. Theoretically, psychotic individuals should not be in penal institutions, but, as noted previously, the percentage of the mentally ill is higher in those settings than it is in the general public. It has also been the universal experience that as civil commitment proceedings have become more difficult, more of the mentally ill have found their way into the penal system. It is also becoming increasingly difficult to obtain hospitalization in a mental institution for those who become psychotic while in detention.

Which of these people are most apt to be dangerous, many times to themselves as well as to others? Primarily it is those who are confused. The cause of the confusion makes little difference, whether it be severe drug or alcohol intoxication, organic brain disorder, or functional psychosis. Any time an individual does not recognize the surroundings, has no clear knowledge of the identity of those in the environment, and is unable to make logical sense of what transpires, that individual is potentially dangerous. Under those circumstances, the most ordinary happenings may be interpreted as a serious threat. Anyone who invades the living space of such an individual may be seen as a potential killer. From the prisoner's view of the situation he must defend himself to the death. (Incidentally, it has been shown that the living space of the impulsively dangerous individual is greater than that of the nondangerous person — approximately four times as great if approached from the rear, twice as great if approached from the front.) A little old man who looks as meek as a lamb but is brought to the jail so drunk that he is not "with it" may fight like a wild bull because he is frightened.

Danger to personnel is minimized if these people are approached slowly and with no sudden moves. Just as with epileptics who are having psychomotor seizures or who are having postictal confused states, there should be no attempt to control motor activity unless there is a grave possibility that the motor behavior will result in serious injury to the person. The slow approach should be accompanied by gentle murmuring speech. It has been suggested it is better to just make soothing sounds to the confused epileptic rather than to utter actual words.

With other confused individuals, cues which foster orientation to the environment should be repeated frequently and gently. It is amazing how often people talking to those who are confused tend to shout, as though shouting would clarify what is being said. In a gentle tone the following type of remarks should be employed. "You're in the Mayton Jail. You've been here for four hours. I am your security guard. My name is

James Johnson. Your name is John Green. It's early morning. You're in the Mayton Jail. Today is Thursday. You're John Green. I'm your guard. My name is James Johnson. It's breakfast time. This is your tray of food. No, it's not a weapon, it's your breakfast tray." Any procedures to be carried out should be repetitively explained in detail, in a soothing tone of voice. Certainly, if it is possible to transfer these people to a mental hospital, an attempt should be made to do so. As has been mentioned this is becoming increasingly difficult in many communities.

In any instance of confusion, whether present at the time of admission, occurring shortly thereafter, or occurring after a few months in an institution, medical aid should be sought immediately to rule out head injury, stroke, toxic delirium, or other nonpsychotic medical reasons for the confusion. Under no circumstances should medication be administered to such an individual without a doctor's orders, and then not unless the doctor has seen the patient first and knows him well. There are many such conditions which are worsened rather than helped by certain medications. Nothing is more distressing to the staff of a penal institution than to find a prisoner dead in his room, and this may happen with the injudicious administration of medicine.

As noted in Chapter 6, manic patients usually make a stop in jail before being sent to the hospital. Although the manic patient is generally quite amusing, jail personnel should be made aware of the irratibility which frequently accompanies the euphoric mood and should conduct themselves accordingly.

The chronically mentally ill patient who is in a penal setting because of administrative choice rarely poses problems if his medication is properly maintained. Certainly, a penal institution does not offer the opportunity for treatment and recovery that an adequately staffed and functioning mental health institution does. Treatment of such an individual with the dignity he deserves as a human being, regardless of how bizarre some of his ideas are or how amusing some of his stereotyped behavior is, will at least give him the opportunity to leave the institution no worse than when he entered.

Dangerousness in Those on Probation or Parole

The identification of the dangerous individual among those on probation or parole is no different from that which has been described in the past two sections. In these instances the probation or parole officer will have already had a considerable amount of historical data available for scrutiny for possible clues as to dangerousness. The problem of prolonged incarceration of those who have a potential for violent behavior because there is no way to guarantee they will not be violent in the future has already been mentioned. It has been suggested that one answer to this problem is more widespread release of these individuals with very careful monitoring. This may increase the number of these persons on parole. Are there any special indicators which may be found in routine reporting, which may alert the officer to the imminence of violent behavior in someone already identified as violence prone? I have no knowledge of any studies which have been done in this area. The material to be suggested has received no experimental validation. It represents an extrapolation to the field of corrections of cues to imminent regression given by mentally ill patients in outpatient status.

The methods of detection are largely those which have been mentioned in the chapters on interviewing. Foremost is observation of behavior. Any changes in habitual behavior patterns, even if that change seems to be for the better, should be carefully evaluated. The man who has complained bitterly about his wife at every reporting session and then fails to do so may have made up his mind that he has taken all he is going to take, and the next time she opens her mouth he is going to let her have it. Once he has reached that decision he is at peace. The client who has had his drinking well under control and starts to drink again is saying, "I'm about to get into trouble." The parolee who has always been clean and neat and now reports in disheveled or dirty clothing must be suspect. In the case of mentally ill offenders, any indication that they are not taking prescribed medication requires prompt attention. The doctor should be notified immediately. Failure to keep medical appointments is an even worse sign of impending trouble.

Equal concern should be shown for those who describe a double-bind situation, where it seems that no action can be taken which is right. Evidence of increasing frustration is also not very difficult to spot. Increasing frequency and intensity of complaints expressing inability to better a situation is another common danger sign. If a really good relationship has been formed, there may even be the overt expression of threats.

How should these threats be evaluated? It is an extremely difficult task to decide when a threat to kill is an empty gesture, a means of expressing a feeling forcefully, or when it should be taken seriously. It must be taken seriously in severely confused and delirious patients, and in acute schizophrenic reactions. While the possibility of dangerousness in the case of a chronically paranoid individual should never be taken lightly, it should cause extra concern if the patient is agitated or feels special provocation. Off-hand statements may need clarification but are usually expressions of fantasy. Solely on a statistical basis, a history of a previous suicidal attempt lessens the seriousness of a homicidal threat. At the same time it must be remembered that Bach y Rita's violent men were covered with self-inflicted wounds. On the other hand, a quiet, determined statement by an antisocial personality should be heard with the greatest respect.

Threats that are conditional, such as, "If the bastard ever does that to me again, I'll kill him," may be taken with a grain of salt. Usually it is wise to ask, "Do you mind if I warn him of that?" It should be realized that whenever a threat against a third person, no matter how serious, is made within the officer-defendant relationship, the unspoken message is, "Please stop me." The officer should respond accordingly.

Defusing Potential Violence

The law looks with disfavor on preventive detention. It is extremely difficult (if indeed it could be justified) to ask for temporary detention on the grounds that the probationer or parolee seems about to blow a fuse. At times, if abstinence has been a condition of probation, revocation of parole or probation on a temporary basis may be requested because of renewed alcohol or drug consumption. This must be used with care since detention might be the final burden on an individual with fragile ego control and might do more harm than good. If the relationship with the probationer or parolee is good enough, the recommendation might be made that the individual see a doctor. Hopefully, temporary medicinal aid will calm the client sufficiently to allow a thorough appraisal and working through of the crisis situation. Hopefully, a more satisfactory alternative to violence may be found.

If the relationship has been previously used properly, there will have been two ongoing mechanisms at work which can now be called on to deal with this sort of uncomfortable situation. The first has been to get the probationer in touch with his own feelings, to identify them specifically, and to talk them out rather than to act them out. Many of those with whom the corrections worker deal have never really sorted out their feelings. If experienced at all, feelings have been divided into "good" and "bad" and the matter has rested there. During the period of probation or parole, serious efforts should have been made to help identify these feelings and define their nature, be they anger, rage, jealousy, hurt, disgust, contempt, loneliness, etc. Attempts should have been made to locate the source of these feelings as well. This can then be followed by attempting to dissipate the feelings by talking about them.

At the same time these attempts should have been supplemented by fantasizing and role playing. Dialogues of this sort should have been taking place:

"I'm angry at my boss, because I think he's taking advantage of me."

"What can you imagine yourself doing?"

"I can see myself going out there and socking him in the jaw."

"How would that make you feel?"

"Good all over. Maybe a sore hand."

"Try to imagine what will happen if you do that."

"I'll probably lose my job."

"What then?"

"Well, my wife said if I lost another job, that was it. She was through."

"Anything else?"

"Yeah, maybe my parole will be revoked."

"You're the one who has the bad feelings. Is it worth it to get rid of them in that way?"

"No."

"All right, what else could you do?"

"I could go out and get drunk."

"How would that make you feel?"

"Probably madder. I'd go out and wreck the joint and come home and wreck the house, and my wife would kick me out for real, and I'd have a nasty hangover."

Such a dialogue might end with, "Maybe I could go out there and try and talk it out with him. Yeah, that's what I'll do. If I don't get anywhere I'll try to remember not to blow my top, and come in and talk to you again before I lose my cool."

SUICIDE

The corrections worker is apt to encounter suicidal attempts and gestures in any phase of the justice system. The greatest emphasis will be placed on those suicidal attempts which are made in jail or prison. This is because the fact of incarceration in a penal institution adds another dimension to the complex motivation which underlies suicidal behavior, and because the supervision of the institution should provide a greater opportunity for prevention. Further, in a penal institution all the ordinary life lines, which might be utilized in rescue, are absent, and the responsibility for prevention rests solely on the shoulders of the custodian. The unequivocal statement can be made that if a person is desperately and inalterably committed to suicide, the act cannot be prevented. Fortunately, it is a rare person who is so driven. It should also be noted that the most intense suicidal preoccupation lasts for only a relatively short time.

This topic is best handled by first considering general knowledge about suicide, and then applying that knowledge to the special situation of penal incarceration. Suicidal attempts may be divided into three types: those which are genuine; those which are gestures; those which are gambles. A large proportion of real attempts are successful. The genuinely suicidal individual, while exhibiting warning signs, does not purposefully reveal his intentions to anyone at the *last* moment. The attempt is generally not made in the actual presence of another or with others in the vicinity. (The father of A. Q. was certainly an exception to this generalization.) There is a genuine expectation that death will follow. Should such people survive the attempt, they express real feelings of disappointment at being still alive.

Suicidal gestures are made after informing someone, "I'm going to kill myself." The gesture is made in the presence of others, or with full knowledge that others are expected in a short period of time. A variant of this is the phone call to say, "I have just swallowed a bottle of pills." Two-thirds of all gestures are made by women. The function of a gesture is different than that of a genuine attempt. Its purpose is to call attention to a particular plight, or to manipulate the environment. It is a call for help, an appeal to the human condition. There are a variety of social effects. particularly on interpersonal relationships, which may determine the eventual outcome following a gesture. If the gesture fails to bring about the desired result, it may be followed by a more serious attempt, or hopefully, a more intelligent way of influencing the environment may be found. That the gesture is more complicated than merely an attempt to modify the environment is demonstrated by the fact that 2 to 10 percent of those who make the attempt, actually do kill themselves within ten years of their original gesture.

A suicidal gamble is conceived of as being midway between a serious attempt and a gesture. The most obvious example of the gamble is Russian Roulette. In a penal setting this would be manifested by an attempt at hanging, two or three minutes before a guard usually, but not always, makes rounds. A gamble is most apt to be seen in the sort of individual who is role-playing. Such an individual was usually the class clown in school and needs to retain the center of the stage. It is sometimes difficult to differentiate between these three types of suicidal behavior. It is, however, of extreme importance in attempting to determine the immediate future of the individual.

Statistics about suicide are very difficult to acquire. That is particularly true of suicide in the penal system. In this country it is generally reported that there are about 12.5 suicides annually per 100,000 population. This works out to 21 to 25,000 suicides a year, although the actual figure could be twice as high as that. It is generally accepted that there are eleven attempts for every successful suicide. This comes out to about 275,000 attempts a year, or roughly one every two minutes. One of the most important predictive factors of a possible suicidal attempt in any person is a history of previous attempts, just as a history of previous violence is important in the prediction of violent behavior.

This can be rephrased. The statement can be made that those who have attempted suicide once will probably try again during their lifetime. I have had several patients with a history of as high as thirty such attempts, obviously gestures.) This implies that there are probably somewhere between 2 and 5 million people in the United States at any one time who have made suicidal attempts and hence are potentially suicidal.

Some of the other known facts about suicide are as follows. As far as age is concerned, the incidence of suicide increases with each decade over thirty, tapering off in women over seventy. The vast majority of attempts are made under the age of thirty-five; the vast majority of successful suicides occur over the age of thirty-five. Suicide is the third leading cause of death in adolescents. Males are three times more successful in committing suicide than females. (The reason for this may be the choice of methods. Men are more apt to kill themselves violently, shooting, hanging, jumping from high places; women by taking pills, by gas, or by wrist slashing.) Whites in our culture kill themselves more frequently than blacks, but the suicide rate in black urban young males is growing rapidly and is already higher than that for white urban males of the same age group. As far as marital status is concerned, the rate rises in this order: married people have the lowest rate, followed by single, divorced, and widowed. The suicidal rate is higher among alcoholics, and particularly during an attempt to abstain from alcohol. As might be expected, the number of suicides amongst the unemployed is greater than in those who are working. One final factor noted is that the greater the presence of physical illness, the higher the rate of suicide.

If a profile of the most likely candidate to commit suicide were to be drawn, it would be that of a white, elderly, widowed, unemployed male, in poor health, and attempting to stop drinking. To this should be added a feeling of depression, which probably could have been assumed from the profile. Not all depressed people attempt suicide, but almost all serious suicidal attempts are made by those who are depressed at the time. This does not imply that depression is necessarily due to mental illness; it may well be due to environmental factors.

There are various ways of looking at suicide. It may be conceived of as a balance of forces among culture, stress, and ego-strength. Cultural factors vary from nation to nation and from era to era. In Japan, cultural suicide in the form of Hari-Kari was expected whenever honor was lost. In the Catholic religion, suicide is a cause for eternal damnation. At one time suicide was a felony and successful suicides were buried at a crossroad with a stake through their hearts. In most states today suicide is no longer a felony, but aiding a suicide is a felonious act. Some stress is external: working conditions, financial problems, the attitudes of others, natural calamities. Other stress is internal: trying to achieve beyond one's capacity; feelings of guilt over behavior; inability to face the consequences of a given action; etc. As for ego-strength, despite the words of the Declaration of Independence, all men are not created equal in this regard. Some people are much better put together than others; they either have a better heredity, or had a more favorable childhood, or have developed better coping capacities.

From this point of view, the possible suicide of an individual in the penal system would depend, among other things, on the way that individual's particular subculture regarded both imprisonment and suicide, on the degree of stress imposed on the individual, the experience — trial, prison, publicity — and on how capable the ego was in coping with these factors. To this might be added how much that ego had been dissolved in alcohol.

Another way of viewing the suicidal act has been called the LAD syndrome. L stands for loss. Almost every suicidal patient has recently suffered a loss. This may be of many kinds: loss of a loved person, financial loss, job, status. The loss may even be symbolic like a loss of self-esteem, but there has always been a loss.

A stands for aggression. In this view suicide represents aggression which has been turned against oneself, rather than against the outside world. This is especially important for corrections. The study of Bach y Rita has already been cited. This was done in a maximum security prison in California. Over 50 percent of these extremely aggressive people have multiple scars of self-inflicted wounds. It might also be noted that suicide is sometimes an extremely impulsive act. Hence, in a prison setting, special attention should be paid to those who have a history of frequent arrests, fights, auto accidents, who like to live dangerously and take chances. The D stands for depression. As has already been stated, this can be either a depressed mood, or the illness, *depression*.

Against this background of epidemiological elements of suicide, certain specific factors precipitate the event. Some common triggers are found to be present in the immediate past of suicidal patients. The more important are, in order, domestic quarrels or difficulties, medical or psychiatric illness in the individual or family, loss or change of job, court appearance, moving to a new home or having a new person move into the home. Any three such significant events, occurring within six months, may precipitate a suicidal attempt, usually within two or three months of the last event.

Unless the suicidal act is completely a matter of impulse, most suicidal people give some sort of warning. Certainly by now it is common knowledge that it is not true that those who talk about suicide never attempt it. This warning may be in words or by behavior. Many suicidal patients act like someone about to leave on a long journey. They put their effects in order, make a will, write a note about what to do. Not infrequently they take out additional insurance. Some begin to lead a really ascetic life. They may withdraw from loved ones as though to make the pains of parting less real.

The most important verbalizations are the following: actual suicidal threats, particularly if details are given as to method and place; discussion of the suicide of others; talk about death and dying in general; and especially talk about being a burden to the family and loved ones.

Since most suicides occur in people who have made attempts, every suicidal attempt must be taken seriously, unless its real meaning is crystal clear. Most gestures are meant to convey one of these meanings: pay attention to me; feel sorry for me; get me out of this; help me; "now, don't you feel bad?" Any gesture might backfire and really work. In this regard many apparent suicides are accidents, just as many seemingly accidental deaths are really suicides. The most serious suicidal potentials are associated with feelings of helplessness and hopelessness, feelings of exhaustion and failure, feelings of "I just want out," and to emphasize once more, feelings of being a burden to one's dear ones.

Suicide in Penal Settings

To translate these generalities into specific suggestions for those responsible for the care of people in the penal setting is not too difficult. As with explosive outbursts, the most likely times for suicidal attempts are within the first forty-eight hours after having been locked up, immediately before or after a court verdict (particularly if the latter has been *guilty*),[6] and immediately after transfer to prison from jail. The risk during the first twenty-four hours is increased if the prisoner has been

---

[9]Suicides have occurred within forty-eight hours after acquittal because of newspaper publicity and embarrassment over facing neighbors.

jailed following a family fight and has been drinking. The risk in this event increases with age and with chronic alcoholism.

Special attention should be paid to those prisoners who talk about having disgraced their families and go into detail about what indignities and deprivations the family has suffered because of them. Many people on first being placed in jail appear quite depressed, and some may become quite agitated. Special care should be given to those who, in addition, seem to have a hopeless and helpless attitude and, even though they may have a personal attorney, refuse to call a lawyer or their families. The outlook is even worse if the family visits and the prisoner refuses to see them. (Unless, of course, there seems to be ample reason for animosity.)

Of special significance are detailed threats to commit suicide, particularly if they contain reference to methods. Obvious signs of depression should not be overlooked. It should be remembered that in depression suicide occurs most commonly at those times when the depressed person is first showing encouraging signs of getting better. Indeed, change of behavior in any direction must be viewed with suspicion. The prisoner who is becoming unduly anxious and agitated, when there has been no change in his life situation to account for the agitation, should be suspect. So should the individual who has suddenly become calm and composed after having been quite worked up. Such calmness frequently indicates a decision to go ahead and die. The chronic alcoholic must be watched carefully, not only because of suicidal potential but also for development of delirium tremens, or for the development of severe physical illness. As was previously stressed the chronic, acting out, impulsive individual who has scars on wrist and neck also bears watching. Finally, any individual who has killed a member of the family, or one who has killed many people in a sort of killing spree, is a prime candidate for suicide.

It should be remembered that a suicidal state of mind is an acute rather than a chronic preoccupation. Sometimes careful watch for twenty-four to seventy-two hours is all that is necessary for the acute period to pass. (This is not true if the suicidal feelings arise from a true inner depression, rather than as a reaction to external circumstances.) This does does not mean that continued surveillance is not indicated beyond the seventy-two hour period, nor that careful evaluation and counseling should not be ongoing. A suicidal attempt occurring in this state should usually not be responded to by the use of antidepressant medication. It should also be remembered that tranquilzers and sedatives have a tendency to increase depressive feelings. If a suicide attempt is made in jail, it can be taken as a rule of thumb that an attempt at hanging represents a more serious suicidal purpose than does one made by wrist slashing (unless the latter is so deep as to cause arterial bleeding). It should also be remembered that an unsuccessful suicide attempt may be quickly followed by a more serious one. Those who make such attempts should be transferred to the prison hospital, if one exists and if around-the-clock observation is available there. In spite of the reality of suicidal attempts, one other possibility must always be kept in mind in a penal setting. There should be an attempt to spot the gestures which are purposely intended to bring about removal to a hospital, from which escape may be more simple.

PART THREE
DRUGS, ALCOHOL, AND CORRECTIONS

Chapter 18

FUNDAMENTALS OF THE PROBLEM

GENERAL CONSIDERATIONS

DSM II lists **Alcoholism** (303) and **Drug Dependence** (304) under the heading of **Personality Disorders and Certain Other Nonpsychotic Mental Disorders.** However, nowhere in *DSM II* is there a description of the acute effects of these substances on behavior. The corrections worker must be familiar with both aspects. It seems logical, therefore, to consider them both at the same time. Understanding of these substances becomes simpler if alcohol is regarded as just another substance, like drugs, susceptible to abuse, for this is what it actually is. In order to address this topic meaningfully it is necessary to understand the terms to be used. For years the study of this area was plagued by fruitless semantic arguments. To avoid this confusion, arbitrary definitions will be assigned.

It is first necessary to differentiate among *use, misuse,* and *abuse. Use* is limited to the medical application of any drug. Some drugs, such as mescaline, hashish, and marijuana have as yet no accepted medical use. The medicinal use of alcohol has almost reached the vanishing point. *Misuse* is the *improper* medical application of a drug. Some examples of misuse are inordinate refills in prescribing sleeping pills for insomnia, the indiscriminate use of narcotics for relief of pain when a nonnarcotic analgesic will serve the same purpose, and the reflex prescription of a minor tranquilizer for the relief of anxiety with no attempt to ascertain the cause of the anxiety. Misuse, which is the responsibility of the physician, is involved in the production of a very small percentage of habituation. *Abuse* is the utilization without medical approval of a substance in order to produce an altered psychological state.

The next two terms to be distinguished from each other are *tolerance* and *dependence.* Tolerance is the process by which the body, particularly the central nervous system, is progressively less affected by increasing quantities of ingested alcohol or drugs. To express this concept from a different point of view, tolerance is said to exist when the same dose of the agent no longer has the same (or any) effect on the consumer. Whether or not tolerance develops depends on a combination of three factors: the characteristics of the specific drug; the mode of consumption, frequency, and span of time over which it is consumed; and the attributes of the specific consumer. Tolerance is never developed to certain drugs. For example, pharmacologists maintain the same quantity of cocaine will produce the same high in a particular individual, no matter how often or over what period of time that individual has been taking it. (Some cocaine abusers deny this.) The question of development of tolerance to marijuana is still unsolved. On the other hand, tolerance develops rapidly to LSD (acid), or Dilaudid® (a narcotic).

In the case of some chronic drug abusers, tolerance is sometimes developed more rapidly than in those who are *using* the substance rather than *abusing* it. This is because the drug-abusers deliberately increase the dose to accentuate the *high*. In this way, they artificially produce a rapid growth of tolerance, which may reach amazing proportions. Some habitual abusers in order to get a *rush* must inject Dilaudid into their veins in a quantity which is forty times the dose normally given intramuscularly for the relief of pain. (The effect of any substance injected intravenously occurs more rapidly and intensely than if administered intramuscularly or taken orally.) Tolerance to other substances such as the barbiturates or alcohol develops more slowly, but can also reach incredible degrees. It is not uncommon for some alcoholics to be able to consume the equivalent of three to four fifths of 80 to 100 proof whiskey in the course of one drinking bout. One offender told of the consumption of eleven fifths of Black Velvet® in twenty-four hours. Tolerance to alcohol is frequently lost with the passage of time, and some notable topers become unable to take more than one or two drinks without obvious manifestations of being intoxicated.

Cross-tolerance develops to many of these substances. This means if an individual develops tolerance to one member of a class of drugs, this tolerance extends to other members of the same class. To use the opium derivates, or narcotics, as an example, an individual who has developed tolerance to heroin will also have increased tolerance for opium, morphine, codeine, Dilaudid, methadone, Percodan®, Demerol®, etc. Cross-tolerance between alcohol and barbiturates is well known. The chronic alcoholic in abstinence will require tremendous quantities of barbiturates to induce sleep. The simultaneous ingestion of both alcohol and barbiturates has an additive effect, and death may result from relatively small quantities of each taken together. This additive effect is called *potentiation*. A small dose of one drug in the group plus a small dose of another will have an effect greater than doubling the dose of either. Cross-tolerance also occurs between the minor tranquilizers and the volatile inhalants (gasoline, glue, anesthetics).

One significant aspect of the development of tolerance is the ability of the lower centers of the nervous system to withstand increasing amounts of the toxic agent without effect. This has important implications. In such a condition, higher functions such as self-criticism, inhibition, judgment, and impulse controls may be severely impaired, without any evidence of muscular incoordination, or any effects on such vital functions as respiration and heart rate. More importantly for corrections, it means the habitual abuser will have to purchase increasingly large quantities of a substance to get the desired effect.

Dependence must not be confused with tolerance. Dependence can be either physical or psychological. The term *physical dependence* refers to the condition in which the functioning of the nervous system is disturbed whenever that system is deprived of the agent of dependence, with a resultant physical craving for that agent. The development of physical dependence is usually closely allied to tolerance. As a general rule, the more rapid the development of tolerance, the more likely and more severe the risk of physical dependence. Tolerance to heroin develops fairly rapidly, and so does physical dependence. Tolerance to cocaine is said never to develop, neither does physical dependence. There are exceptions to this correlation between tolerance and dependence. Tolerance to LSD develops very rapidly; physical dependence never does. Tolerance to alcohol and barbiturates develops slowly; physical dependence, once it develops, is severe. Physical dependence can best be substantiated by the presence of the *withdrawal syndrome*.

In the withdrawal syndrome, specific physiological manifestations occur when an individual is deprived of a chronically abused drug to which physical dependence has developed. In the public mind, withdrawal symptoms are most commonly associated with heroin. There is no question there are physical symptoms associated with sudden abstinence from heroin, and they are unpleasant, but the rigors and dangers of stopping *cold turkey* have been greatly exaggerated. Such withdrawal is rarely life threatening. On the other hand, as noted in Chapter 3, one of the withdrawal syndromes in alcoholism, Delirium Tremens, carries a substantial risk of death even with proper medical management. The withdrawal syndrome in barbiturates is likewise extremely severe. It is very risky to withdraw barbiturates suddenly from someone who has become physically dependent on these substances. The *craving* mentioned in the definition of physical dependence grows out of body awareness of the onset of the withdrawal syndrome and the attempts to avoid it. Although rarely considered in this sense, nicotine and caffeine are the two most widely abused substances to which physical dependence develops. It might be possible to bring about physical dependence by repeatedly injecting certain drugs against a person's will. While this may have happened, it is certainly rare. Both relatively and absolutely, the number of those made physically dependent by the *misuse* of drugs is quite small.

The one factor common to all abused drugs, and the reason that they are taken, is that they change the mental state of the user because of the effect on the central nervous system. This change may be in the direction of increased relaxation, increased stimulation, or in the production of alterations in sensory experience. Some abusers attempt to experience all of these changes simultaneously. This change in mental state is considered by the user to be preferable to the normal state of consciousness. It is seen as an improvement, a *high*. In psychiatric terminology this state of being high is called *euphoria*. The attainment of this state is the primary motivation for the initiation of abuse of the drug. Abuse is perpetuated and made chronic by *psychological dependence*.

Psychological dependence is the need to continue taking a drug to maintain a state of mental well being. It is the end result of the interaction of a complex system which includes social, cultural, and economic, as well as psychological, factors. It is a truism that there is no personality type which can be specified as prone to alcohol or drug dependence. It is equally a truism that a reasonably well-adjusted individual may experiment with drugs, and not become dependent, even though the abuse is relatively frequent. It has been demonstrated that, even when the drug under consideration is heroin, there are many who confine its abuse to weekends and other special occasions, just as 80 to 90 percent of the population use alcohol. Such heroin abusers are referred to as *chippers*.

There is still considerable arguments as to whether a person who has been dependent on heroin can ever become a chipper, just as there is disagreement as to whether an alcoholic can ever become a social drinker. Some writers talk of *susceptible individuals*. I have some doubt about using this term, since in the public mind this conjures up a picture of an individual eternally *hooked* after one exposure to a drug. Actually, this term refers to those in whom there is a greater than average risk of becoming drug dependent. This is brought about by a combination of factors. In terms of personality patterns, those who are inadequate, dependent, passive, or hedonistic are more apt to become drug dependent. Other factors are equally as important and are quite diverse. In the inner city there may be an increased danger of drug dependence because of a combination of circumstances, including but not limited to, the following; chaotic family conditions; inadequate living space; poverty; unemployment; feelings of rejection and hopelessness; cultural patterns, including peer pressure and the convivial atmosphere in which the drug is taken; role modeling after the successful pusher. In the suburbs similar sets of predisposing factors emerge: equally disturbed family patterns expressed less openly; peer pressure; parental expectations; feelings of failure and discouragement; general tension; boredom; the need to assume a *tough guy* facade. In other individuals, particularly in late adolescence, the chief factor may be *anhedonia* (inability to achieve feelings of pleasure) arising from inner discontent due to identity diffusion.

What is common in all these instances is an emotional state which is painful, whether that pain is manifested by anxiety, tension, insecurity, depression, or boredom, for which no alternative satisfactory relief has been found. The substance of abuse offers temporary relief of such pain. As the effects wear off, the pain returns. Psychological dependence may then be created. In that sense there are susceptible people. If the substance abused is one to which tolerance rapidly develops, then physical dependence is soon added to the psychological dependence. If, like alcohol and barbiturates, the substance is one to which tolerance develops more slowly, then physical dependence develops more slowly. In either instance, the need for relief from the physical craving is added to the desire for relief from psychological suffering. The result is the heroin addict who needs a fix every eight hours, or the alcoholic who cannot start the day without a drink.

This entire process can be conceptualized as a conditioned response. In the early stages, the pleasurable state, the high, acts as a positive reinforcer for taking the drug. Later, as physical dependence commences, the unpleasant state of the early symptoms of withdrawal acts as an aversive reinforcer against abandoning the drug. The development of dependency might also be conceptualized as a paradigm of the Freudian postulate of the *pleasure principle,* which states that the organism tends to seek pleasure and avoid pain. Wikler feels that the setting in which the primary conditioning takes place (the physical environment, peer presence, conviviality) acts as a secondary reinforcer and explains why an addict, drug free for months or years in the penitentiary, resumes the habit almost as soon as there is a return to the old environment.

EXTENT OF THE PROBLEM

It is impossible to estimate the extent of the problem of drug and alcohol abuse, whether acute or chronic to the point of dependency. An AP dispatch published in the *Toledo Blade* on 11/18/76 had the headline:

HALF OF ARMY ENLISTEES
USE DRUGS, STUDY SHOWS

In this particular study of seven hundred enlisted soldiers, 47 percent admitted using drugs regularly. This contrasted to 27 percent found in a similar study in 1969.

The National Institute on Drug Abuse recently released the results of an extensive study completed in 1974 and quoted in the *APA News*. This survey revealed the following information:

> That experience with marijuana in the age group 12 to 17 had jumped from 14 percent in 1972 to 23 percent in 1974.
>
> That people were trying marijuana at an earlier age. In 1972, 10 percent of the 14-15 year-olds had had experience with marijuana; in 1974, 22 percent of them had.
>
> That from 1969 to 1975 there was a three-fold increase in marijuana use, a four-fold increase in barbiturate use, and a three-fold increase in amphetamine use by male high school seniors.
>
> That 53 percent of all 18 to 25-year-olds have experimented with marijuana and more than six percent of all 18-year-olds used it daily.
>
> That Vietnam veterans are using more amphetamines and alcohol than they once did, while only 2 percent of them who returned to the U.S. more than three years ago have reported addiction to heroin at any time since their return.
>
> That 13 percent of the adult and 10 percent of the youthful population make some nonmedical use of tranquilizers, sedatives, stimulants, and over-the-counter drugs.

Figures as to the extent of the legitimate production of abused substances are relatively easily obtained. It is, of course, impossible to know what percentage of these substances are diverted to the black market, but it is obvious that this tremendous quantity is not being legitimately used. For example, in 1973 enough barbiturates were legitimately produced to fill 10 billion capsules, equivalent to about fifty capsules per person in the United. States. The great bulk of that undoubtedly finds its way into the black market for use as street drugs. The figure for 1970 for the legal production of amphetamines was almost identical to those just reported for barbiturates in 1973. It must also be remembered that amphetamine is easily produced clandestinely in basement laboratories. Various studies have shown amphetamines to be consumed by as many as 25 percent of high school students, while other surveys reveal amphetamine usage in college students to go as high as 33 percent. It has been estimated that about 100 million Americans use alcohol. Figures as to the production and use of narcotics and hallucinogens are more difficult to arrive at.

One of the factors which makes it so difficult to estimate the actual number of those who abuse drugs is the increasing group of those who abuse multiple drugs simultaneously. One possible reason for the increase in this polyvalent drug abuse is the increasingly youthful age of those who experiment with the drugs. In most metropolitan communities this experimentation is now beginning in junior high school, in the twelve to fourteen age group, although even younger subjects have been reported. There are certain important considerations implicit in this fact. One of these is that children of this age exercise little judgment. They will experiment with anything given, sold, or touted to them, or that they find in the family medicine chest, or even in other peoples' garbage pails. Thus, their early conditioning is to a wide variety of drugs, rather than to one single drug. In addition, since their experimentation is so widespread and their judgment is so poor, they are apt to experience the more potent euphoriants early in their drug careers.

Frequently, in this youthful suggestibility, they get high on substances which have no possibility of producing such effects. In fact I have had twelve- and thirteen-year-olds ask me to identify pills they bring in, because they have made them feel so stoned they wanted to be able to get them again. These turned out to be medications as varied as birth control pills or asthma remedies, not to mention many vitamin preparations. This ignorant experimentation may frequently lead to serious overdosage with very toxic substances, such as digitalis, atropine, thyroid compounds. These substances have no euphoriant affects, but are found, sold, or given to young children and taken blindly.

Attempts to arrive at any statistical evaluation of the number of *drug dependent* individuals have been very unsatisfactory. In part, this is due to the difficulty in differentiating between those who abuse drugs and those who are truly drug dependent. To an even greater degree, this may be due to the legal implications. The drug dependent person has, until very recently, been subject to legal sanctions for use, or even possession, of substances on the Drug Enforcement Administration (DEA) Controlled Substances List. Hence, only a small proportion of those involved have been registered as dependent. The figure has been advanced that 4 to 600,000 narcotic addicts alone are present in the United States. This does not include dependence on any of the nonnarcotic agents. The total of those drug dependent may be as high as one and a half million people, to which must be added the 9 million estimated alcoholics.

DRUG DEPENDENT PERSONS

Many states now have special laws which apply to those who are drug dependent or in danger of becoming drug dependent. The specific nature of these laws varies from state to state, but their general intent is to provide an alternative method for dealing with the drug dependent individual. Under such a law, an individual guilty of certain types of offense (the particular offenses vary from state to state) may be given an option of accepting sentence to a drug treatment program rather than to a penal institution.

The problem posed by the greater number of these laws is that they fail to define the terms *drug dependent* or *in danger of becoming drug dependent*. This puts a burden on those who are expected to make this diagnosis. In some states the law specifies that these labels be affixed only after examination by a psychiatrist and/or psychologist; in other states the means by which the judge is to make this determination are left unclear. Under those circumstances the probation officer may be asked to address this question in the presentence report.

There is usually little difficulty in identifying the drug dependent individual. As a usual rule, the entire life-style is built around the acquisition and utilization of drugs. Any specific signs which may be available, such as the persistence of the constricted pupil in the narcotics user, will be noted in the specific section devoted to each class of drug. The difficulty is far greater when an attempt is made to denote the person in danger of becoming drug dependent. It is my own belief that this question can only be answered in the affirmative if a qualifying phrase is added by the individual making the determination: unless there is a radical change in current behavior patterns.

It has already been noted that there is no such thing as a personality profile specific for the drug user. There are danger signs in those who are already using drugs but are not as yet drug dependent. These signs include lack of obvious goals in life, poor employment record, association with known drug users, orientation toward pleasure-seeking behavior, lack of obvious sources of personal gratification, and lack of any close personal relationships. The two most favorable prognostic signs are a good work record, including a current stable job, and a long standing close personal relationship with someone of the opposite sex.

PROBLEMS IN STUDYING ACUTE EFFECTS

The following statements are frequently heard while conducting a presentence evaluation:

"Maybe I did do it. I don't know. I can't remember anything after I took that last hit."

"I've been drunk before, but never like that. Someone must have mickeyed me."

"I wouldn't have ever done anything like that if I hadn't had that acid."

Anyone of these statements may be a con or may be true. It is important that corrections workers be able to recognize, if possible, when one of these statements is probably true, possibly true, or probably false. It is also important to be aware of all the effects of the acute ingestion of any one of the many substances of abuse. Attention will also be called to those occasions when the addition of a second drug changes the clinical picture. In the last chapter of this part of the book there will be a discussion of what happens when a street drug is taken by someone already using antipsychotic medication prescribed by a physician.

The possibility of full awareness of the effects of taking a substance of abuse is complicated by several factors. These are concerned with the problem of knowing exactly what drugs have been taken. As will be seen, this is always a matter of conjecture unless urine and blood have been extensively analyzed by many complicated techniques. Most of those heavily into the drug scene are apt to abuse many different drugs, whether sequentially or simultaneously. At times, even when the user believes that only one drug is being ingested, two or more may actually have been taken. Many street drugs contain contaminants left as the residual of the manufacturing process. This was responsible for a rash of deaths in Chicago attributed to contaminated sopers. It is also common for the street drugs to be cut by deliberate dilution with a cheaper drug. Furthermore, in many instances the drug is not what the user believes it to be. To give just two examples: most street *mescaline* is actually a weak hit of LSD with strychnine (a powerful poison above a certain level) added to give a *buzz;* most THC sold in the streets is actually PCP in a weak dosage form, since most tetrahydrocannabinols (THC) disintegrate into other compounds unless refrigerated.

A final factor which may complicate efforts to unravel the effect of specific drugs on behavior is the difficulty imposed by imprecise street names for these substances. These names may vary from location to location, or even from time to time. Thus, *angel dust* may refer to PCP in Toledo, Ohio, at the same time it designates cocaine in Tacoma, Washington. It is necessary to keep all these factors under consideration when talking to the person under presentence investigation, or even when reading this book.

The simplest way to attempt to make some sense out of the effect of street drugs is to divide the drugs into classes according to their effects on the central nervous system. The main groups in each class can be discussed, both as to the acute effects when abused and the result of dependence on that drug and the exceptional effect of any drug in that group noted. There are five such classes: the central nervous system depressants, commonly called *downers;* the narcotics, sometimes referred to as *dope;* the central nervous stimulants, commonly called *uppers;* the hallucinogens; those drugs which do not seem to fall specifically into any of these groups. The one factor common to all these drugs, and the reason that they are taken, is that they do change the mental state of the user because of their effect on the central nervous system.

This change may be in the direction of increased relaxation, stimulation, or the production of alteration in sensory experience. This change is considered by the user to be preferable to the normal state of consciousness. This change produces the high previously referred to. It must also be noted that personal idiosyncrasies to ingested substances may exist. At times, these idiosyncrasies are present on first exposure to a drug, as in Pathological Intoxication. At other times they occur only after repeated ingestion, as in the LSD user who suddenly starts having *bad trips* after having had a series of pleasant experiences.

Chapter 19

CENTRAL NERVOUS SYSTEM
DEPRESSANTS (PART ONE)

DOWNERS — GENERAL CONSIDERATIONS

THIS group is composed of alcohol, the barbiturates, the nonbarbiturate sedatives, and the volatile inhalants. The minor tranquilizers, or anxiolytics, which also belong in this group, will be discussed in the last chapter of this section of the book. Tolerance develops rather slowly to all of these substances, with the exception of the inhalants (particularly glue) where it develops at a rapid rate. The significance of the development of tolerance is important enough to bear repeating. Once tolerance has developed, it is possible to ingest doses large enough to have a profound effect on higher centers without impairment of muscular coordination and strength. Development of tolerance explains why some people can drink tremendous amounts of alcohol and appear superficially to be sober.

Downers are so called because their action is to depress the function of the central nervous system. This may seem surprising to some since in low concentrations the effect resembles stimulation. This is because the depressant effect is exerted first on higher cerebral functions, those which have to do with critical judgment, impulse control, and inhibition of behavior. The self-observing function of the ego is impaired. With the loss of critical judgment, ordinary events become quite amusing. Because of the damping of inhibitions, the expression of previously forbidden impulses is permissible. During this phase in the consumption of the downer, individuals may see themselves as charming, witty, polished, skillful, the life of the party, the most powerful person in the world, etc. Other people, too, seem to take on a sparkle they do not normally possess. The whole world tends to seem rosy. It is much more easy to be open with others, and there is less concern for their good opinion. Loss of impulse control may also lead to aggressively antisocial behavior.

At times toward the end of this stage *sensory hyperacusis* occurs. All sensory modalities seem to be functioning at a higher pitch. Bodily sensations are experienced more intensely (this may account for the often reported heightening of sexual enjoyment due to drugs), light seems brighter, and the slightest sounds are heard with great clarity.

As the concentration of the drug in the blood (and brain) increases, the centers controlling motor function are the next to be affected. This may lead to a feeling of estrangement from the body, accompanied by a pleasant feeling of giddiness. As this progresses, reflexes become slowed, coordination and equilibrium are impaired, and speech becomes increasingly slurred, at times almost unintelligible. At the end of this stage, motor weakness has become apparent. The combination of weakness and disturbance in equilibrium first produces staggering and then a series of falls. Frequently at this point the pleasant giddiness is replaced with severe vertigo, nausea, and vomiting. As still lower centers become involved, there is increasing sleepiness which, if the concentration of the substance in the brain is sufficiently high, may go on to stupor and then to coma. Finally, the vital centers are involved; respiration ceases; the heart beat falters; death supervenes. What features are present in any individual at any given moment are the product of the specific depressant, the quantity taken, the level within the bloodstream, and the degree of tolerance.

ALCOHOL

Acute Effects

The behavioral manifestations caused by the ingestion of alcohol fit very well into the picture just described. The effect on reflex time and motor coordination is recognized by the law in the statute covering driving while under the influence. In most states, a blood alcohol level of 0.10 percent is considered proof of intoxication. The behavior under the influence of alcohol which is of significance for corrections is that described in the first stage of ingestion of a downer, particularly in those who have developed tolerance. The results of loss of drive, inhibition, and self control have already been commented on. Two factors, unique to alcohol, are of importance. It is almost possible to divide those who drink into two groups depending on their reaction in this first stage.

The first group is composed of those in whom underlying character pathology is released by alcohol. There is an old Latin maxim, *in vino veritas,* in wine there is truth, which applies to this group of individuals. Repressed character traits are expressed while in the first stage of alcoholic intoxication. Casper Milquetoasts may become roaring tigers; latent homosexuals become overt; compulsive individuals may become very sloppy in appearance, and their speech reeks of the toilet; the sexually repressed tell obscene stories and may make passes at strangers; explosive personalities may lose all control over aggressive behavior during this stage. It has been truly said that alcohol is a solvent, and the first thing which dissolves is the *superego* or conscience.

The second group is made up of those in whom the effect of the first stage of alcohol is to intensify and extend the mood which had been present when drinking started. If the person was irritable or upset before the first drink, these conditions are worsened by the third or fourth. Anger may turn into rage; sadness into suicidal depression; a pleasant feeling into exuberance; mild sexual desire into strong lust. When taking a history in which alcohol consumption is given as a justification for antisocial behavior, it is important to be able to differentiate these two groups. (Legally, of course, the voluntary consumption of alcohol does not decrease responsibility. Indeed, in some jurisdictions, when the alcohol is taken deliberately to facilitate a mood in which action is possible, it adds to the degree of felonious behavior.) If the individual has a consistent pattern of being more withdrawn when drinking, intoxication is a poor justification for assaultive behavior. In an individual whose behavior under the influence of alcohol cannot be predicted unless the mood preceding the drinking is known, it is important to be able to obtain a description of that mood. A very small group of people seem to combine these two modes of reaction. That is, acts of behavior of the early phases of this first stage conform to the type in which there is accentuation of the underlying mood, but as this stage begins to merge into the stage of early motor involvement, there is a sudden emergence of basic character traits. It cannot be repeated too often that in the individual who has developed a high degree of tolerance to alcohol, extreme first stage behavior may go unrecognized as a release phenomenon of alcohol because of the complete lack of evidence of any motor impairment.

There is a second factor to be mentioned in discussing the matter of alcohol ingestion and its effect on behavior. In certain individuals, after repeated instances of consumption of large quantities of alcohol, a phenomenon known as the *alcoholic blackout* begins to occur. This must not be confused with Pathological Intoxication, where after one or two drinks the individual blacks out and does not know what is happening. In the usual alcoholic blackout, the effect happens only when many drinks have been taken and, as noted, in an individual in whom tolerance has developed. Under those circumstances, at some point in any particular bout of drinking, the individual continues to act as though sober, but literally is no longer in control and the next day does not remember what has occurred. Telling a story such as this would indeed be a convenient out for many alcoholics to excuse antisocial behavior. The validity of such a state would have to be questioned if it only occurred when antisocial behavior had taken place. However, far more commonly an alcoholic wakes up the next day in bed at home with no recollection of getting home or of getting into bed, and with no knowledge of behavior beyond a certain instant in time. It is even difficult to pinpoint that instant precisely. Only by asking others who were present at the time can the nature and extent of the behavior be learned. In the vast majority of instances, no truly antisocial behavior is involved. In rare instances, serious antisocial behavior may very well be.

For example, Mr. B. B. was examined for competency to stand trial. Mr. B. B. is a thirty-six-year-old white male with a long history of alcoholic consumption. He states that at one time there were short periods everyday which were fuzzy in his mind. That frightened him a little and he had begun to cut down on the consumption of alcohol but had never cut it out. The quantities he continued to take were those which would make an ordinary person quite intoxicated. He felt, however, that he did not show any such signs. Mr. B. B. was accused of murder. He had been drinking in a bar in the cheap hotel in which he lived. He had been sitting in his own booth paying attention to no one. Three or four men were sitting at the bar talking with each other. Mr. B. B. seemed to be paying no attention to them. On two occasions he left the bar and apparently went to his room in the hotel, only to return very shortly thereafter.

After the second such trip he moved over to the bar and stood next to the end of the group sitting there. He did not enter the conversation, nor was the conversation in any way directed toward him. After approximately ten minutes of standing there he drew a gun, held it against the man next to him, and killed him with a single shot. He then remarked to no one in particular, "I think I'll go to bed now," and calmly walked out of the bar, through the hotel lobby, upstairs to his room, and went to bed. Shortly thereafter the arresting officers found him there sound asleep.

Mr. B. B. did not deny the event, but stated that he had absolutely no memory of it. He was able to give a fairly good account of the entire day up to a short time before the murder. He remembers going to his room once to take some Anacin® for a headache; he does not remember going to his room the second time, although he presumes that if he did it was to get the gun. It must be noted that Mr. B. B. stated that he was somewhat suspicious of people because two weeks earlier, when he had been drinking, he felt that he was perfectly all right, but just as he crossed the lobby to go to his room, his legs gave way under him and he fell heavily. This behavior would not seem unusual in an alcoholic, but he had the suspicion that he had been mickeyed. He does not state that he had this same suspicion the night of the killing but that it might very well have been the case. At any rate, the next thing he remembers, after having returned to his seat in the booth, is being questioned in the police station by police officers.

This is a typical picture of an alcoholic blackout. It can be differentiated from pathological intoxication due to the facts that (1) it occurs in a chronic alcoholic and (2) there is no wildly excited behavior accompanying it, although the behavior was certainly irrational and bizarre.

Alcoholism

It has been estimated that between 9 and 10 million Americans suffer from alcoholism. It has also been estimated that, prior to the recent movement toward decriminalization of alcoholism, 40 to 60 percent of all arrests in the United States were alcohol related, i.e. drunk and disorderly, public intoxication, and similar offenses. Various studies have reported that up to 75 percent of assaultive crimes are committed while the offender has been drinking. A recent study[1], focused on the victim rather than the offender, reported that of 214 cases of homicide, two-thirds of the victims had been under the influence of alcohol when killed, and one-third precipitated their own murder.

Many definitions of alcoholism have been proposed. No single definition is satisfactory. There is now quite a general consensus that alcoholism is a disease. The author subscribes to this concept but feels that it is a disease which should be more the concern of general medicine than of psychiatry alone. *DSM II* reserves the category, Alcoholism, "For patients whose alcohol intake is great enough to damage their physical health, or their personal or social functioning, or when it has become a prerequisite to normal functioning." The last phrase seems to imply there is a compulsive component to alcohol intake, but otherwise the definition does not touch on etiology.

Other descriptions of alcoholism focus completely on behavioral phenomena with a division into social drinkers, problem

---

[1]Herjanic, Marijan, M.D. and Meyer, David A., as reported in the *Newsletter* of the American Psychiatric Association, 8/4/76.

drinkers, and chronic alcoholics. They are concerned with such behaviors as inability to face a social situation without a drink, loss of work due to drinking, alcoholic blackouts, total amount of alcohol consumed, development of tolerance, etc. These descriptions are more comprehensive than that of *DSM II*, but they too neglect etiology.

Any comprehensive picture of severe alcohol dependence (alcoholism) must include several features. In its extreme form, alcoholism is comparable to any form of drug dependence. The entire life style of the individual is built around drinking and the need to obtain the next drink. The social and cultural environment of the alcoholic is important, both during the individual's formative and developmental years and during the period of drinking. Heavy drinking is more apt to develop in a culture where excessive consumption of alcoholic beverages is the rule, but it may also develop as a reaction against excessively rigid parental standards. Teetotalism may even be one of these standards. Alcoholism is apt to happen in those who have a life history of unmet dependency needs, or in those who habitually run from problems rather than trying to solve them. Drinking patterns tend to continue even though they are self-destructive, both in terms of health and of the quality of life. Loss of control, both over further consumption and over behavior, is frequently seen. Personal relationships, employment security, and life goals may all be sacrificed to the drinking pattern. All of this is generally punctuated by periods of resolve to stop drinking, ambivalent attitudes toward the use of alcohol, and by frequent guilt, commonly overcome by denial and bravado.

The question of the inheritance of alcoholism, or the predisposition thereto, is still unsettled. The differing rate of alcohol consumption in different countries is just as easily attributable to cultural factors as to genetic ones. Even those patterns change. For years, France was used as an example of a country where daily use of wine with meals was almost universal, but intoxication and alcoholism were rare. However, in the last decade, the French government has expressed concern at the rising rate of intoxication and alcoholism. Studies on direct parent-child inheritance are contradictory. They would suggest that where two generation alcohol abuse is present, it may be as much a matter of identification as of heredity. Certainly, many children of alcoholic parents are completely abstinent as a result of their childhood exposure to the effects of drinking. It is possible that they fear that if they started to drink, they too would be unable to stop.

One theory holds that while dependence on alcohol may be psychosocially determined, a tendency to physical addiction is inherited. According to this theory, when such a person has sampled alcohol, the brain cells are sensitized, leading to a state of distress when alcohol is not in the system. This distress can only be alleviated by the consumption of more alcohol. A variant of this theory suggests that in certain individuals alcohol acts to excite rather than depress the nerve cells. This excitation initiates the consumption of further alcohol to allay the excited state until a level is reached at which stupor occurs.

Alcoholism spares no social class. The metamorphosis from respectable businessman to skid row character is well known. What is not so widely disseminated is the information that alcoholism is also a common problem for women. This is not directly a concern of the corrections worker, since a majority of female alcoholics confine their drinking to their own homes and never come in contact with the law. However, its indirect influence may be tremendous. More and more studies confirm that a chaotic home, with either one or both parents alcoholic, is a prominent feature in the childhood of those who later commit aggressive and assaultive offenses. Evidence is also beginning to accumulate that alcoholism in the mother during pregnancy may contribute to the development of a mentally retarded child.

While the majority of female alcoholics do not come in contact with the legal system (other than through traffic offenses), those who do are apt to prove troublesome to both law enforcement and corrections workers. The association of alcoholism and prostitution has been known for a long period of time. Recently, there has been an increasing tendency for alcoholism in females to be associated with aggressive and assaultive behavior. The exact reason for this is still speculative, but it is probably due more to changing sociological factors and the changing role of women in society than to any psychiatric causation.

In either sex, chronic alcoholism, even when it does not lead to psychosis, is accompanied by far-reaching physical effects. As is well known, the chief of these is the effect of alcohol on the liver, with the eventual outcome of severe cirrhosis of the liver, a condition which may cause invalidism and death. In addition, stomach ulcers are not uncommonly seen. The combination of excessive alcoholic intake and vitamin deficiency may well lead to severe degeneration of heart musculature. Weakness in general bodily musculature, almost to the point of being unable to serve the needs of the individual, has also been reported. It has been suggested that with each drink a certain number of cells in the brain are poisoned and die. This may be the basis for the development of the alcoholic psychosis, Alcoholic Deterioration (291.5), discussed in Chapter 3. Certainly, many chronic alcoholics exhibit deterioration, even if not to a degree which would permit a diagnosis of psychosis to be made. At times, definite changes in personal appearance are almost pathognomonic of alcoholism. These changes are, in addition to the generalized appearance of lack of personal care, a combination of bloodshot eyes, ruddy complexion, dilated (at times broken) capillaries in the nose, reddened palms, and rhinophyma, an irregular bulbous swelling of the tip of the nose, which is almost never seen except in alcoholism.

DSM II differentiates three types of alcoholism. This differentiation is made on the basis of the type of consumption rather than the quantity or the effects thereof.

Episodic Excessive Drinking

Episodic Excessive Drinking (303.0) is used as a diagnostic term when, "Alcoholism is present, and the individual becomes intoxicated as frequently as four times a year . . . Intoxication is defined as a state in which the individual's coordination or speech is definitely impaired, or his behavior clearly altered." At first glance this definition might apply to the great majority of people who drink at all. If, however, the referent phrase, "when alcoholism is present," is kept in mind, then it can be seen to apply to those who drink habitually, but become intoxicated infrequently. As might be expected, these are the people who are most reluctant to admit they are alcoholic. They presumably fall in the category of *problem* drinkers. They are rarely arrested for being drunk and disorderly, but are frequently involved in crime.

Habitual Excessive Drinking

Habitual Excessive Drinking (303.1) is also a diagnosis which depends on the frequency of intoxication. "This diagnosis is given to persons who are alcoholic, and who either become intoxicated more than twelve times a year or are recognizably under the influence of alcohol more than once a week, even though not intoxicated." In the author's opinion, the inclusion of these two subtypes (303.0 and 303.1) is more an evidence of how difficult it is to classify the myriad types of alcoholics than it is of any practical help in management. It may be that they are two steps in the development of **Alcohol Addiction (303.2)**. Relatively few who suffer from alcoholism remain as either Episodic Excessive Drinkers or Habitual Excessive Drinkers throughout their careers.

Alcohol Addiction

It is the category of **Alcohol Addiction (303.2)** about which most of us think when we think of the chronic alcoholic. It is interesting that this classification in *DSM II* was published in 1968, at the time when a debate was raging over whether there was a difference between *addiction* and *dependence*. As will be seen, the definition of Alcohol Addiction fudges this distinction by coming down squarely on both sides of the fence simultaneously. According to *DSM II*, alcohol addiction "should be diagnosed when there is direct or strong presumptive evidence that the patient is dependent on alcohol. If available, the best direct evidence of such dependence is the appearance of withdrawal symptoms. The inability of the patient to go one day without drinking is presumptive evidence. When heavy drinking continues for three months or more, it is reasonable to presume that addiction to alcohol has been established.''

In the discussion of alcoholic psychoses in Chapter 3, the need to insist on the sobriety of the abstinent offender is stressed. Certainly, this need is equally as great in the management of the alcoholic offender who has not developed psychosis. Alcoholism is a complicating factor in a large number of those with whom the corrections worker deals. There are many individuals who have never committed an offense unless they were under the influence of alcohol at the time. Mr. B. C. illustrates this, as well as many other facets of alcoholism.

Mr. B. C. was only twenty-one years old when seen on charges of aggravated robbery and kidnapping. He had run out of gas in his car at almost two o'clock in the morning, had walked to the nearest bar, pulled a pistol on the sole barmaid, emptied the cash register, and then at gunpoint made her drive him across a state line in her car. At that point he was apprehended.

Mr. B. C. had started drinking at about twelve years of age. He had always run with older boys and started drinking with them to make an impression on them. Soon he was drinking more than they did. His first brush with the law came at age thirteen, when he and an older friend, while drunk, stole his uncle's car, and ended up about fifteen hundred miles from home. Since the car was undamaged, the uncle did not press charges. Two years later, again while drunk, he and a group of other youths stole a large, empty, tractor trailer. He was driving and during a high speed chase in an attempt to evade the police turned the truck over. Incredibly, all the boys walked away from the crash unharmed. For this offense he was sent to a Youth Rehabilitation Center. He adjusted well enough to be allowed to go home for weekends and was confined for only six months. (At the time of the examination he told me that he had been drunk every weekend that he had been home.) His drinking continued on release from the institution.

He quit school shortly thereafter, having turned sixteen.

With his parents' collaboration he falsified his age and enlisted in the Army. After completing basic training successfully he applied for a special school. In checking his past school records for eligibility, his true age was discovered, and he was discharged from the service.

Mr. B.C. used that discharge as a rationalization for continued drinking. His tolerance increased consistently to a point where he could drink two to three fifths of liquor without showing any ill effects. He himself was aware (or at least purported to be during the examination) that his judgment and critical functions were impaired, even though it might not be obvious to others. Many subsequent arrests for disorderly conduct, assault and battery, and resisting arrest stemmed from this impairment of judgment. On one occasion, for example, he attempted to remonstrate when an officer was arresting a friend of his for creating a disturbance. When the officer asked him who he was, he answered, "What the hell business is it of your's?" with the fairly predictable result that he too was arrested.

Because of his drinking he was unable to keep a job for any length of time. He alternated between living alone when employed and moving back in with his parents when out of work. He had many drinking companions, but no "friends." He had never had a steady relationship with a woman. He had had one hospital admission for an overdose of pills while drinking. On another occasion members of Alcoholics Anonymous (which he had attended sporadically) had brought him to a hospital for detoxification, as they thought he was on the verge of Delirium Tremens. He also had experienced several blackouts in which he would wake up in strange communities with no idea of how he got there.

At the time of the latest offense, he was working as a security guard at a large plant and had been issued a revolver. (The lack of checking on background of security personnel is somewhat frightening.) About noontime on his day off he had started drinking with a friend encountered in a tavern they both patronized. They drank and played cards together until about eleven o'clock that night. Mr. B.C. estimated he had had about thirty shots and a dozen beers by that time. The friend went home. Mr. B.C. met a girl he knew and took her to another bar where they had a few more drinks. When the bar closed he took her home. He decided he was not yet ready to go home himself. He picked up a six-pack of beer at an after hours spot and headed for a neighboring metropolis, drinking the beer as he went. He always carried the gun in his trunk, but now he took it out and put in on the seat. According to him, this was because he was headed for a rough part of town and, "You never know."

Just as he reached the outskirts of the city he ran out of gas. He stated this was a rough neighborhood so he, "Tucked the gun in my belt just in case." He could not spot a gas station open at that time of night so he walked to the nearest bar. After paying for a beer he discovered he had only twenty cents left. It occurred to him that it was quite a sensible idea to hold up the barmaid and get some money. He was aware of his intention to do so and waited until the last customer had left. The idea to have her drive him in her car, since his was out of gas, was apparently impulsive and spontaneous. Once they were in her car his first thought was to have her drive him to the airport. That thought did not seem to lead him anywhere, so he told her to just get on the highway and drive. A couple of hours later, incidentally after they had crossed the state line, he said he had to use the toilet and suggested that they pull off at the next exit. They pulled up at a motel. Once inside she lost no time in attracting a clerk's attention. The police were called.

At no time did he attempt to molest the barmaid nor were there any such implications. At no time during the examination did he mention the he could not remember or that he was fuzzy as to the thought processes which led to his suggesting they leave in her car. Interestingly, the police who arrested him did not take a blood or blood alcohol test, and indeed, did not suspect that he was intoxicated.

In this instance, his attorney had requested an examination, even though he was aware voluntary consumption of alcohol is in no way exculpatory in respect to crime. He was hoping to establish diminished capacity to form intent in the kidnapping. It is interesting to speculate as to whether recent federal court decisions decriminalizing chronic alcoholism will have any effect on this matter of responsibility of the intoxicated individual who commits a felony. The ruling in these federal cases is that since alcoholism is a disease, and the sufferer is unable to control the drinking, then drunkenness cannot be considered a crime. As of now I do not know of any attempt to show that an individual is not responsible for an offense under the influence of alcohol on the grounds that because of chronic alcoholism it was impossible to refrain from drinking.

Dipsomania

I should like to add a fourth class of drinker to those three already listed in *DSM II*. Dipsomania should probably be classified under **Other (and Unspecified) Alcoholism (303.9)**. Dipsomania is the condition commonly referred to as *spree drinking*. In this type of drinking behavior, the individual is completely abstinent for periods of time varying from months to years. Suddenly, seemingly inexplicably and with no apparent environmental stimulus, such an individual will start to drink and will continue to drink until either one of two conditions occurs. One, all available money is used up in drinking, there is nothing left to pawn and no one left from whom to borrow. At this point, some individuals turn to panhandling, others to stealing. Some just quit. In the second condition, the individual continues drinking until so physically ill that it is impossible to drink any more. This latter pattern may be repeated two or three times after recuperating from any one bout, until the entire spree is finished. Either of these types of spree may last from several days to weeks (rarely months) until it has run its course.

If this pattern is examined closely, it can be seen that it resembles the sudden and inexplicable mood swings seen in manic-depressive reactions (see Chapter 6). Three bits of evidence would seem to attest to this hypothesis. One is the finding of alcoholism in a high proportion of first degree relatives of patients suffering from manic-depressive disease. The second is that many spree drinkers find they can take a drink with impunity on some occasions, while on others the whole sequence starts anew. The third is that some preliminary tests with the use of lithium[2] indicate it may be used to abort or prevent sprees in some individuals who have dipsomania.

---

[2]See Chapter 6 for discussion of the use of lithium in the treatment and prevention of manic reaction.

Chapter 20

BARBITURATES AND OTHER CENTRAL NERVOUS SYSTEM DEPRESSANTS (PART TWO)

BARBITURATES

Acute Effects

THERE is relatively little association between barbiturates and antisocial behavior, with three exceptions which will be detailed below. The barbiturate user is seeking either a *down*, the vague, floating, detached feeling which comes in the first stage of barbiturate intoxication, or the giddy, released feeling occurring with the loss of inhibition. If the dose taken is great enough to cause severe loss of inhibition and dissolution of critical faculties, it is generally large enough to be sleep inducing to the point where it is difficult to act on these impulses. Indeed, the user, to enjoy the desired feeling to its greatest extent, must fight the desire to sleep. Naturally, people in this state are more suggestible (barbiturates are also classed as hypnotics), and they go along with proposed antisocial behavior with little thought of consequences. That is, if they are still able to navigate.

On rare occasions, in sensitive individuals, a paradoxical stage of excitement and disinhibition may precede the onset of the floating and drowsy stage of the barbiturate intoxication. When this occurs, behavior may be quite bizarre and at times highly assaultive. The first of the three mentioned exceptions occurs with the ingestion of Seconal® (reds or red devils) or Tuinal® (rainbows). Tuinal is a mixture of Seconal (secobarbital), an extremely rapidly acting barbiturate, and Amytal® (amobarbital), a longer acting barbiturate. Because of its extremely rapid action, Seconal may cause dissociation in some individuals which is similar to that seen in hysterical dissociative states. This may also be complicated by paradoxical excitement during the first stage. These individuals may be truly dangerous. In Tuinal, the Seconal reaction of this combination is meant to induce sleep rapidly, while the Amytal component prolongs it. In certain individuals, particularly if the sleep-inducing properties of the drug are fought, the Amytal potentiates the paradoxical excitement of the Seconal.

The second instance in which barbiturate ingestion may lead to antisocial, acting out behavior is in the combination of barbiturates and alcohol. This is particularly true in a individual with a high tolerance level for this class of drugs when alcohol has first been consumed for two or three drinks and then the barbiturate added. Due to the mechanism of potentiation, the effect of adding the barbiturate is greater than that of doubling the alcohol, while at the same time individual tolerance permits much more acting-out behavior without motor involvement than would otherwise be the case. This combination also is much more apt to lead to the blackout stage which was mentioned under alcohol, and hence the claim of, "I can't remember anything after having taken the downer," may be a valid one.

The third exception to the general statement that barbiturate users are as a rule quite peaceful while under the influence of the drug occurs when it is combined with an upper. This most commonly takes place in the combination known as Dexamyl® in which Dexedrine (dextroamphetamine), an amphetamine, is combined with Amytal, a barbiturate. These two drugs are not in the same group, and hence each counteracts the effects of the other, rather than potentiating it. In some individuals in whom tolerance to both drugs has developed, the effects of this combination is to reduce irritability and tension because of the presence of barbiturate, while continuing the increased drive and goal-directed behavior produced by the amphetamine. As a result, antisocial activity may be planned and carried out with great efficiency. At the same time, the dissolution of inhibitions and of critical judgment, common to first stage barbiturate intoxication, may very well permit more violent acting out behavior without the proper checks and controls which the normally integrated personality would employ.

There is such a multiplicity of barbiturates they will be listed separately with their street names[1] where applicable. The most widely used barbiturates will be marked with an asterisk. All of these drugs are labeled by their trade names.

Alurate®, Amytal®* (blues, downers, blue jackets), Brevital®, Butisol®, Carbrital®* (blue and whites, carbs), Cyclonal®, Cyclopal®, Cyclopen®, Delvinal®, Dial®, Evipal®, Gemonil®, Ipral®, Lotusate®, Luminal®* (phenobarb), Mebaral®, Nembutal®* (yellow jackets, yellows, nembies), Neonal®, Nerval®, Ortal®, Pernocton®, Pharodorn®, Pentothal®, Sandoptal®, Seconal®* (reds, red devils, seggys), Surital®, Sombulex®, Tuinal®* (reds and blues, rainbows, double-trouble, tooies), Veronal®* (barbiturate).

In addition to this, there are over forty different medications, normally available only on prescription, which contain barbiturates in combination with other substances. These products may be intended for relief of pain, for relief of certain gastrointestinal conditions, for relief of high blood pressure, and for the relief of asthma. When an attempt is made to ingest one of these combinations in a large enough quantity to get the desired barbiturate effect, a quantity of the other components high enough to be toxic may result.

It should also be pointed out that certain short acting barbiturates, notably Seconal and Nembutal, can be injected intravenously. Under these circumstances extremely bizarre, and at times violently antisocial, behavior may occur. Fortunately, depending on the amount injected, this stage may last for only fifteen to forty-five minutes, following which sleep may supervene. On awakening there is usually complete or partial amnesia for the event. One other illegal use of barbiturates occurs with sufficient frequency that it is worthy of mention. In any community when the supply of narcotics suddenly dries up there is frequently a rush to obtain some sort of substitute which may appease the pangs of drying out cold turkey. The barbiturates are often chosen as such a substitute, albeit a poor one.

---

[1]As has been noted, street names vary from location to location and from time to time. Hence, only those most widely and currently used will be included.

Drug Dependence, Barbiturates (304.2)

From the decade of the thirties to that of the sixties, the barbiturates as a class were the most widely misused and abused drugs in this country. Intended to replace the previously misused chloral hydrate and bromides, the barbiturates were eminently successful for the task for which they were introduced, namely to combat insomnia. When it was found that in small doses they also tended to relieve tension and anxiety and through this relief to aid indirectly in certain psychosomatic problems, their use increased widely, particularly in combination with other medications. Misuse was manifested by too great a reliance on their use, by indiscriminate prescribing, by prescribing in larger doses or quantities, over longer periods of time than were indicated or were safe. As with most drugs on which people can become psychologically dependent, tolerance develops with the need for larger doses to produce the same effects. As the dosage increases over time, physical dependence then develops.

A chronic barbiturate abuser, like the chronic alcoholic, shows definite evidence of continued abuse. Speech is slow and slurred, thought processes are slowed down. This is frequently accompanied by confusion. Sleep patterns become reversed. The stage of REM sleep, in which most of our dreaming is done, is shortened markedly. For some reason, adequate REM sleep is essential to maintain psychic equilibrium. Thus, toxic delirum may result when it has been suppressed over a long time. The withdrawal syndrome of the barbiturate abuser is not too dissimilar from that of the alcoholic. For a brief period of time, lasting from eight to twelve hours, there may seem to be improvement. Confusion clears, speech is more distinct. Slowly at first and then more rapidly, symptoms develop. Headache and anxiety become prominent. Nervousness, feelings of weakness, even tremor and twitching in large muscle groups appear. Sweating may become profuse. Insomnia is the usual rule. Within sixteen to twenty-four hours, all symptoms are intense and vomiting may be present. A single, isolated convulsion, rarely two, may occur from sixteen hours to eight days after the onset of abstinence. Several hours of confusion may follow the convulsion, or a confused, delirious state may occur which resembles Delirium Tremens and remits spontaneously, usually within five days. While the death rate is not as high as in Delirium Tremens, deaths do occur. The abstinence syndrome of barbiturate addiction is treated by administration of a short acting barbiturate, which is carefully withdrawn over a long period of time. Treatment of the psychological dependence lies in removal of the underlying cause and may be extremely difficult.

Barbiturates, as is well known, are common agents of suicide. Their ready availability and the relatively painless quality of the death is what makes them so attractive. Because of a specific phenomenon in chronic abusers, it is sometimes very difficult to tell whether death was intentional. This phenomenon occurs when the individual takes the usual dose of barbiturates and then, because of developing tolerance, does not get the desired effect. Some clouding of consciousness has occurred at that point however. The individual then cannot remember whether or not the original dose was taken, and repeats it. This same pattern repeats until a lethal dose has been ingested. Another possibility of unintentional death with barbiturates occurs when absorption from the stomach is delayed, possibly because of large quantities of food in the stomach. Under these circumstances, the desired effect is not obtained and a greater quantity is then ingested. When absorption finally takes place, the blood concentration is far greater than the vital centers can stand and death ensues.

NONBARBITURATE HYPNOTICS AND SEDATIVES

Acute Effects

In addition to the anxiolytics, or minor tranquilizers, which will be discussed in the last chapter of this section, there are a large number of medications in this category which must be listed. All of the drugs were introduced to replace the barbiturates, because of the danger of dependency associated with the use of the latter. Unfortunately, those medications which are effective as sedatives, are as apt to be chronically abused as are the barbiturates. The great majority of these products require prescriptions. Only two of them have found any wide popularity on the streets, but the remainder are seen with sufficient frequency to justify listing the names of those most frequently prescribed. These include: Aquachlor®, Noctec®, and Somnos® (all of which are chloral hydrate), Quaalude®, and Sopor® (both of which are methaqualone), Noludar®, Placidyl®, Triclos®, and Valmid®.

Of the over-the-counter drugs sold to produce sleep, only those containing the bromides truly belong in this group. Nervine® is the outstanding example of this class. The remainder of the over-the-counter drugs will be included in the fifth group of drugs to be discussed.

Cross-tolerance exists between this group and the other central nervous system depressants, and potentiation occurs within the group, particularly when used with alcohol.

Of this group of nonbarbiturate sedatives, the two most commonly abused are glutethimide (Doriden®) and methaqualone (Quaalude or Sopor). These are commonly referred to as ludies, sopers, or 7-14's, after a manufacturer's code mark. The reason for their popularity is not hard to find. Both medications, when taken in small doses or during the early stage of higher dosage action, produce the floating, dreamy state so much desired by those whose life-style is organized around drugs. Methaqualone was not introduced into this country until 1972, although it had been widely used in England prior to that time. It gained instant popularity on the college campuses as the Love Drug, and that misnomer has clung to it on the streets, even though it was quickly learned that it had no aphrodisiacal properties. It is easily produced in home chemical laboratories, but unfortunately elimination of chemical impurities with highly toxic properties is not as simple. One widely disseminated, illegally produced batch of sopers was responsible, when only single tablets were taken, for producing severe urinary bladder hemorrhage and gangrene of the bladder wall. Knowledge of this tragedy seemed to stop illegal manufacture and use of sopers for a while, but they are again being produced.

The other widely abused drug in this group is glutethimide (Doriden). As was noted, early stages of action of this drug include the floating stage which is widely sought by illegal drug users. It is one of the first drugs to be sought by the narcotics user when the supply of narcotics dries up. One physiological action that sets Doriden apart from the majority of the downers is that it has a tendency to cause low blood pressure when large quantities are ingested at one time. At times this may go on to a condition known as *shock*, in which the individual becomes quite weak, the pulse is rapid and thready, cold clammy skin is common, and syncope or fainting occurs.

Tolerance develops quite rapidly to both of these drugs and larger and larger doses are required to produce the desired effect. Potentiation of these large doses by the addition of relatively small quantities of alcohol may cause near fatal results.

One other type of drugs in this group is rarely taken voluntary by drug abusers, since its sedative action is not preceded by much of a high. These are chloral hydrate (Aquachlor, Noctec, and Somnos) and its derivative Triclos. Their effectiveness in potentiating alcohol has been known for over a hundred years. Over that time chloral hydrate has gained notoriety under the name of *knockout drops*. These were the original *Mickey Finns*, slipped surreptiously into a drink to cause rapid and prolonged unconsciousness.

Drug Dependence, Nonbarbiturate Sedatives, and Hypnotics

There is little difference between barbiturate dependence and dependence on the nonbarbiturate sedatives and hypnotics. Two minor exceptions might be noted. Glutethimide (Doriden), taken either over long periods of time or in a single overdose with suicidal intent, may cause a paralysis of the nerves of the extremities. The upper extremities are affected more commonly than the lower, and a condition known as wrist drop may result. In this state, the afflicted individual is unable to extend the wrist. Fortunately, this condition is rarely permanent, although it might be so.

The other condition is seen only rarely nowadays, since this drug is almost never prescribed any longer. Its use is limited almost completely to over-the-counter purchase (quite legal incidentally) by those who have difficulty sleeping. It is being brought to the attention of correction workers because their non-drug abusing clients are more apt to seek relief from insomnia at a drugstore than through a physician's prescription. This condition is known as *bromism* and develops after long term use of the bromides, found most commonly now in Nervine. The bromides are common chemicals which were some of the earliest known, naturally occurring sedatives. They are excreted from the body at a very slow rate. Hence, when taken regularly, the concentration of bromide in the bloodstream increases slowly. Once it passes a certain level, symptoms of bromism occur.

When a probationer or parolee, known not to use alcohol or the usual drugs, is seen to be slowed down, with slurred or thickened speech, staggering gait, and difficulty in staying awake, bromism should be suspected. The simple way to make the diagnosis is to ask if the client is using Nervine. If the answer is "Yes" quick confirmation can be obtained by referral to a doctor for a blood bromide level. Treatment, under medical supervision, consists of replacing the bromide ion with chlorides by continuous slow drip, intravenous infusion of salt water. If unrecognized and untreated, bromism may be fatal.

THE VOLATILE INHALANTS

Acute Effects

One other group of substances of abuse which fits the category of downers are the volatile inhalants. Historically, it is interesting that two of the earliest anesthetics, nitrous oxide (laughing gas) and ether were both abused as euphoriants for a short time after their introduction into medicine. During the prohibition era, spiking near beer (which has no alcoholic content) with ether was a common practice. Today, the most widely used substances in this group are plastic glue, paint thinner, and gasoline, although almost any volatile substance has been used. Many of these inhalants are highly toxic and even fatal. Like all depressants, they produce a euphoriant effect through depression of the higher centers of the central nervous system. Tolerance develops rapidly and the dose has to be increased progressively. Originally, sniffing the fumes from one squeeze of airplane glue placed in a plastic bag will induce the desired high. Ultimately, many tubes of glue must be used to achieve the same effects. Apparently, physical dependence does not occur.

The volatile inhalants seem to be abused most commonly by children and young adolescents. This is probably because, at least until recently, they were the most easily available of all substances of abuse. National figures are not available, but I am daily becoming more convinced from the children and adolescents whom I see, that the number of sniffers is decreasing in direct relationship to the increase in the number of younger children abusing other substances.

The effects of sniffing are due to the rapid permeation of the cells of the brain by the inhaled substance, which is absorbed by the lungs. From there it is quickly picked up by the blood and carried rapidly to all parts of the body. The acute effects are those of a giggling, laughing high. Everything seems funny. Because of the rapid permeability of the blood-brain barrier by these substances, many centers of the brain are affected simultaneously. Hence, incoordination and lack of equilibrium occur rapidly.

Drug Dependence on Inhalants

Drug dependence on the volatile inhalants probably should be classed in *DSM II* under **Drug Dependence, Other (304.8)**. Almost invariably, the sniffers are looking for the relief of deep feelings of depression, which might not be recognized as such by them. For this reason, psychological dependence is marked, and the condition is extremely difficult to treat. The majority of those who are still sniffing glue in the mid to later teens will almost universally switch to abusing alcohol. After the age of twenty-one, habitual sniffing of volatile substances is rare but has been reported. In the older person, occasional use of the volatile inhalants as a temporary substitute when the supply of narcotics has dried up is sometimes seen. It is relatively common in penal institutions where other substances of abuse are either difficult to obtain or too expensive.

While glue is the most commonly abused of the volatile inhalants, gasoline sniffing seems to start at the youngest age and is the most persistently difficult habit to alter. Rural children seem to abuse gasoline more than urban children do. This would appear to be another case of using the most available substance.

> B.D., a fourteen-year-old whom the author had the opportunity to observe, had been sniffing gasoline since the age of six. He was the fourth of six children brought up on a farm by an alcoholic father and mentally defective mother. He was the least intelligent in a family of retarded children. He was subjected to his father's brutality, his mother's ineffectiveness, his siblings' persecution, and to his classmates' teasing when at the age of six he started school. How the gasoline sniffing started is not known, but probably it began with the first time he found an open container and accidentally achieved a blissful feeling of being above his suffering. From then on he could not refrain from unscrewing the caps of gasoline tanks and inhaling until he reached the desired state. Red eyes, chronically running nose, hacking cough, nothing deterred him. He had been hospitalized in three different hospitals for mentally disturbed children. He improved in each instance, but resumed sniffing shortly after return home. He was currently improving during this hospitalization, but at last report his mother had refused to allow him to return home. Present plans call for foster home placement when it is thought he is able to leave the hospital. It is hoped that an improved environment will lessen the need for an anodyne to relieve his unhappiness.

There has been a great deal of discussion of the toxic effects of the solvents. An intensive scare campaign was carried on about the dangers of sniffing glue. This proved as futile as did the later campaign about the dangerousness of marijuana. It is true that most of the volatile inhalants are fat solvents, and there is always the possibility of damage to the central nervous system which contains a high percentage of lipids (fats). Certainly, also, a high concentration of carbon tetrachloride (the chief ingredient of many cleaning fluids), naphtha, benzine, or toluol (called tullio by youngsters) can be extremely destructive to the nervous system. To the best of the author's knowledge, no one has demonstrated permanent brain damage as a result of glue sniffing. Apparently, the concentration of toluol, the active ingredient of glue, does not reach a high enough level in the brain to be severely toxic. A psychosis resembling the delirium of Delirium Tremens has been reported, but recovery takes place in forty-eight to seventy-two hours. Damage has been reported to the blood forming organs and to the liver, but this too is reversible. In addition to fostering patterns of escape through drug dependency, the chief dangers in glue sniffing are suffocation, because of the method of inhaling from a plastic bag, and accidental death, arising from the temporary delusion of being able to fly like Superman from a high building or of having Superman's power to stop a speeding car.

Chapter 21

NARCOTICS AND STIMULANTS

GENERAL CONSIDERATIONS

THE narcotics are so called because of their ability to produce a pleasant, dreamy, drowsy, lethargic state. They differ from the central nervous system depressants in that the pain centers and the sleep centers seem to be specifically affected without any affect on the cortical centers controlling inhibition, critical judgment, and impulse control. As the narcotic action increases, the respiratory centers are involved prior to those controlling blood pressure and heart rate. Death due to narcotic overdosage comes about because of failure in respiration. The narcotics share two other properties in common. They are constipating in their effect on the intestinal system, regardless of whether they are smoked, sniffed, swallowed, or injected. They also cause constriction of the pupils of the eyes, a constriction which is even present in the dark.

The naturally occurring narcotics are found in opium. Opium is the dried residue obtained from the milky substance excreted by the seed pod of the opium poppy. Opium abuse is no longer common in this country, although still widespread in the Far East. The dreamy effect of opium is obtained by smoking the substance in a special pipe. Its constipating properties are utilized when it is dispensed as paregoric, which is a camphorized alcoholic extract of opium. Paregoric addiction was relatively common at one time. Presently, however, it can only be obtained on prescription and then only in small quantities. The two most important natural alkaloids of opium are morphine and codeine. Slight changes in the chemical structure of morphine produce heroin, the narcotic which is currently abused most frequently, and hydromorphone (Dilaudid) which is becoming increasingly popular as a drug of abuse.

Two completely synthetic substances which have actions

403

similar to the opiates but which have quite dissimilar chemical formulae, are methadone (Dolophine®) and meperidine (Demerol). Dextropropoxyphene (Darvon®) is similar to methadone in chemical structure, but has only the pain-killing properties and none of the lethargy-inducing ones.

ACUTE EFFECTS OF NARCOTICS

The effect sought by those who abuse narcotics is a pleasant, drowsy, floating state. Heroin abusers refer to this state as the *floats*. When the drug is taken by intravenous injection, the floating feeling is preceded by a *rush*, a sensation difficult to describe. It would appear to be a sudden feeling of relaxation, of relief of tension, coupled with an euphoric elevation of mood. In the neophyte this may be followed by nausea before the onset of the floats. In the habituated individual, the rush is an especially significant experience because it signals the relief of symptoms of the withdrawal syndrome. In heroin injection, the floats last for from eight to twelve hours. Dilaudid is said to give the more satisfactory rush when injected as a single specific drug. Its chief disadvantage is that the subsequent floating sensation lasts only two to three hours. For those whose goal is the experience of the rush, the simultaneous injection of heroin and cocaine (a stimulant) is said to give the greatest pleasure. Morphine, methadone, Demerol, and codeine, in the order named, are effective pain relievers, and in the same descending order are less effective in producing either a rush or the floats.

If the effects of the acute reactions to narcotics were used as the only criteria, it could be stated confidently that narcotics are associated with antisocial behavior with less frequency than any other group of drugs. A floaty, dreamy feeling is not conducive to criminal effort. In those countries where free narcotics are supplied to habitual abusers, the crime rate is said to be lower for this group of people than for the general population. The high association between narcotics and crime in this country is partially due to the cost of keeping up with the need for an ever increasing amount of these expensive substances. Much of the violent crime associated with narcotics has to do with rivalry over territory, retaliation against informers, arguments over nonpayment of large amounts of money, etc.

Narcotics are rarely taken intentionally in doses large enough to produce stupor. Overdosage sometimes occurs as a deliberate suicidal attempt. More frequently, it is the result of a sudden change in the concentration of the purchased drug. Narcotics sold on the street are purposely cut in strength by addition of adulterants in order to increase the profit from the sale. Occasionally, a quantity of the drug is sold in an unadulterated state, and the unsuspecting user injects what appears to be the usual amount into the vein. This may be up to ten times the normal strength and may well be fatal. The statement, "I didn't know what I was doing, I was too strung out on heroin," is rarely heard. When it is, it should be discounted, unless there is evidence of a severe alteration of the level of consciousness just prior to the criminal act, or unless there has been coincidental use of alcohol. This latter is becoming increasingly frequent.

DRUG DEPENDENCE, OPIUM, OPIUM ALKALOIDS AND THEIR DERIVATIVES (304.6)

If the ordinary individual is asked to describe a drug addict, the answer will almost invariably be in terms of addiction to heroin or some other member of the narcotics group. During the 1920s there were still lingering tales of legendary opium dens, where not only was the drug smoked to attain some blissful nirvana, but it was also said to be accompanied by unspeakable debauchery, followed by the most heinous crimes. Today, opium smoking is practically unknown. Paregoric use is now carefully controlled. Morphine addiction was fairly common in the thirties. It must be stated in all honesty that this was generally the result of misuse rather than abuse. Today, addiction to both morphine and Demerol is confined almost entirely to the medical and nursing professions, those who have ready access to these drugs. Codeine and its derivatives Hycodan® and Percodan® are abused much less frequently than any of the other narcotics. The degree of euphoria attained is relatively mild, and physical dependence develops much more slowly. For these reasons, dependence on codeine is relatively rare. One commonly used cough medicine, Elixir of Terpene Hydrate with codeine, contains 12 percent alcohol as well as a small quantity of codeine. Since rare addiction to this combination has occurred, it is no longer sold as an over-the-counter medication, and dependence on it is almost unknown.

Currently, opiate dependence is confined almost solely to heroin and Dilaudid. The reason for this is easily found in the degree of both *float* and *rush* which they provide. Tolerance develops rapidly and both psychological and physical dependence follow quickly. Continued ingestion of the opiates apparently does not cause psychosis. In this respect they stand out amongst the various categories of drugs abused. As with many alcoholics, the chief behavioral change is the reorientation of life to the preoccupation with the drug. To the person truly dependent on an opiate, the chief motivation in life appears to be, "How do I get my next fix?" It is this need for the next dose of the drug which turns so many heroin dependent individuals to crime or to becoming dealers or pushers themselves. Criminal behavior is generally against property rather than person, although an armed robbery may always have tragic consequences.

Physical changes in narcotic addicts are not so pronounced as in alcoholics. Constipation is almost universally seen. Amenorrhea (failure of menstruation) is common in females, as is impotence in males. The constricted pupils are well known, and this symptom may persist months after the last abuse. Needle tracks in the arms, abscesses and bluish markings in the veins are also seen. Many opiate addicts do die. This is generally not attributed to the chronic use of the drug. The most common cause of death is the infectious reaction caused by dirty needles — pneumonia, septicemia (blood poisoning), hepatitis (inflammation and infection of the liver), and endocarditis (infection of the lining of the heart). Even tetanus has been reported. As noted, death from accidental overdosage is relatively common.

People have cured their own narcotic habit and, as was stated, some people continue sporadic use for years without being "hooked." One of the most troubling aspects of narcotic addiction is that long time abstinence (years) may be no guarantee against relapse, particularly if the addict returns to old surroundings. Methadone maintenance programs have proved helpful in fighting habituation, but it has been shown that the success of methadone clinics is as much a function of the entire program, social, vocational, educational, and psychological counseling, as it is of the administration of methadone alone. The two non-drug related factors believed to be of most importance for successful outcome in opiate addiction are a good work record and a stable marriage. More recently, a long acting methadone (LAAM) is being used. It has the advantage of no longer requiring daily reporting for medication. (Some feel this to be a disadvantage.) Community based treatment programs on the Synanon model have had a moderate amount of success, particularly if the ex-abuser can become an employee of the community and use his recovery to help others. As with alcoholism, relapse followed by further abstinence is the most common picture seen.

DRUG DEPENDENCE, SYNTHETIC ANALGESICS WITH MORPHINE-LIKE EFFECTS (304.1)

The three most commonly used synthetic analgesics with opiate-like effects are Dolophine, Demerol, and Darvon. Dolophine is more widely known as methadone and has its greatest use as a heroin antagonist. It has the advantage that when used orally it does not produce a high, but does block the craving for heroin. (Methadone injected intravenously will produce a high, but it is made only in the form of tablets which cannot be dissolved for purposes of injection.) Almost the only methadone-dependent individuals seen are those who have been purposely made that way as a substitute for heroin dependence. In a well-run clinic, dosages of methadone are given daily to those under treatment, crushed in orange juice or some other palatable medium so that they can not be secreted for resale. Spot urine checks are done to be sure that heroin usage has not been resumed. Once this has been satisfactorily established, an effort is made to withdraw the dependent individual from methadone as well.

As has already been noted, Demerol is a drug of habituation and dependence almost exclusively for those involved in either medicine or nursing. This is probably because they have easier access to the drug than do others. It is quite uncommon for the nonprofessional individual with psychic pain to seek surcease in Demerol. Symptoms of chronic abuse of this substance are similar to those of other narcotics.

Darvon is a widely used pain killer. Theoretically, it is only available on a doctor's prescription. It is only prescribed to be taken orally. Darvon is chemically very closely allied to methadone. From the point of view of the DEA, Darvon is not considered a narcotic. However, both physical and psychological dependence have developed to this drug. Alone of the narcotic drugs, Darvon possesses the property of causing a toxic psychosis if taken in large doses over a long period of time.

CENTRAL NERVOUS SYSTEM STIMULANTS

General Considerations

The central nervous system stimulants, or uppers, include two classes of drugs. These are the amphetamines and their analogues, and cocaine. These drugs work directly on the alerting centers in the central nervous system to produce a state of increased awareness and drive. The original *rush* of these substances is said to lead to an increasingly heightened sense of pleasure. Due to their stimulant properties, there is a marked increase in psychomotor activity and behavior. Hence, the common street name of the amphetamines is *speed*. Everything is speeded up. This does not result from an alteration in time sensation, but from an actual heightening of reaction time and facilitation of thought processes. This can also lead to a hyper-irritability which in turn may produce impulsively aggressive behavior.

The Amphetamines

The chief forms of amphetamine are: amphetamine sulfate

(Benzedrine), dextroamphetamine (Desoxyn®), and metamphetamine, the most widely used intravenous form. A combination of Dexedrine and amobarbital is marketed as Dexamyl. Biphetamine® an ethically produced combination of both amphetamine and dextroamphetamine, has attained wide recognition as a street drug under the name of *black beauty*, so called because the highest dosage form comes in a black capsule. The other most widely used stimulant is methylphenidate (Ritalin).

Currently, the only recognized medical uses for these drugs is in the treatment of *narcolepsy* (a relatively rare condition which is manifested by pathological sleepiness), minimal brain damage in children, and the short term treatment of obesity. Since some people have been made amphetamine dependent because of continued misuse in the treatment of obesity, a drive is currently under way to ban the prescription of these drugs for this purpose. While this is a step in the right direction, it is doubtful that this will make any dent on the black market availability or usage of the amphetamines. Amphetamines are widely, if illegally, used by over-the-road drivers to keep them awake and by students pulling an all-nighter before an exam. Athletes also sometimes use amphetamines just before a competitive event.

Because of the physiological effect of these drugs, the alarm system is activated (the amphetamines are quite similar chemically and physiologically to adrenaline which is the hormonal messenger of the alarm system). Through this mechanism, a temporary state of panic sometimes accompanies or quickly succeeds the rush. At times this panic becomes translated into a paranoid view of the environment, and behavior may become unpredictable. (See case of Mr. D. in Chapter 3 which illustrates this mechanism.) Those who are dependent on downers tend to shun the *speed freaks* because of this unpredictability.

The amphetamines are more widely used than cocaine because of easier accessibility and lower cost. Antisocial behavior is associated with amphetamines in many different ways. The increased state of alertness leads to a false sense of heightened ability. Hence, attempts may be made to carry out dangerous antisocial acts that would not be attempted without such false courage. The increased irritability leads to impulsive acting out. This irritability may be seen when *crashing* from a prolonged high, as well as shortly after the original rush. The acute paranoid psychoses, seen with overdosage or too prolonged continuous usage, are also fertile soil for acting out behavior.

It has already been noted that a combination of barbiturates and amphetamines may increase the antisocial behavior of the amphetamine abuser. A particularly potent combination in this regard is that of amphetamines and alcohol. In no matter what combination the amphetamines are taken, any claim of amnesia for antisocial behavior must be taken with a grain of salt. Even the great preponderance of those who develop psychoses with amphetamine usage remain clear and with unimpaired memory.

Drug Dependence, Other Psychostimulants (Amphetamines, etc.) (304.6)

Tolerance to amphetamines develops rapidly if the dosage is progressively increased. The usual medical dose is five to ten milligrams, two to three times a day. Amphetamine-dependent individuals have been reported to maintain a habit of over one-thousand milligrams a day, a dose which would kill the non-abuser. Tolerance for these stimulants follows the same course as does tolerance to all the other drugs discussed so far. The vital systems, in this case the cardiovascular system, can tolerate increasing quantities of the drug long after higher cerebral centers can. Thus, the chronic speed freak does not show the high blood pressure, rapid pulse rate, and pupillary dilatation that might be expected. The other effects of chronic stimulation are shown.

The state sought by the amphetamine abuser is quite the opposite of the goal of the heroin, barbiturate, or alcohol abuser. It is the euphoriant, stimulating, activating effects of the drugs that are sought. Speed freaks say they feel alive, they can function better over a longer period of time. In a sense this is true, but no one can be driven beyond endurance. With the continued abuse of the stimulants, euphoria tends to change to dysphoria and irritability, but the stimulation persists and so does the craving. As might be imagined, the chronic abuser of stimulants shows evidence of severe weight loss. At times nausea, and even vomiting, accompanies any attempt to eat. Restlessness and over-activity are chronic. Behaviorally, there is little delay between stimulus and response.

For a long time a debate raged similar to that waged over cocaine as to whether withdrawal symptoms were or were not present on abstinence from amphetamines. That debate has now been settled in the affirmative. The stimulant abuser who *crashes* after long continued abuse has a definite withdrawal syndrome. The two to three days of sleep which occur are not as peaceful as they seem. The sleep is restless, intermittent, and filled with horrible nightmares. This period of sleep is followed by headaches, fever, nausea, muscle cramps, and exhaustion. Depression may be severe; weakness is extreme. The driven irritability of the high is replaced with a chronic irritability and petulance. Unlike alcohol, psychosis is not a part of the withdrawal syndrome following long term stimulant abuse, although confusion may exist. Psychosis caused by stimulants occurs either with toxic overdose or as a result of continued abuse. It is marked by the presence of paranoid delusions, sometimes with auditory hallucinations in the presence of a clear sensorium.

Since the most common medical use of the amphetamines has been in the treatment of obesity, it was only logical that as the problem of widespread amphetamine abuse became known, an attempt would be made to find chemical derivatives which would have appetite suppressant properties without the stimulant effect. Exactly the same thing has happened as with the attempt to replace the barbiturates with other substances. Almost all of the substitutes are like amphetamine, in that if taken in large enough doses, they will produce the desired high. Some of the drugs in this category are Vontril PDN®, Fastin®, Preludin®, Pre-Sate®, Tenuate®, and Tepanil® Of these, the most widely abused has been Preludin®, presently known on the street, as *ludies*. Tolerance and dependence develops to all these drugs as it does to the amphetamines.

Cocaine

Cocaine is an alkaloid obtained from the leaves of the plant erythoxylon coca. Cocaine is either sniffed as a powder (this is sometimes referred to as *snorting*) or dissolved and injected intravenously. The acute effects of taking cocaine differ little from those described for the amphetamines. Since tolerance does not develop, it is not possible to increase the quantity of cocaine taken at one time beyond a certain point without serious physical signs of overdosage. As with amphetamines, the increased physiological and psychological hyperirritability may lead to impetuous violence. Muscle twitching may be seen in high intake cocaine abuse, and a twitching trigger finger is not conducive to increased self-control in an armed robbery. Cocaine is currently quite expensive and antisocial behavior frequently results in an attempt to obtain the necessary money to purchase the drug. Unlike heroin users, such attempts by cocaine abusers are much more apt to be violent. It cannot be stated too often that alcohol, amphetamines, and cocaine are the three drugs whose immediate use is most closely associated with criminal behavior.

Drug Dependence, Cocaine (304.4)

Tolerance to cocaine does not develop, nor is there any evidence of physical dependence. There is no withdrawal syndrome. However, psychotic-like reactions do occur, both with continued use and in acute overdosage. Cocaine, like the amphetamines, depresses the appetite. The chronic cocaine user is markedly underweight, at times to the point of emaciation. Because of chronic overstimulation, the cocaine abuser is tense, overactive, and quick to respond to stimulation. Mildly suspicious ideation is frequently seen, even in the absence of psychosis. Not uncommonly, muscle twitching and even jerkiness on motion is quite obvious. The original euphoria of early abuse gives way to an almost chronic irritability, a sort of drivenness in the habituated individual. Chronic sniffers may develop perforation of the nasal septum (the vertical divider of the nose). Cocaine psychosis is characterized by widespread hallucinations, auditory, visual, and olfactory. Paranoid delusions are common. They are often bound up with the drug usage itself, i.e. onlookers are all narcotic agents about to pounce; friends and acquaintances are informants who are poised for betrayal. Confusion may or may not be present. Treatment of the acute psychosis is relatively simple requiring sedation, supportive measures, and withdrawal of the drug. Treatment of the psychological dependence is much more difficult.

Chapter 22

EUPHOROHALLUCINOGENS AND DRUGS
NOT OTHERWISE CLASSIFIED

EUPHOROHALLUCINOGENS

General Considerations

THE hallucinogens as their name implies are those substances which when abused possess the potential to produce hallucinations. They may be divided into two groups: the naturally occurring hallucinogens and the synthetic hallucinogens. There are many naturally occuring substances which belong in this group. The most widely known are marijuana (including hashish and ghanj), LSD (acid), psylocybin, peyote, organic mescaline, morning glory seeds, and jimson weed. Of the synthetic hallucinogens, the most widely used are synthetic mescaline (the chemically produced alkaloid of peyote), the tryptamines (DET, DMT, DPT), and the amphetamine derivatives (DOM, STP, and MDA). There is definite disagreement as to whether marijuana belongs with the euphorohallucinogens. This will be discussed in detail later. The naturally occurring hallucinogens all have actions similar to LSD; the synthetic hallucinogens differ in many ways.

Marijuana

Acute Effects

Marijuana (grass, weed, pot, tea, MJ) is the name given to the leaves, stems, and seeds of the hemp plant *(cannabis sativa)*. The strength varies according to what parts of the plant are used and where the plant is grown. In Jamaica a particularly potent form of the substance is known as ghanj (called ganja in the Far East). The most potent of the marijuana products is

414

hashish. It is from the association of hashish with a band of Middle Eastern brigands called the assassins (hasheeshins) that marijuana got its undeservably bad reputation of being a drug which was mixed with violence and sex. Indeed, marijuana had received such a bad name that until recently it was thought of by the public as a narcotic, which it definitely is not.

Marijuana can be smoked (as is most commonly done in this country) or swallowed, generally in a liquid extract or in sweets. In the movie, *I Love You Alice B. Toklas* it was baked in brownies. The active ingredients which are responsible for the effects on the central nervous system are the cannabinols. Over sixty of these compounds have been isolated, and it is generally agreed that the ingredient responsible for the active effect of marijuana is one of the tetrahydracannabinols (THC). However, there is even disagreement over which particular one it is, whether it is the Δ^6 or the Δ^9 form. Synthetic THC is extremely unstable. As a result, while frequent reference is made by drug abusers to THC (also called T), it is never possible to be sure this is the drug which was actually taken. Much so-called THC, as well as much street mescaline, is actually weak LSD mixed with a little strychnine. (More recently PCP has replaced acid.)

At present, marijuana has no known medicinal indication so one cannot talk about its use or misuse. At one time it had many medical applications (including use as an antidepressant) for all of which more effective medications have been found. Because of difficulties with the legal aspects of its use, little experimentation in possible applications has gone on. One recent study suggests its possible effectiveness in markedly enhancing other agents used for the relief of pain in cancer. Still more recently, it has been reported to have a beneficial effect on glaucoma (a very serious ocular condition, producing an increase in the pressure within the eyeball, which may lead to blindness).

Next to alcohol, marijuana is the single, most widely used substance of abuse in this country, if not in the world. In November 1976, the DEA announced that the results of a survey of 17,000 high school seniors revealed that the percentage of those who had sampled marijuana had risen in one year from 47 percent to 52 percent. This same survey revealed that regular use in this group had increased in that year from 16 percent to 19 percent, and that daily use had gone from 6.1 percent to 8.1 percent. At the same time there was a definite drop in consumption of other substances of abuse, excluding alcohol. There is a general tendency to consider that marijuana is not a drug, just as in the mind of the general public alcohol is not a drug. The sale of marijuana is illegal throughout the country, and in the great majority of states possession and use are still crimes.

The effects of inhalation of marijuana last from two to four hours although they may be prolonged almost indefinitely by inhaling another *joint* as the effects of the first wear off. As a general rule, marijuana smoking is a social event, and the cigarette is passed around, much like the old Indian peace pipe. The smoke is inhaled deeply and held in the lungs an appreciable period before exhaling in order to attain the maximum effect. Frequently, first time users are unable to *get off*, to obtain the desired high. Practice generally remedies this. When the drug is ingested, effects usually last five to eight hours. Tolerance does not develop to marijuana.

Many users report an original period of anxiety lasting ten to fifteen minutes before the euphoriant effect of the drug is felt. In some the mildly paranoid effects of this anxiety persist in an altered form throughout that and all subsequent experiences. This usually takes the guise of suspecting all in the vicinity of being narcotic agents or spies for the narcotic agents. Usually, however, the period of anxiety is quickly replaced with a pleasant, light-hearted state. At times there seems to be dissociation in which the participant is also the observer. Everything is amusing. Laughter, even giggling, is a common response. Some people report a sensory hyperacusis in which even minimal stimuli are perceived to the fullest extent. There is a distortion of the time sense, generally in the direction of an almost infinite extension of time. Two or three minutes might seem like ten or twelve. Indeed, this is the reason often given that jazz musicians prefer marijuana to alcohol. Under the influence of the distortion of time it is possible to squeeze an incredible number of notes rhythmically into one bar. (I have not heard of a scientific experiment which has settled the question as to whether that statement is or is not apocryphal.) It is the distortion in the color sense, present in some who smoke marijuana, which leads to its being classed with the hallucinogens. For some people objects glow in vivid and beautiful colors which come and go. (This is said to be one of the chief characteristics of mescaline intoxication as well.) One final quality which the effects of marijuana share with some other hallucinogens is a peculiar periodicity of effect. Objects, experiences, sensations tend to fade in and out of consciousness. There is also claimed to be a heightened sense of self-awareness.

Here the resemblance to the hallucinogen ceases. The true hallucinogens, natural as well as synthetic, tend to have stimulating and awakening qualities. Marijuana usage produces a dreamy, relaxed state, which tends to inhibit action. Certainly this is true of action of an aggressive nature. Evidence would seem to indicate that, except for the illegality of its possession, use, and sale, there is little direct connection between marijuana and crime, particularly aggressive crime. Antisocial behavior to raise money to buy the drug is minimized by the almost universal experience of shared usage.

This is not to neglect the problem of the multiple drug user for whom marijuana is just an incidental drug, nor the problem of the antisocial individual who may happen to smoke marijuana as a part of his particular culture. It has been the author's experience on examining those who are involved in violent crimes while smoking marijuana that investigation usually revealed one of two circumstances. The first was that the offender was basically an explosive personality; the second was that alcohol was generally consumed in large quantities along with the marijuana.

Drug dependence, Cannabis Sativa (hashish, marijuana) (304.5)

It may be stated without equivocation that more controversy has occurred about the abuse of marijuana than about any other drug mentioned in this book. In spite of the fact that marijuana has been used in one form or another for well over 2,000 years, there is still no agreement that such a state as Drug Dependence, Marijuana exists. There is universal agreement that physical dependence does not exist and that tolerance does not develop. Beyond that, there is not even agreement as to how it should be spelled, with a "j" or an "h." There have even been claims that reverse tolerance occurs, i.e. that after the first few experiences with smoking marijuana, it requires a lower rather than a greater quantity to produce the same effects. This certainly is not a universal phenomenon, and its significance is questionable. The two major arguments raised are: Does psychological dependence exist; Is long term use harmful?

The argument over whether there is or is not such a thing as psychological dependence on marijuana, particularly as it is used in this country, has generated more sound and fury than it has thrown light on the subject. It has been agreed generally that the overwhelming majority of abusers (some writers place the figure as high as 90 percent) will limit their smoking to periods of social relaxation, even if this involves one or two joints several times a week. For these people there seems to be no problem in abstention over long periods of time. Not only is there no withdrawal syndrome, but there is no psychological craving. It would seem that these people use marijuana as the social drinker uses alcohol, with even less danger of increasing the quantity and frequency or of becoming *pot heads*. Pot heads are the analogue of alcoholics. There is also fairly general agreement that the social abuser suffers no lasting effects from that abuse.

The situation of the chronic abuser is somewhat different. Many of these people seem to suffer what has been referred to as an amotivational syndrome. They are listless, emotionless, have no drive, no interest, and accomplish nothing. There is no argument as to the existence of the syndrome. The question at issue is whether the excessive marijuana smoking is a result of a personality disorder, or whether the personality disorder is the result of the smoking. Evidence has been adduced from Far and Near Eastern countries where hashish and ganja (more potent forms of marijuana) are widely used. This purports to prove that large proportions of the population are reduced to that amotivational state. There is, however, a real question as to whether the poverty stricken, hopeless existence of these people does not lead to the excessive marijuana use as a way to avoid their miserable lives, just as opium smoking flourished at one time in China.

The other question is as to whether prolonged, heavy marijuana use leads to psychosis. The brief toxic psychosis seen in American servicemen on their first exposure to marijuana in South Vietnam has been mentioned. Occasional marijuana users also complain of a paranoid feeling when high or stoned. As a rule, once this occurs, it will recur with each subsequent usage, disappearing in the intervals between. Many people who are in remission from paranoid schizophrenia relapse whenever marijuana is smoked. As with cocaine, most of the paranoid ideation centers around the matter of drug usage.

As far as physical change from chronic abuse of marijuana is concerned, this too is still undecided. Some evidence has accumulated to indicate chronic marijuana abuse may cause abnormal lung conditions, although marijuana has not been indicted as a possible carcinogen. A recent large scale collaborative study was done in Jamaica by Harvard University scientists and Jamaica physicians. This study compared the physical state of chronic heavy users of ghanj, the strong Jamaican marijuana, with those who had not used it or used it only occasionally. The subjects were hospitalized for a week for comparison. The only difference found afzer intensive and exhaustive physical, psychological, and laboratory testing was found in the nurses' notes which indicated smokers were, as a rule, more pleasant patients.

The following case illustrates the difficulty in making a clear statement as to the relative cause and effect relationships between marijuana use and symptom production.

B. E. was a nineteen-year-old college junior when first seen. A child prodigy, he was the only child of a refugee couple who had fled from Europe. His father had deserted the family when B. E. was seven years old. The mother had then placed him for a year in a foster home in the country until she could reestablish her life. In this country less than one year, and barely able to speak English, he felt deserted and rejected. After his mother found work, she was able to bring him back to live with her. During the daytime he would be under the care of his mother's sister-in-law who lived in the same building. This aunt watched him after school until the mother would return from work.

Because of his virtuosity on the piano, he was eventually sent to a special high school devoted to music as well as academic subjects. Between the need to practice and the vigilance and overprotectiveness of his aunt, he had little time for friends. An all-A student, he was admitted to a prestigious school of music but at the last moment decided that this was too uncertain a career. His subsequent choice of college was influenced by his desire to get out of town and away from all of his hovering relatives. He did relatively well during his freshman year. In his sophomore year he joined a fraternity, lived for a while in the fraternity house, and then moved off campus into an apartment. At this point he started smoking marijuana socially. Music had been such an integral part of his life that he now felt lost without it so he started to teach himself the violin. As his interest in the violin grew, he spent less time on studies and began to cut classes. He began to believe he could play better when under the influence of marijuana. Hence he started to smoke more heavily. He failed two courses during the third quarter of his second year and stayed on for the summer to make up the work.

At this point he began to feel guilty about what he was doing to his mother. He had avoided going home at holiday time during the school year and now he was away all summer. To assuage his guilt he began to smoke more heavily. He punished himself by stopping his violin playing, but still continued to smoke, cut classes, and stopped studying completely. One week before the summer session ended he managed to stop smoking. With his intelligence it was not too difficult to learn enough in the last week to slip by in both courses.

The first quarter of his junior year he avoided marijuana assiduously. Now instead of attending classes he read omnivorously. Again, he got barely passing grades. At the beginning of the winter quarter he began to feel that maybe he was meant to be a musician. He took up the flute. Shortly thereafter the most intense smoking of his life started. He was literally stoned throughout every day. He moved around in a daze. He became completely indifferent to his personal appearance. His apartment, as he described it later, would have been condemned by the health department had they known of its condition. He failed every course he took and was placed on probation. A psychology instructor became interested in him, and he was referred to my office in the middle of the spring quarter.

At the time he was first seen he could only be classified as a *head*. He was stoned during several therapy sessions, and would ramble on at length about the way he saw himself, his world, and his relationships. At the next session he could not remember what had transpired the session before. All sorts of future goals were explored: businessman, musician, social worker, philosopher, drug pusher. None of them fit. He had difficulty deciding whether he was heterosexual or homosexual. (He was a virgin.) He masturbated almost compulsively. His masturbatory fantasies contained elements of identification with both homo- and heterosexuality.

It was decided it would be necessary for him to drop all his classes to avoid being expelled. This seemed to make no difference to him. In spite of promises to both himself and also to me, he continued to smoke heavily. Finally, with his permission, his mother was informed of his difficulties, and it was arranged for him to return home to enter a private hospital. After four weeks in the hospital, he seemed to have gained some focus and purpose and was released. He was readmitted two weeks later because of again smoking marijuana excessively with a return to his slovenly indifference. At this time he seemed to regain his energy and was discharged to reenter school.

He reentered therapy. After several stormy weeks of exploration of his feelings about the central figures of his early life, and several weekends spent in a continuously stoned state, he seemed to make a series of discoveries about himself. He set a goal of bringing his grade point average up to where he could enter graduate school. He took a different apartment and acquired first a dog and then a girl. It was almost as though he had to prove by way of the dog that, if he trusted, the trust would be returned. His smoking became confined to single joints on an occasional social weekend.

In retrospect, it is impossible to say which came first, the identity diffusion or the marijuana. However, his identity probably could never have crystalized if the heavy marijuana usage had continued.

The Natural Hallucinogens

Acute Effects

The wide variety of naturally occurring hallucinogens has already been listed. This list is constantly expanding as sensation seekers search for a new high. At one time the hallucinogens, particularly LSD (d-lysergic acid dyethylamine) were touted as consciousness expanding (psychedelic) drugs. Attempts were made to use them in psychiatric treatment of some of the functional conditions and alcoholism. These attempts have been abandoned, partially because they were not entirely successful and partly because they seemed to encourage widespread abuse and misuse of the drug. A whole cult of abusers sprang up who felt that repeated use of the drug allowed them to "get into themselves" and become more integrated and more at one with the universe. This sort of abuse has diminished markedly and these drugs are now used largely for the effect of the experience, the *trip*.

As was previously explained, tolerance develops extremely rapidly to LSD, and if the drug is taken in increasing quantities for four or five days, it would be impossible to get any effects on the next day. After a rest of a few days the original tolerance will return. LSD, commonly referred to as *acid, windowpane, pink dot, blue dot, blotter,* to give it only a few of its street names, is currently taken largely for the thrill of the experience. The chief component of this experience, or trip, is a bombardment with sensory stimulation, real and fancied. Synesthesia, the combination of sensory experiences is a common phenomenon. People see sounds and hear colors. Multiple emotions are experienced simultaneously, and one bizarre experience seems to fuse with another. Panic may sometimes occur acutely even in a good trip, only to be replaced immediately by an amusing situation. Hallucinatory experiences are intensified by their vividness and transitory nature.

While testing new hallucinogens for clinical use I had the opportunity to spend six to eight hours with several patients while they described their experiences as they occurred. One woman literally screamed in delight as she told of approaching a beautiful tropical island, bathed in a brilliant light, colored in vivid greens, blues, and oranges. Beautiful nude tropical maidens came swimming out to meet her ship, singing indescribably beautiful melodies. Suddenly the scene changed. She was in the kitchen of her home; the maidens were still there, but now she had to duck and dodge as they emptied her cupboards and threw all the available crockery and canned goods at her. This was just as quickly replaced by the picture of a beautiful mansion, sheathed in solid gold. As she approached the door the whole place seemed to slither and melt, like a figure in a reflecting mirror in an amusement park fun house.

Another patient had a bad trip, filled with huge black hairy spiders, constantly about to devour him. This was succeeded by seeing his own face, as in a reflecting mirror. It was a pastiche of nauseating colors, each of which hummed with a particularly unpleasant sound. As he watched and listened, the flesh fell away and the bare bones of the skull were clearly visible.

Because of the possibilities of such a bad trip, most of those who ingest acid nowadays do so only in the presence of an experienced individual who does not ingest the drug at this time. If the trip is bad, the unaffected guide can talk the sufferer down, even though this may take several hours. The rare offenses connected with the hallucinogens occur generally in conjunction with a bad trip, and the need to defend against imaginary aggressors or to respond to auditory hallucinations. The other naturally occurring hallucinogens react roughly as does LSD, except to a lesser extent dose for dose.

LSD and alcohol form a peculiar combination. Both are metabolized at the same site in the liver. The result, instead of potentiation, as in alcohol and barbiturates, is a prolongation of effect. If the LSD has been ingested before the alcohol, it will frequently appear as though no effect were taking place as drinks are added. However, the trip, instead of lasting the usual eight to ten hours, may last from twelve to sixteen.

From time to time an individual who is already experiencing some problems with ego identity may disintegrate completely while under the influence of LSD. It would seem as though the disturbance in consciousness and awareness were more than the personality could stand. This disintegration tends to be relatively short lived, two to three months, and in some instances it is harmed more than helped by antipsychotic medications.

One other important phenomenon associated with the hallucinogens is the occurrence of *flashbacks*. A flashback is a reoccurrence during a drug free interval of an experience while under the influence of the drug. These may occur as long as a year after the last usage. Sometimes they reflect only an emotional state; at others the full hallucinatory experience is relived. At times they are transient, some have been known to last for hours.

The Synthetic Hallucinogens

For the most part, the action of the synthetic hallucinogens, DOM, STP, DET, DMT, DPT, are very much like those of LSD. It is said that the euphoriant, laugh-producing qualities of some of these is greater. It has also been claimed that they are more stimulating, and wakefulness lasts longer. Unfortunately, the inaccurate labels under which most street drugs are sold makes any meaningful conclusions impossible.

Drug Dependence, Hallucinogens (304.7)

The same questions must be asked about the remainder of the hallucinogens as were asked about marijuana. Because of the peculiar nature of tolerance to the natural hallucinogens physical dependence cannot develop. Whether psychological dependence occurs is open to question. The general consensus is that that question should be answered in the negative. The attempts to use hallucinogens as treatment modalities in the mental disorders have generally been disappointing. To the contrary, there seems to be convincing evidence that repeated abuse of the synthetic hallucinogens may lead to long term psychiatric decompensation. There would appear to be little evidence linking long term abuse to crime.

DRUGS OTHER THAN THOSE PREVIOUSLY CLASSIFIED

PCP

There is some discussion as to whether this compound is so called because of its chemical formula, PhenylCyclohexyl Piperidine, or from its earliest street name, PeaCe Pill. Its two most common current names are "angel dust" and "elephant tranquilizer." Some twenty other names have been applied to this compound. The ordinary corrections worker may think, "Why is this drug being included? I don't see one person a year who is on PCP." That is probably true as far as the client's description of current drug abuse is concerned. Actually, however, PCP is probably one of the most ubiquitous and widely used of all the chemicals. Almost all substances sold as THC are PCP. The same is true for mescaline, and at times even for "acid." Under some circumstances, small quantities of PCP may be added to other drugs. This generally occurs when the vender is afraid that the original drug has been cut to such an extent that the purchaser will complain of the weak effect. Since in reality its use is widespread, and since it is such a dangerous drug, the corrections worker should possess knowledge about it.

PCP was originally given a clinical trial in medicine under the trade names Sernyl or Sernylan. It was developed as a general anesthetic, and indeed did have excellent properties in that regard. Unfortunately, a majority of patients on whom it was used developed postanesthetic confusion, delirium, or agitation. Some became actually psychotic. Its use was quickly discontinued. At present its only legitimate use is as an anesthetic in animal research. It may find another use in pharmacological research since it is able to produce a schizophreniform psychosis almost indistinguishable from schizophrenia. Hence, medication intended to treat the latter condition can be given to animals to determine its effectiveness in blocking the action of PCP.

Many of its qualities make it attractive to the drug abuser. It must also be remembered that a large number of drug users ingest PCP while unaware that they are doing so. In very low doses, the floaty euphoria so earnestly sought is produced. Early numbness may be experienced. There are rapid mood swings. Associative processes are facilitated. The tongue is loosened. The general effect is not unlike that produced by three or four drinks.

As the dosage increases, the effect begins to resemble that of LSD. There are distortions of the body image. Restlessness and wakefulness is common. However, as the effects continue to increase in severity there is disruption in communication; disorientation may take place. Eventually, a withdrawn, almost stuporous state may be seen.

Higher doses produce a clinical picture that is practically indistinguishable from schizophrenia. Complicating the difficulty is the fact that such conditions do not follow the usual pattern of drug-induced psychosis, which generally clears up completely in a few days. Schizophreniform psychosis resulting from a single large dose of PCP may last for months. The difficulty in diagnosis is further compounded by the fact that small doses of PCP may reactivate florid disease in an individual who had previously had schizophrenia but who had been in a state of complete remission. To make matters even more difficult, the ordinary antipsychotic drugs frequently worsen, rather than help, the PCP-induced psychosis.

PCP psychosis may resemble any of the varieties of schizophrenia. Of most interest to corrections workers are those states which resemble the excited phase of catatonic schizophrenia, and those which resemble paranoid schizophrenia. The former may be manifested by senseless lashing out against the environment during the excitement. This may lead to damage both to person and to property. In the paranoid type, the common problem of the need to defend oneself against fantasied attack comes to the fore. Since PCP-induced psychosis of this sort is most apt to be marked by complete inability to distinguish fantasy from reality, it is particularly dangerous. I have already seen five clearly authenticated cases of PCP-induced schizophreniform psychosis, and many in which there was suggestive evidence, but it could not be definitely proved that PCP was actually involved.

Two other manifestations of PCP are of importance. The first is the fact that there may be a cumulative effect of taking small doses of PCP repeatedly. Actual Organic Brain Syndromes have been reported in which there have been permanent disorientation, speech difficulty resembling the aphasia of Cerebral Vascular Disease, and patchy memory loss. The second fact involves a flashbacklike possibility in which there are sudden outbursts of unprovoked aggression including antisocial behavior.

As far as is known tolerance does not develop to PCP. Hence, physical dependence does not occur. I have not yet known of an individual who could be described as psychologically dependent on this drug, although certainly our information about it is far from complete. It must be considered the most dangerous of all the drugs of abuse insofar as its adverse effects on the individual are concerned. The total story of its relationship to antisocial behavior needs further clarification.

ABUSE OF OVER-THE-COUNTER DRUGS

With the number of more potent chemicals available on the street, abuse of over-the-counter medicine is not common, but does occur. Naturally, it is the sleeping medicine which gets the widest play. Of these, Sominex®, Sleep-Eze®, Quiet World® and Compoz®, are the best known. Each contains a certain amount of a substance called scopalamine, an antihistamine, and a salicylate (aspirinlike substance). The first two named substances have definite central nervous system effects. Scopalamine is one of the belladonna alkaloids and is the substance responsible for the toxic reactions from jimson weed. Medically, scopalamine found its widest use in obstetrics, where for years a combination of morphine and scopalamine was administered to the mother in labor. The scopalamine produced a dreamy state with subsequent amnesia for the painful event of labor. Hence, the name "twilight sleep" by which this combination was known. Taken by itself in sufficient quantities, scopalamine will cause a toxic delirium with hallucinations, disorientation, loss of body boundary, and occasionally severe excitement.

The antihistaminic component, such as Benadryl®, or Pyribenzamine® also produces drowsiness in small doses but in larger doses may rarely induce delirium. (Pyribenzamine has been called *blue opium* and is often added to narcotics or cocaine to prolong the effect when shooting up.) The additive effect of the scopalamine and the antihistamines is sufficient in large enough overdosage to produce an excited delirium before the onset of sleep. One other over-the-counter product, Asthamador®, sold to be smoked for the relief of asthma, contains a mixture of belladonna alkaloids including scopalamine. It, too, may produce delirium in overdosage. None of these substances produces physical dependence. Not enough is known about their use in combination to be aware of whether true psychological dependence may occur.

DRUGS AND ANTISOCIAL BEHAVIOR

In one sense, it may be said that abuse of drugs in itself constitutes antisocial behavior. Beginning with the Harrison Narcotics Act of 1921, continuing with the Registration Act of 1937, and developing through the successive changes in that act, the use of almost all the substances discussed heretofore in Part Three have been rendered illegal except under strict medical supervision and prescription. Specific drugs and combinations of drugs have been singled out as triggering antisocial behavior. In this regard, special emphasis has been placed on alcohol, the amphetamines, and cocaine. The frequent need to steal for profit in order to maintain a drug habit has also been mentioned.

What has not been stressed to this point, and which certainly deserves comment, is the relationship between the drug culture and crime. The hippies and the flower children, the members of the counterculture as they originally came to public attention in the sixties, represented those who were turning their backs on a culture which they felt had failed. They shunned all forms of violence. Peace and love were their watchwords. However, their high public visibility attracted a great many people to drug abuse, people who did not share the same social and ethical values, people whose chief goal was the kick, the high. Both of these groups were composed largely of young people. Actually, their members seem to get younger each year. In respect to these groups, the public reacted first with amused condescension, and then with increasing fright as it was seen that suburban youngsters were involved as deeply as those from the inner cities.

Unfortunately, the thrust of the educational campaigns mounted at that time was organized around a "scare them to death" theme, replete with half truths and palpable untruths. The result was to produce a feeling of mistrust about all drug information emanating from grownups. This tide has begun to turn only recently. A "truth in advertising" theme is finally beginning to make a little headway, at least in the eighteen- to twenty-three-year-old group.

Long before the hippies, there has always been a small drug subculture. This was not in any way connected with any philosophical movement, but was composed largely of those whose lives were so impoverished that alcohol or other drugs were the only way out. The larger subculture of which they were a part had no strong taboos against antisocial behavior, and crime either when drug free, under the influence of the drug, or in need of the price of a fix was a way of life. Unfortunately, over the past few years there appears to have been a strange amalgamation of these latter two groups. What may have occurred is the same sort of change in national attitude toward the law which followed the halfhearted, graft-ridden, unsuccessful attempt to enforce the prohibition of alcohol. Without wanting to seem to offer a too simplistic viewpoint on a very complicated problem, it would almost appear that there is now a large group of people, ranging in age from the early teens to the late forties, in whom antisocial behavior and drug usage are parallel, and at times interchangeable, facets of the same problem. People who take drugs tend to commit crimes. People who commit crimes tend to take drugs. The existence of any causal relationship, if it does exist, is unclear. The fact remains that the corrections worker will obtain a history of regular or intermittent drug abuse in a large number of clients.

THE ROLE OF THE CORRECTIONS WORKER IN ALCOHOLISM AND DRUG DEPENDENCE

The decriminalization of public alcoholism will not lead to reduction in the involvement of the corrections worker with the alcoholic. The number of crimes in which alcohol plays a contributing role shows no evidence of diminishing. The same may be said of crimes linked to drug abuse, although this would probably not be the case were marijuana to be decriminalized, since it is now generally conceded that the use of marijuana and crime are not directly linked. The management of alcoholism or drug dependence is a complex problem. To some extent this has been described in discussing the management of the alcoholic psychoses (Chaper 3). If there are community resources available, the corrections officer will probably be working as a member of a multidisciplinary team.

It is generally agreed that the most important part of the treatment of the drug-dependent individual is to instill the feeling that someone really cares, someone is concerned, someone is interested. Ideally, that interest should be shown by someone who has no personal stake in the outcome, someone in addition to a close relative or a business partner. This someone may be a representative of society (the corrections worker), a member of a group (Alcoholics Anonymous or a drug clinic), or from an institution (a halfway house, Synanon). That interest must be tempered with the knowledge that permanent abstinence is a goal which may never be obtained. The great majority of alcohol- or drug-dependent individuals may be expected to have shorter or longer periods of relapse punctuating periods of success. (The recent conclusion by the Rand Foundation that social drinking is a possible successful outcome for some recovered alcoholics has raised a storm of outraged protest from Alcoholics Anonymous and other experienced workers in this field. The recent finding that "chipping" is possible in heroin abusers tends to reinforce this finding of the Rand Institute as to alcohol.) Without the knowledge that relapse is to be expected from time to time, there will inevitably be discouragement when working with the alcoholic or drug-dependent individual.

In spite of this knowledge, total abstinence may well be made a condition of probation.[1] It may act as a strongly positive reinforcer of the resolve to continue clean and interpose a moment's needed reflection between impulse and action, in the same way the knowledge of the presence of Antabuse in the system does. It can be anticipated that this particular probation condition will be violated sooner or later. Care must be taken that this anticipation does not produce a self-fulfilling prophecy. If this condition is broken, a weekend detention (with the court's assent) may be utilized. This should be implemented without preaching, moralizing, or conveying any lack of faith in the capacity for future self-control. More than in any other area, the attitude of, "There but for the grace of God go I," is needed for success in working with the alcoholic or drug-dependent person. This does not imply a sentimental approach, but an understanding and realistic one.

This realistic approach is particularly important with the narcotic-dependent individual. Constant contact with all other agencies involved is a must. The worker should know the strengths and weaknesses of the particular clinics being utilized. In some clinics the mechanics of monitoring urine and carefully supervising the distribution and ingestion of methadone is well controlled, but ancillary services are weak. In other clinics, counseling in all fields is excellent, but the technical aspects of medical management are poor. In the first instance, the worker must make up for the deficiencies in counseling. This may be by direct service or by referral. In the second

---

[1]See footnotes, Chapter 3, p. 31.

instance, it is incumbent on the worker to order spot urine checks to make sure the client remains *clean*. Surprisingly, if this checking is done with a show of interest rather than in an atmosphere of mistrust, the client may be grateful rather than resentful.

The chief dilemma for the worker is posed by those people mentioned in the last section, those in whom antisocial behavior and drug abuse are alike symptoms of the same problem. There may be no drug dependence, either physical or psychological, and yet the use of drugs as a way of life parallels other antisocial activities. Many of these people pose the familiar problem of which came first, the antisocial behavior or the drug abuse. Others, particularly juveniles, will have been in flight from impossible situations, whether at home, in the community, or both, long before drug abuse commenced. In some of these instances, the abuse of drugs or alcohol may be the presenting problem, which has to be solved before any progress can be made. In others, the environmental situation must be resolved before any headway can be made in changing the drug habit. In the largest number, the most important aspect of the situation is the willingness of the corrections worker to maintain an attitude which keeps the drug aspect of the problem in its proper perspective. The fact that an individual smokes marijuana does not indicate an advanced degree of criminality any more than the presence of long hair or a straggly beard does.

Certainly, if the subject is an upper lower or middle class youth, both of these topics will have been emphasized by near relatives to the point where they almost become a rationalization for antisocial behavior. "I have the name, why not the game?" This applies to females as well as males. A willingness to meet these people halfway, to admit that no automatic conclusions can be drawn from either their habits or their attire helps get the corrections worker off dead center and started on the right foot.

Chapter 23

MEDICATIONS USED IN PSYCHIATRY

GENERAL CONSIDERATIONS

A KNOWLEDGE of the medications commonly used in psychiatry is important to the corrections worker for several reasons. Many of the clients who are being seen are, or have been, on these medicines and the worker should know what the possible effects of these substances may have been. The great majority of these medications are not used as street drugs, since they do not produce the desired high no matter how large the dosage. It may come as a surprise to learn that psychiatrists do not commonly prescribe barbiturates or the other drugs described as downers any longer. Also, the use of amphetamine-like substances is limited sharply to the treatment of Minimal Brain Damage in children, and to the treatment of a very rare condition called *Narcolepsy*. As the use of downers and amphetamines has declined in psychiatry, they seem to have become increasingly popular on the street. Many offenders may be taking both classes of drugs (street drugs and drugs used in the practice of psychiatry) simultaneoulsy, and it is important to be aware of the interactions between these differing chemical substances. Frequent reference is made to these medications, whether in the professional journals or in the lay press. Therefore, the worker should have some familiarity with them in order to read with greater understanding. The chemical, or generic, name rather than the proprietary name is beginning to be used more commonly so these names will be included in the material to follow.

These medications can be divided into four large groups according to the purpose for which they are prescribed. These groups are the anxiolytics (minor tranquilizers), the antipsychotic drugs (major tranquilizers), those drugs prescribed to counteract possible side effects of the antipsychotic drugs; and the antidepressants. The term tranquilizer has been relegated to parentheses. It is such a widely used term that it must be included. However, this name carries the unfortunate implication that the calming, sedative, tranquilizing effects of these medications are the sole reasons for their use. This common misconception has led to the mistaken belief that all patients on these medications are reduced to the state of zombies, unresponsive to the environment. This is far from the truth, as will be apparent when these substances are discussed at length.

ANXIOLYTICS

These substances have become the most frequently prescribed medications in this country. They were introduced to replace the barbiturates in the symptomatic treatment of anxiety and tension. As has been so often the case, it did not become apparent until quite a long time after their introduction that tolerance and physical dependence could develop to these agents as well as to the barbiturates. Fortunately, both of these reactions to the anxiolytics develop extremely slowly. Equally fortunately, these substances do not evoke either a rush or a high, no matter how they are introduced into the system and no matter how great the dosage. Knowledge of tolerance and addiction has come about only through the misuse of these substances rather than through their abuse. Numerous studies have shown that over 98 percent of those for whom these medications have been prescribed have discontinued their regular use within sixty days, long before either tolerance or physical dependence can develop. Therefore, physicians see relatively few people dependent on these drugs.

There are two main groups of anxiolytics: the meprobamates (Equanil® and Miltown®); and the benzodiazepides (chlordiazepoxide, Librium®, diazepam, Valium®, and clorazepate dipotassium, Tranxene®). Abuse of these substances is confined almost exclusively to the twelve- to fifteen-year-old group, experimenters who will take any substance they can get their hands on. In some people small doses produce mild giddiness; with most people the original effect is slight drowsiness, which generally disappears after using the medicine for two or three days. Only rarely do youngsters take a sufficiently high dosage to show any significant manifestations. Since all of these drugs are central nervous system depressants, high dose intake resembles intoxication with alcohol or barbiturates. Also, since they are central nervous system depressants they have a mild tendency to potentiate the actions of other drugs in the same class. For example, combining one of these drugs with alcohol will cause the same behavioral patterns as when the barbiturates are taken with alcohol, but to a lesser extent. There is little effect on behavior when the anxiolytics are taken in conjunction with other drugs we have discussed.

The worker should be aware of two, rarely occurring, specific effects of these substances. Librium, because of its basic pharmacological properties, tends to reduce aggressive drives and behavior. For this reason it is frequently administered to calm people who are upset. However, a rare individual exhibits a pathological rage reaction on ingesting Librium and may lash out wildly against the environment. This is not a function of overdose or intoxication but occurs, when it does, at the standard dosage range. This is not a manifestation of overdosage, as in the adolescent who has taken the drug for kicks but occurs in those who are beginning to take the medication under a physician's orders. On extremely rare occasions, an individual may be seen following arrest for assault and battery, or malicious destruction of property, in whom the behavior was induced by beginning to take prescribed Librium. This is not a toxic reaction, there will be no signs of confusion or delirium. For some still unexplained reason, the normal mechanisms for inhibiting hostility temporarily cease to function in these people.

The other phenomenon to be noted as far as the anxiolytics are concerned has to do with Valium. Overdosage with Valium, particularly if taken in conjunction with small quantities of other central nervous system depressants such as alcohol or barbiturates, may produce a retrograde amnesia. This is completely analogous to what is seen in an alcoholic blackout or in a Pathological Intoxication. The individual remembers what happened up to a certain time and then remembers nothing more until awakening, even though functioning may have appeared to be adequate for several hours after this last memory.

B. F., a fourteen-year-old white male, was remanded to detention after he had been apprehended trying to remove a ship-to-shore radio from a docked motorboat. This was at 6:50 AM. He was well enough coordinated at that time so that he was able to remove three of the four bolts which secured the radio to the boat. By 7:00 AM when he was received at the detention home, he was staggering, incoordinated, and his speech was almost unintelligible. Within the next ten minutes he was obviously lapsing into a state of unconsciousness and was sent to a hospital emergency room for treatment.

When B. F. recovered consciousness he could remember almost nothing of what occurred from 12:15 AM that morning. The evening before he had been visiting his brother and sister-in-law with a friend of his. About 11:00 PM the couple retired. He and his friend spotted a bottle of "Roche 10's" (Valium, 10 mg.) on the piano. Apparently, they continued to dare each other to take a couple. This behavior alternated until each had taken somewhere between ten to fifteen capsules. At that point the brother came out and asked if the friend had permission to stay overnight. On learning that he did not, the brother said that under those circumstances he would have to drive the friend home. B. F. said that if his friend went, he would go also. The brother then dropped them off at B. F.'s home at about 12:15 AM. From then on B. F.'s memory is very vague. He is not sure whether he went into his home or not. He has a hazy memory of walking with his friend along some railroad tracks. There is then a vague recollection of standing alongside the boat with his friend next to him. He has no other impressions until he came to in the hospital about noontime the following day. There is no evidence that his friend had ever been near the boat with him.

THE ANTIPSYCHOTIC DRUGS

The antipsychotic drugs have two main functions. The first is to control the excitement, agitation, excess motor activity, and aggression that may occur in such major psychoses as schizophrenia, manic reaction, or severe involutional melancholia. It is this tranquilizing function which forms the popular image that these drugs are being used solely for this purpose. Certainly this function of the drug is an important one during times of acute disturbance in major psychoses. Their greatest usefulness, however, lies not in the acute calmative action, but rather in long term, continued administration for exactly what the appelation implies, their antipsychotic properties. Given regularly over a period of time, they ameliorate the psychotic process going on within the individual. In some instances, administration of these agents may bring about a complete restoration of functioning. At other times there may be only partial restoration. In some cases the medication may be capable only of halting the disease process at the level at which medication was begun.

Three interrelated features of these medications should be kept in mind. The first is that tolerance does not develop. Thus, the same dosage level can be maintained indefinitely with no increase in the desired effect. The second feature is that massive doses are sometimes needed to bring about the desired response. If the same dosage were to be given to a normal individual, even if that level were attained over a long period of time, that normal individual would be unable to tolerate the medication and would be in a continuous stupor. The medication could easily be fatal. This is one reason for the opinion given about the impropriety of using these medications for behavior control in penal institutions. The aggressive behavior is controlled but at the cost of making an automaton of the individual.

As might be expected from this reaction of nonpsychotic individuals to the medication, patients, once they begin to improve, require progressively smaller doses of medication. In the case of schizophrenics, it is eventually necessary to determine the smallest dosage level necessary to maintain the improvement.[1] The third feature to be noted is that unless that dosage

---

[1]There is no guarantee that relapse will not occur with continued drug administration, but repeated, carefully controlled studies, covering what by now are literally thousands of patients, have demonstrated that recurrence of active disease is much less likely to occur if maintenance chemotherapy is continued.

level is maintained, relapse will almost inevitably follow.

There are many antipsychotic drugs.[2] Obviously, the ideal one has not yet been found or they would not exist in the number they do. For purposes of simplicity we shall divide these drugs into two classes, the phenothiazines and the non-phenothiazines. These drugs are listed in Table I. The indications and contraindications for the use of any specific drug is of no significance to corrections. The side effect of the medication, and the result of combining these medications with street drugs are roughly the same for all the substances listed. These drugs also tend to be central nervous system depressants, although the sites of action and mechanisms of action differ from the central nervous system depressants already discussed. Hence, while they do potentiate the effects of alcohol and downers, they do not do so to the extent to which those substances potentiate each other.

If large quantities of alcohol or barbiturates have been taken prior to the ingestion of antipsychotic drugs, coma or stupor may result. If small quantities of downers have been taken the effect of the antipsychotics will be to increase motor dysfunction mildly. Generally, the phenothiazines tend to counteract the effects of the hallucinogens. Until recently, individuals brought to an emergency room with a bad trip were administered large doses of Thorazine®. Actually this is now felt to be contraindicated, and "talking the person down" is the approved method of treatment. The use of phenothiazines has been discontinued because street drugs are commonly contaminated with other chemical substances. These substances are byproducts which were not properly removed during the manufacturing process. Phenothiazines react strikingly with certain of these impurities to bring about a severe toxic delirium. The usual response to this is to administer more phenothiazines in order to calm the patient. This worsens the situation.

---

[2]Lithium carbonate, which is specific only for manic reactions and bipolar depression has already been discussed in Chapter 6 and will not be included in this chapter. It should be noted that lithium for some reason markedly decreases the response to LSD, natural hallucinogens, and marijuana.

TABLE I

Class	Trade Name	Generic Name	Description
			(Tablets Unless Specified) (Numbers, Initials and Names
Phenothiazines			indicate Manufacturer's Code)
	Thorazine®	Chlorpromazine	Beige and White Capsules SKF T63, T64, T66, T67, T69 Brown SKF T73, T74, T76, T77, T79
	Stelazine®	Trifluoperazine	Blue SKF S03, S04, S06, S07
	Mellaril®	Thioridazine	Blue, Lavender, Beige, White, Yellow Sandoz 78-2, 78-3, 78-4, 5, 6, 7, 8
	Trilafon®	Perphenazine	Bluish White SCH, ADH, ADJ, K, M, X
	Sparine®	Promazine	Green, Pink, Peach, Salmon, Red 28, 29, 200, 201, 202
	Serentil®	Mesoridazine	Red, Brown B120, B121, B122, B123
	Permitil®	Fluphenazine	Yellow, Green, Peach, Violet, Pink WKJ, WBK, WDR, WFF, WFG
	Prolixin®	Fluphenazine	Coral Yellow, Green 863, 864, 867
	Repoise®	Butaperazine	Yellow, Green, Peach AHR
Other			
	Taractan®	Chlorprothixene	Peach, Salmon, Roche, 46, 47, 49
	Navane®	Thiothixene	Capsules: Peach and Yellow, Blue and White, Blue and Green Roerig 571, 572, 573, 574, 577
	Haldol®	Haloperidol	White, Yellow, Lavender, Green, Blue, 1/2, 1, 2, 5, 10
	Loxitane®	Loxapine Succinate	Capsules: Green and Yellow, Two-Tone Green, Green and Blue
	Daxolin®	Loxapine Succinate	Capsules: Blue and White, Blue and Maroon, Light and Dark Blue

For this reason, even though the phenothiazines and the hallucinogens are antagonistic drugs, an occasional case of uncontrolled, severely confused behavior may occur when an antipsychotic is taken in conjunction with a street hallucinogen.

Two of the more common side effects of the antipsychotic drugs should be noted. One is a tendency to produce low blood pressure. If a client on a worker's caseload complains of occasional blackouts and persistent weakness, questions should be raised as to whether one of the antipsychotic medications is being used. If so, the client should be referred to his physician immediately for checking of blood pressure and adjustment of dosage.

The other common side effect is to produce changes in the motor system which resemble those seen in Parkinson's Disease, a condition which occasionally affects older people. It is this side effect which is partially responsible for the zombielike state referred to earlier. The affected individual's muscles become increasingly rigid, bodily movement tends to be in one piece, the face takes on a masklike quality, and there may be a coarse tremor of the hands. The corrections worker who is unfamiliar with this condition might believe the client who presents this picture to be under the influence of a street drug.

One other motor condition sometimes attributed to the antipsychotic medications is worth discussing. This may be quite baffling, and even upsetting, if seen by the worker who is unaware of the possibility of its existence. It is called *akisthisia* and is the predecessor of the Parkinsonlike state just described. Briefly stated, it consists of motor restlessness. The sensation felt by the patient is analogous to the common experience of lying in bed and feeling that a leg has a will of its own and wants to move or jerk. If it is not moved, an almost indescribable feeling of discomfot occurs. So too in akisthisia, the individual feels impelled to move with no clear feeling of volition or understanding why the feeling occurs.

DRUGS USED TO PREVENT SIDE EFFECTS

Because the antipsychotic drugs are apt quite commonly to

produce these side effects on the motor system, it is not at all unusual to administer medications to a patient in order to prevent, or correct, these troublesome states. It is now considered better medical practice to wait until symptoms have developed before prescribing these ameliorating medications. They are then discontinued a few weeks after the motor symptoms are under control. In spite of this, many patients receive these antiparkinson drugs routinely.

The most commonly used medications in this group are Akineton® (a white tablet with an inscribed shield), Artane® (a white scored tablet or a blue capsule), Cogentin® (a white tablet marked MSD 60, 635 or 21), or Tremin® (a white tablet marked AKH or AKJ). Many patients, especially those seen in corrections, seem to consider these medications to be another variety of mind-blowing drugs. Accordingly, they may be taken in large quantities for this purpose. Under these circumstances, they may produce a severe toxic delirium with visual hallucinations and extreme confusion. The same pharmacological aspect of these drugs which is responsible for this toxic delirium is also responsible for the adverse reaction produced when phenothiazines are taken in conjunction with contaminated hallucinogens. Since these antiparkinson drugs are almost always taken simultaneously with antipsychotics[3] their effect is additive when taken with an impure hallucinogen, and extremely bizarre behavior may result. With these two exceptions, overdosage or mixture with an impure street drug, these substances have no bearing on the mental state of an offender and furnish no sufficient reason for disturbed behavior or amnesia. A combination of these antiparkinson drugs and downers (including alcohol) should have no potentiating effect.

THE ANTIDEPRESSANTS

For the most part the antidepressant medications have little significance to the corrections worker. However, some knowl-

---

[3] I have seen patients who have discontinued their antipsychotic drugs but have continued the antiparkinson drugs under the mistaken notion that these were the medications helping them.

edge about them should be available since clients will be seen who are taking these medications. The worker should be aware of one life-threatening situation in conjunction with their use. The possible existence of the background for this situation might be better known to the worker than to the physician. For this reason, these drugs will be briefly discussed.

The first statement to be made about the antidepressants is that they are not uppers, or stimulants. Unknowing youngsters from time to time ingest increasing quantities of antidepressants in the expectations of getting a high. Depending on the substance ingested, the resultant reactions may range from toxic delirium to stupor or death. The antidepressants do little to help the *mood* depression; they are effective only in the *illness* depression. They have no effect when taken as a single dose, but must be taken daily in sufficient doses over a period of one to three weeks, at which time there is a relatively sudden, dramatic reversal of the illness.

The antidepressants are composed of two groups. The drugs in one group, the tricyclic antidepressants, are related to each other by their chemical formula. The most commonly used drugs in this group are the following:

Imipramine (Tofranil®, reddish brown, labeled Geigy, numbers 21, 11, 74).

Amitryptylin (Elavil®, blue, labeled MSD 23; yellow, lab-eled MSD 45; tan, labeled MSD 102).

Desipramine (Norpramin®, yellow labeled L 11, green labeled L 12). (Pertofran® capsules, pink or pink and red, labeled USD).

Nortryptyline (Aventyl® capsules, yellow and white labeled Lilly H17 or H19).

Protyptryline (Vivactil®, lozenge shaped tablets in peach or yellow labeled MSD 26, 47).

The tricyclic drugs do have the effect of potentiating alcohol, which means that those taking tricyclics show greater effects to lesser amounts of alcohol. No effect on behavior or memory has been noted in combination with tricyclics and street drugs.

The second group is known as the mono-amine-oxidase inhibitors. They differ from each other in chemical structure but have the same function of hindering the effects of the enzyme monoamine oxidase, which is necessary to break down certain chemical substances called biogenic amines as they occur in the system. There are three chief monoamine oxidase inhibitors.

Trancylpromine (Parnate®, red tablets, labeled SKF N71).
Isocarboxazid (Marplan®, peach colored scored tablets).
Phenelzine (Nardil®, red tablets, labeled WC).

It is this class of drugs in which fatal reactions may occur if taken in combination with other substances. The most dangerous of these other substances are the amphetamines. A physician treating a depressed patient may have no history of the fact that the depression was incurred while crashing from prolonged use of speed or that the depressed individual had been using street drugs. The worker, knowing that this client was a speed freak, should warn the client against any use, orally or intravenously, of any of the amphetamines for at least two weeks after the last dose of a monoamine oxidase inhibitor has been taken. This time span is necessary because the medication remains in the blood for a long period of time after ingestion. The resultant combination of MAOI and an amphetamine may lead to what is called a *hypertensive crisis,* a sudden rise in blood pressure to a level high enough to possibly cause a sudden rupture of a blood vessel inside the skull and bleeding into the brain.

On rare occasions, a corrections worker may see a client who complains of a sudden tremendously painful headache. The client is known to abuse speed. If inquiry reveals that that client has been taking one of the MAOI antidepressants, the client should be rushed to the nearest emergency room. A similar crisis may occur on drinking certain alcoholic beverages, taking certain medicines for the common cold, or eating certain foods such as broad pod beans, pickled herring, raisins, or liver. The combination of MAOI and Demerol may be immediately fatal. The action of the barbiturates, the narcotics, and alcohol are all potentiated when the MAOI agent is ingested. Thus a story of, "I only had two drinks, but I was real stoned," may be true if one of these medications is being taken.

One final quality of the MAOI drugs is important. They increase resistance to the action of LSD and of marijuana, so that an individual may find himself increasing the dosage of these drugs tremendously to get his accustomed high. In the case of acid, this is not so significant since, as was pointed out, tremendous tolerance develops rapidly only to disappear when the drug is discontinued for three or four days. In the case of marijuana, however, once the individual goes off the MAOI any attempt to smoke the same quantity of marijuana will lead to a markedly increased marijuana effect.

The final section of this book has emphasized once more the necessity of a thorough history. The effects of drugs on an individual client can only be assayed properly when there is a thorough knowledge of that client's drug usage. Not only the kind of drug, but also the quantity, the combinations, and the duration of usage must be known before any definite statement can be made as to the effect of those drugs on the behavior of that particular person.

SELECTED READINGS

Encyclopedic

American Handbook of Psychiatry, Arieti, S., Ed.; Vols. 1-6, Basic Books, New York, 1974, 1975.
Comprehensive Textbook of Psychiatry II, Freedman, A. M., Kaplan, H. I., and Sadock, B. J., Eds.; Vols. 1 and 2, Williams and Wilkins, Baltimore, Maryland, 1975.
The Theory and Practice of Psychiatry, Redlich, F. C. and Freedman, D. X.; Basic Books, New York, Second Edition, 1975.
Encyclopedia of Sexual Behavior, Ellis, A. and Abarbanel, S., Eds.; Vols. I and II, Hawthorn Books, Inc., New York, 1961.
Second Edition, Diagnostic and Statistical Manual II, American Psychiatric Association.

Mental Retardation

Handbook of Mental Deficiency, Ellis, N. R., Ed.; McGraw-Hill, New York, 1963.
Mental Retardation, American Medical Association, Chicago, 1964.

Organic Brain Syndromes

Epileptic Seizure Patterns, Penfield, W. and Kristiansen, K.; Charles C Thomas, Springfield, Illinois, 1951.
Episodic Behavioral Disorders, A Psychodynamic Neurological Analysis, Monroe, R.; Harvard University Press, Cambridge, 1970.
Violence and the Brain, Mark, V. and Ervin, F.; Harper and Row, New York, 1971.
Late Effects of Head Injury, Walker, A., Caveness, W., and Critchley, M. Eds.; Charles C Thomas, Springfield, Illinois, 1969.
Mental Disorders in Later Life, American Psychiatric Association, Washington, D.C., 1973.
Cerebral Vascular Disorders, Toole, J. T. and Patel, A. N.; McGraw-Hill, New York, 1967.
Postpartum Psychiatric Problems, Hamilton, J. A.; C. V. Mosby, St. Louis,

446   *Basic Psychiatry for Corrections Workers*

Missouri, 1962.

Neurosyphilis, Merritt, H. H., Adams, R. D., and Solomon, H. C.; Oxford University Press, New York, 1946.

The Mind of the Injured Man, Fetterman, J. L.; Industrial Medicine Book Company, Chicago, 1943.

Brain Injuries in War, Goldstein, Kurt, M.D.; Grune and Stratton, New York, 1942.

Psychotic Reactions

Manic Depressive Illness, Winokur, G., Clayton, P., Reich, T.; C. V. Mosby, St. Louis, Missouri, 1969.

Affective Disorders, Greenacre, P., Ed.; International University Press, New York, 1950.

Depression in Medical Practice, Enelow, A. J.; Merck, Sharp and Dohme, West Point, Pennsylvania, 1970.

Psychopathology of Schizophrenia, Hoch, P. and Zubin, I., Eds.; Grune and Stratton, New York, 1966.

Dementia Praecox or the Group of Schizophrenias, Bleuler, E.; International University Press, New York, 1950.

Language and Thought in Schizophrenia, Kasanin, I. S., Ed.; University of California Press, Berkley, 1946.

Paranoid and Paranoiac Psychoses, Retterstol, N.; Charles C Thomas, Springfield, Illinois, 1966.

The Paranoid, Swanson, D. W., Bohnert, P. J., and Smith, J. A.; Little Brown, Boston, 1970.

The Origin and Treatment of Schizophrenic Disorders, Lidz, T.; Basic Books, New York, 1973.

Neurotic Reactions

Amnesia, Whitty, C. M. and Zangwill, O. L., Eds.; Butterworth and Company, London, 1966.

The Dissociation of a Personality, Prince, M.; Longmans, Green and Company, New York, 1906.

The Obsessive Personality, Salzman, L.; Science House, New York, 1968.

Personality Disorders

The Mask of Sanity, Cleckley, H.; C. V. Mosby, St. Louis, Missouri, 1964.

Deviant Children Grown Up: A Sociological and Psychiatric Study of Sociopathic Personality, Robins, R. L.; Williams and Wilkins, Baltimore, 1966.

Psychopathy, Theory and Research, Hare, N. D.; Wiley, New York, 1970.
In the Shadow of Man, Van Lawick-Goodall, J.; Houghton Mifflin, Boston, 1971.
The Borderline Syndrome, Grinker, R. S., Werble, B., and Drye, R. C.; Basic Books, New York, 1968.
Personality Disorders, Diagnosis and Management, Lion, J. R., Ed.; Williams and Wilkins, Baltimore, Maryland, 1974.

Sexual Deviations

Sex and Gender, Stoller, R. J.; Random House, New York, 1968.
Patterns of Sexual Behavior, Ford, C. C. and Beach, F. A.; Ace Books, New York, 1951.
Sexual Identity Conflicts in Children and Adults, Green, R.; Basic Books, New York, 1969.
Transsexualism and Sex Reassignment, Green, R. and Money, J., Eds.; John Hopkins Press, Baltimore, 1969.
Man and Woman/Boy and Girl, Money, J. and Eberhardt, A. A.; John Hopkins Press, Baltimore, 1972.
Contemporary Sexual Behavior, Critical Issues in the 1970s, Zubin, J. and Money, J., Eds.; John Hopkins University Press, Baltimore, 1973.
Homosexuality, Bieber, I., et al.; Basic Books, New York, 1962.
Rape, Offenders and Their Victims, MacDonald, J. M.; Charles C Thomas, Springfield, Illinois, 1971.
The Sexual Offender and His Offenses, Karpman, Benjamin; Julian Press, New York, 1954.
Pedophilia and Exhibitionism, Mohr, J. W., Turner, R. E., and Jerry, M. B.; University of Toronto Press, 1964.
Sexual Behavior in the Human Male, Kinsey, A. C., Pomeroy, W. B., and Martin, C. E.; W. B. Saunders Company, Philadelphia, 1948.
Sexual Behavior in the Human Female, Kinsey, A. C., Pomeroy, W. B., and Martin, C. E.; W. B. Saunders Company, Philadelphia, 1953.
When the Laughter Died in Sorrow, Rentzel, L.; Saturday Review Press, New York, 1972. (The autobiography of an exhibitionist.)
Sexual Behavior and the Law, Slovenko, R., Ed.; Charles C Thomas, Springfield, Illinois, 1965.

Adolescent Behavior Disorders

Toward a Typology of Juvenile Offenders, Glueck, S. and Glueck, T.; Grune and Stratton, New York, 1970.
Searchlights on Delinquency, Eissler, K. R., Ed.; International University Press, New York, 1949.
Behavior Disorders of Childhood and Adolescence, Jenkins, R. L.; Charles C

Thomas, Springfield, Illinois, 1973.
Temperament and Behavior Disorders in Children, Thomas, A., Akers, H., and Birch, H. G.; New York University Press, New York, 1968.
Child and Juvenile Delinquency, Karpman, B., Ed.; Psychodynamics Monograph Series, Washington, D.C., 1959.
Modern Developments in Adolescent Psychiatry, Howells, John G., Ed.; Bruner/Mazel, New York, 1971.

Interviewing

The Diagnostic Interview, Stevenson, I.; Harper and Row, New York, 1971.
Interviewing Techniques in Probation and Parole, Hartman, H. L.; Bureau of Child Welfare, 1963.
The Initial Interview in Psychiatric Practice, Gill, M., Newman, R., and Redlich, F. C.; International University Press, New York, 1954.
The Psychiatric Interview, Sullivan, H. S.; W. W. Norton, New York, 1954.
The Clinical Interview, Deutsch, F. and Murphy, W. F.; International University Press, New York, 1955.

Alcohol and Drugs

The Disease Concept of Alcoholism, Jellinek, E. M., Hillhouse Press, New Haven, Connecticut, 1960.
To Know the Difference, Ullman, A.; St. Martin's Press, New York, 1960.
The Road to Narcotics, Delinquency and Social Policy, Chein, I., Gerald, D. L., Lee, R. S., and Rosenfeld, E.; Basic Books, New York, 1964.
National Committee on Marijuana and Drug Abuse: Marijuana, a Signal of Misunderstanding, First Report of the National Commission on Marijuana and Drug Abuse, United States Government Printing Office, Washington, D.C., 1972.
Drug Abuse in America: Problem in Perspective, Second Report of the National Commission on Marijuana and Drug Abuse, United States Government Printing Office, Washington, D.C., 1973.
The Varieties of Psychedelic Experience, Masters, R. E. L. and Houston, J.; Holt, Rinehart and Winston, New York, 1966.
Psychopathology and Psychopharmacology, Coles, J. O., Friedman, A. M., and Friedhoff, A. J., Eds.; John Hopkins University Press, Baltimore, 1973.
Psychotropic Drug Side Effects, Shader, R. I. and DiMascio, A., Eds.; Williams and Wilkins, Baltimore, 1970.
Drugs and Youth, Wittenborn, J. R., Brill, H., Smith, J. P., and Wittenborn, S. A., Eds.; Charles C Thomas, Springfield, Illinois, 1969.
Opiate Addiction, Origins and Treatments, Fisher, S. and Freedman, A. M., Eds.; V. H. Winston, Washington, 1973.

Amphetamine Psychosis, Connell, P. H.; Chapman and Hall, London, 1958.
Desk Reference on Drug Abuse, American Hospital Association, 1972.
Drug Dependence, American Medical Association, Chicago, Illinois, 1969.

INDEX

definition of safe person and, 341-342
developmental factors and, 339-344
lack of validity of, 336-338
mental illness and, 337-339
previous behavior and, 336
Dangerousness in probationers and pa-
rolees, 352-355
behavior patterns, significance of change
in, 352
double bind, significance of, 353
feelings, identification of, 354
management of
medication in, failure to take, 352-353
role of detention in, 353-354
threats in, evaluation of, 353
use of relationship in, 354-355
Darvon (*see* Drugs, Darvon)
Defense mechanisms, 304
Delirium tremens (*see* Alcoholic psychoses, delirium tremens)
Delusions, 7, 25, 26, 32, 33, 35, 41, 42, 45,
48, 75, 78, 81, 82, 85, 86, 88, 89, 90,
96-97, 101, 109, 113, 114-115, 118, 119,
120, 339, 411, 426-427
definition of, 75f
Demerol (*see* Drugs, Demerol)
Desoxyn, 409
DET, 404
Deterioration, alcoholic (*see* Alcoholic
psychoses, alcoholic deterioration)
Deterioration, epileptic (*see* Epilepsy,
deterioration)
Deterioration, post-traumatic (*see* Psy-
choses with brain trauma, post-
traumatic deterioration)
Dexamyl, 409
Dexedrine, use in hyperkinetic reaction of
childhood, 242
Dilaudid, (*see* Drugs, Dilaudid)
Dipsomania (*see* Alcoholism, Dipso-
mania)
DMT, 424
Dolophine, (*see* Drugs, Methadone)
DOM, 424
Doriden, (*see* Drugs, Doriden)
Double bind
in probationer and parolee, 353
in schizophrenia, 68
Downers, (*see* Drugs, downers)

Down's syndrome (*see* Mental retardation,
other causes)
Doyle, Sir Arthur Conan, 302f
DPT, 424
Drag, dressing in, 190
Drugs
Amytal, 392, 393
abuse, definition of, 365
abuse, multiple drugs, 372-375
alcohol, as, 365
amphetamines, 408-412
abuse of, 409
alcohol and, effects of, 410
antisocial behavior and, 410
barbiturates and, effects of, 393, 410
MAOI anti-depressants and, 443
physiological actions of, 409
production of, 1970, 372
psychological actions of, 411
psychosis, 411
psychosis, dangerousness in, 338
substitutes for, 411-412
tolerance to, 410
use, increase in, 371, 372
withdrawal syndrome in, 411
antisocial behavior and, 428-430
drug culture and, 429
importance of need for fix, 428
barbiturates
alcohol and, effects of, 393
alcohol and amnesia in, 393
alcohol, cross tolerance to, 367
amphetamines and, effects of, 393, 410
antipsychotic drugs and, effects of, 438
as central nervous system depressants,
377
death, accidental, due to, 396
effects of, acute, 392-395
heroin withdrawal, use as substitute in,
394
MAOI antidepressants, potentiation by,
443-444
misuse, 395
names of, proprietary and street, 394
production of, 1973, 372
suggestibility, increased by use of, 392
suicide and, 396
tolerance, development of, 368
use, increase in, 371